PATHOLOGY
PRACTICAL BOOK

System requirement:

- Operating System—Windows XP or above.
- Web Browser—Internet Explorer 8 or above, Mozilla Firefox and Safari.
- Essential plugins—Java and Flash player:
  - Facing problems in viewing content—it may be your system does not have Java enabled.
  - If Videos do not show up—it may be the system requires Flash player or need to manage Flash setting.
  - You can test Java and Flash by using the links from the troubleshoot section of the CD/DVD.
  - Learn more about Flash setting from the link in the troubleshoot section.

Accompanying CD/DVD-ROM is playable only in computer and not in DVD player.

CD/DVD has autorun function—it may take few seconds to load on your computer. If it does not work for you, then follow the steps below to access the contents manually:

- Click on my computer.
- Select the **CD/DVD drive** and click open/explore—this will show list of files in the **CD/DVD**.
- Find and double click file—"launch.html".

The photographs on the cover of the book depict images of following diseases:

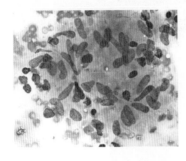

FNA in tuberculous lymphadenitis

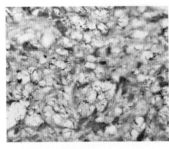

Lepra bacilli in lepramatous leprosy

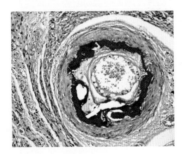

Monckeberg's arteriosclerosis

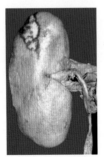

Infarct kidney

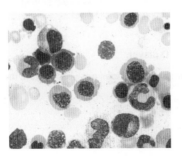

Bone marrow in megaloblastic anaemia

PATHOLOGY PRACTICAL BOOK

THIRD EDITION

Harsh Mohan MD, FAMS, FICPath, FUICC
Professor and Head
Department of Pathology
Government Medical College
Sector-32 A, Chandigarh-160 030
INDIA
e-mail: drharshmohan@gmail.com

JAYPEE BROTHERS MEDICAL PUBLISHERS (P) LTD

New Delhi • Panama City • London • Dhaka • Kathmandu

Jaypee Brothers Medical Publishers (P) Ltd.

Headquarters

Jaypee Brothers Medical Publishers (P) Ltd.
4838/24, Ansari Road, Daryaganj
New Delhi 110 002, India
Phone: +91-11-43574357
Fax: +91-11-43574314
Email: jaypee@jaypeebrothers.com

Overseas Offices

J.P. Medical Ltd.
83, Victoria Street, London
SW1H 0HW (UK)
Phone: +44-2031708910
Fax: +02-03-0086180
Email: info@jpmedpub.com

Jaypee-Highlights Medical Publishers Inc.
City of Knowledge, Bld. 237, Clayton
Panama City, Panama
Phone: +507-301-0496
Fax: +507-301-0499
Email: cservice@jphmedical.com

Jaypee Brothers Medical Publishers (P) Ltd.
17/1-B, Babar Road, Block-B, Shaymali
Mohammadpur
Dhaka-1207, Bangladesh
Mobile: +08801912003485
Email: jaypeedhaka@gmail.com

Jaypee Brothers Medical Publishers (P) Ltd.
Shorakhute
Kathmandu, Nepal
Phone: +00977-9841528578
Email: jaypee.nepal@gmail.com

Website: www.jaypeebrothers.com
Website: www.jaypeedigital.com

Inquiries for bulk sales may be solicited at: jaypee@jaypeebrothers.com

This book has been published in good faith that the contents provided by the author contained herein are original, and is intended for educational purposes only. While every effort is made to ensure accuracy of information, the publisher and the author secifically disclaim any damage, liability, or loss incurred, directly or indirectly, from the use or application of any of the contents of this work. If not specifically stated, all figures and tables are courtesy of the author. Where appropriate, the readers should consult with a specialist or contact the manufacturer of the drug or device.

Pathology Practical Book

First Edition : 2000
Second Edition : 2007
Third Edition : **2013**

Assistant Editors : Praveen Mohan, Tanya Mohan, Sugandha Mohan

ISBN 978-93-5090-266-0

Printed at Replika Press Pvt. Ltd.

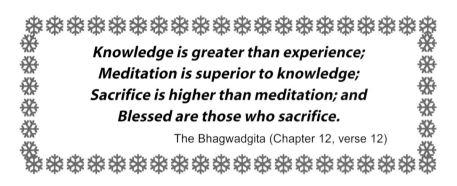

Knowledge is greater than experience;
Meditation is superior to knowledge;
Sacrifice is higher than meditation; and
Blessed are those who sacrifice.

The Bhagwadgita (Chapter 12, verse 12)

Dedicated to
My wife Praveen,
for her profound love and devotion;
and our daughters: Tanya and Sugandha,
for their abiding faith.

Preface to the Third Edition

Since the last revision of the *Pathology Practical Book* in 2007, many technological advances have taken place in diagnostic pathology; therefore the students have to keep pace with the rapid strides and hence revised edition became necessary. While revising the book, however, well-accepted basic style of both the previous editions of the book as exercise-based learning akin to teaching in a practical class of pathology has been retained. The emphasis throughout the revised edition has been on effortless and focused learning by the students on practical points in various sections of pathology and simultaneously preparing them for viva voce in diagnostic pathology such as on slides, specimens, instruments, normal values, similes, etc. Thus, the revised edition in a small package encompasses abundant practical knowledge of immense value.

Some of the *highlights* of the revise edition are as under:

Reorganised and updated contents: The revised edition is reorganised into 8 sections, each section having certain number of practical exercises (in all 61 compared to 58 in the last edition) patterned on the format of practical class of students. These are: Techniques in Pathology (Exercise 1-5), General Pathology (Exercise 6-20), Systemic Pathology (Exercise 21-38), Cytopathology (Exercise 39-41), Clinical Pathology (Exercise 42-45), Haematology (Exercise 46-59), Autopsy Pathology (Exercise 60-61) and Appendices (I-III compared to one in the last edition). All these exercises have been updated in their textual content and newer images added at several places while redundant information and older images have been deleted, taking care that the volume of the book does not grow much bigger.

Additional exercises: Besides rational reorganisation of the exercises in various sections, the revised edition has three totally new exercises. These include exercises on topics of immunohistochemistry (Exercise 4), surgical pathology request form (Exercise 5) and types of blood samples, anticoagulants and blood collection (Exercise 46). Learning and practice of these contemporary topics by the students during their formative years in pathology were considered essential.

Newer appendices: While the appendix on normal values of the previous edition has been retained and updated, present edition has two new appendices: Common Instruments in Pathology (Appendix I) and Common Similes in Pathology (Appendix II). Both these appendices are profusely illustrated with fairly catchy and helpful legends for quick learning.

CD on CPCs and museum review: Ten CPCs (including organ images and their photomicrographs) on the self-learning CD given in the previous edition were found quite useful and user-friendly and have been retained and updated. Besides, the CD in the revised edition also contains a quick review of pathology museum with images and legends of over 100 museum specimens of common conditions considered *must know* for students.

Although the revised edition of the book is primarily prepared for undergraduate students of pathology, it is also expected to be useful for practising clinicians and other students of medicine such as those pursuing course in dentistry, physiotherapy, pharmacy, nursing, laboratory technology and alternate systems of medicine.

ACKNOWLEDGEMENTS

In preparing the revised edition, I have been helped and supported by various friends, colleagues and my family, which is gratefully acknowledged. I owe a word of special thanks to Ms Agam Verma, MSc (MLT), Senior Laboratory Technician, for liberal and skillful technical assistance and her valuable suggestions in chapters on laboratory technology.

I thank profusely the entire staff of M/s Jaypee Brothers Medical Publishers (P) Ltd, New Delhi, India, in general for their constant support and cooperation, and Mrs Y Kapoor (Senior Desktop Operator) and Mr Manoj Pahuja (Senior Graphic Designer) in particular, in layout of the text and organising the large number of figures as per my requirements, ungrudgingly and smilingly. My special thanks are due to Shri Jitendar P Vij (Group Chairman) and Mr Ankit Vij (Managing Director), M/s Jaypee Brothers Medical Publishers (P) Ltd, New Delhi, India, for their constant co-operation and for being so supportive for getting the best final product for the users.

Finally, although sincere effort has been made to be as accurate as possible, an element of human error is still likely. I shall humbly request users to continue giving their valuable suggestions and feedback as they have been doing before for my all books; this helps me greatly to learn from the experience of users, improve further and carry out correction, wherever required, at the earliest possible opportunity.

Government Medical College **Harsh Mohan,** MD, FAMS, FICPath, FUICC
Sector-32 A, Chandigarh-160030 Professor & Head
INDIA Department of Pathology
e-mail: drharshmohan@gmail.com

Contents

SECTION 4: CYTOPATHOLOGY

SECTION 5: CLINICAL PATHOLOGY

SECTION 6: HAEMATOLOGY

Section One

TECHNIQUES IN PATHOLOGY

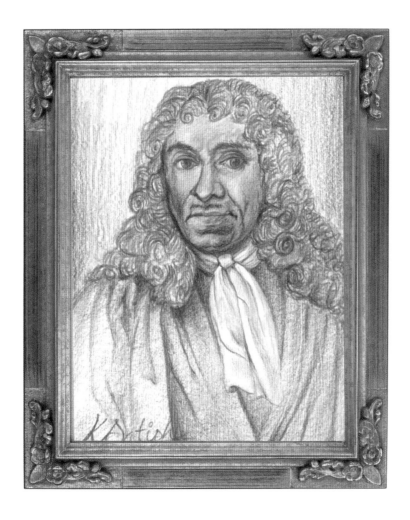

ANTHONY VAN LEEUWENHOEK (1632–1723)

**Born in Holland, draper by profession, during his spare time invented the first
ever microscope by grinding the lenses himself and made 400 microscopes.
He also first introduced histological staining in 1714 by
using saffron to examine muscle fibre.**

Section Contents

Microscopy

Objectives

➢ To understand the working of various parts of a light microscope and learn how to maintain and operate a light microscope.
➢ To enumerate various other types of diagnostic microscopy and understand the basic principles of their working and applications.

Microscope is the most commonly used apparatus in the diagnostic laboratory. It produces greatly enlarged images of minute objects. Most commonly used is a light microscope; this is described first, followed by various special types of microscopy.

Light Microscope

The usual type of microscope used in clinical laboratories is called light microscope that employs visible light as source of light. A light microscope can be a simple or a compound microscope.

Simple microscope. This is a simple hand magnifying lens. The magnification power of hand lens is from 2x to 200x.

Compound microscope. This has a battery of lenses fitted in a complex instrument. One type of lens remains near the object *(objective lens)* and another type of lens near the observer's eyes *(eyepiece lens)*. The eyepiece and objective lenses have different magnifications (described below). The compound microscope can be *monocular* having single eyepiece (Fig. 1.1), or *binocular* which has two eyepieces (Fig. 1.2).

A usual compound microscope has mechanical, electrical and optical parts. These include: stand, body, optical system, and light/illumination system.

STAND

This is horseshoe-shaped in monocular microscope and gives stability to the microscope. Binocular microscopes have a variety of shapes of stand.

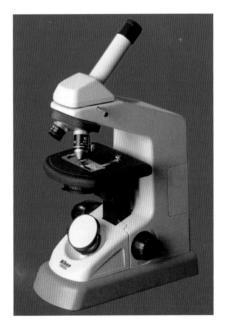

FIGURE 1.1 ◆ Monocular light microscope, Model YS 50 (Photograph courtesy of Nikon, Japan through Towa Optics India Pvt. Ltd., Delhi).

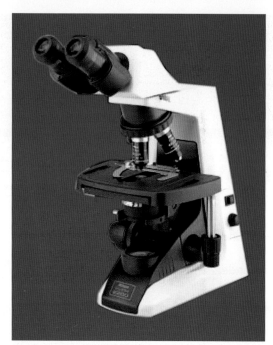

FIGURE 1.2 ◆ Binocular light microscope, Model E 200 (Photograph courtesy of Nikon, Japan through Towa Optics India Pvt. Ltd., Delhi).

BODY

Microscope body consists of a limb which arises from the joint with the stand. It helps in moving microscope in comfortable position from one place to another. Nowadays, microscope body is built in an ergonomic shape to avoid excessive strain on the back and neck of the user.

The stand and the limb of the body carry the following parts: body tubes, mechanical stage, and knobs for coarse and fine adjustment.

Body tubes. There are two tubes for optical path of the microscope. *External tube* at its lower end has a revolving nosepiece having slots for screwing in objective lenses of different magnifications. According to the number of objective lenses required to be fitted on the nosepiece, it may be triple, quadruple (4 slots), quintuple (5 slots) or sextuple (6 slots) nosepiece. The other end of the optical tube has an *internal tube* which is a draw tube with eyepieces placed at the upper end.

Mechanical stage. This is a metallic platform having slide holder that accommodates glass slide having object to be seen. Stage is attached to the limb just below the level of objective lenses. It has an aperture in its centre which permits the light to reach the object. Movement of the glass slide on the stage is regulated by two knobs attached to slide holder on the side of the stage. By this, the slide can be moved forward-backwards as well as left-right sides; it is also possible to make measurements on the object in the slide by graduated scale provided on the stage in both x and y axis.

Just below the stage is substage which consists of *condenser* through which light is focused on the object. The substage can be moved up and down. The substage has an *iris diaphragm*; its closing and opening controls the amount of light reaching the object with maximum resolution and minimum glare. Viewing object under higher magnification of objective lens requires more light and hence opened up diaphragm, and vice versa while viewing under lower magnification of objective lens.

Knobs for coarse and fine adjustment. For focusing of the object, knobs are provided on either side of the body—bigger knobs for coarse adjustment and smaller knobs for fine adjustments. In earlier models of microscopes, in order to focus the object on the glass slide to be viewed, coarse and fine adjustment knobs moved the body tube along with objective lenses up and down, while the microscope stage remained fixed. However, currently available models of microscopes provide for up and down movement of the microscope stage in order to bring the glass slide in focus near the objective lens, while the latter remains fixed. The fine focus is graduated and by each division objective moves by 0.002 mm.

OPTICAL SYSTEM

Optical system is comprised by different lenses which are fitted into a microscope. It consists of eyepiece, objectives and condensers.

Eyepiece. A monocular microscope has one eyepiece while a binocular microscope has two. Eyepiece has two planoconvex lenses. Their magnification can be 5x, 10x, or 15x. Commonly, 10x magnification is used.

Objectives. These are made of a battery of lenses with prisms incorporated in them. Their magnification power provides varying range. Usually 4x, 10x, 40x and 100x (oil immersion) objectives are used. However, other magnifications such as 2x and 20x are also available. These lenses are of various types, e.g. achromat, apochromat, planapoachromat, etc.

Condenser. This is made up of two simple lenses. As discussed above, it condenses light on to the object on the slide by up or down movement, and by opening or closing of the diaphragm.

LIGHT/ILLUMINATION SYSTEM

For daylight illumination, a mirror is fitted at the base of the microscope which is plane on one side and concave on the other side (Fig. 1.1). Plane mirror is used in sunlight while concave in artificial source of light. Currently, most of the microscopes have in-built electrical illumination fitted in the base with illumination ranging from 20 to 100 watts (Fig. 1.2).

MAGNIFICATION AND RESOLVING POWER OF LIGHT MICROSCOPE

Magnification power of the microscope is the degree of image enlargement. It depends upon the following:
  i. Length of the optical tube
  ii. Magnifying power of the objective lens used
  iii. Magnifying power of the eyepiece

With a fixed tube length of 160 mm in majority of standard microscopes, the magnification power of the microscope is obtained by the following:

Magnifying power of objective × Magnifying power of eyepiece.

Resolving power represents the capacity of the optical system to produce separate images of objects very close to each other.

$$\text{Resolving power (R)} = \frac{0.61\,\lambda}{\text{NA}}$$

Where
* λ is wavelength of incidental light; and
* NA is numerical aperture of lens which is generally engraved on the body of the objective lens.

Resolving power of a standard light microscope is around 200 nm.

HOW TO USE AND MAINTAIN A LIGHT MICROSCOPE?

1. The microscope should be kept on stable even surface and in comfortable position.
2. It should be kept dust free, taking care to use separate cleaning paper/cloth for mechanical and optical parts.
3. Obtain appropriate illumination by adjusting the mirror or intensity of light.
4. When examining colourless objects, condenser should be at the lowest position and iris diaphragm closed or partially closed.
5. When using oil immersion, 100x objective should dip in oil.
6. After using oil immersion, the lens of the objective should be cleaned with tissue paper or soft cloth.

NEWER APPLICATIONS OF LIGHT MICROSCOPE

In the recent times, computers and chip technology have helped in developing following newer applications of light microscope:

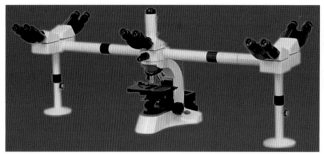

FIGURE 1.3 ◆ A penta-headed light microscope, for simultaneous use by one primary user and 4 other users seated nearby.

Teaching Microscopes

It is possible to modify a modern light microscope by various attachments for the purpose of teaching, training and group discussions (Fig. 1.3). These include attaching multiple viewing stations for simultaneous viewing by more users seated across or on the side (dual headed, multiheaded). Alternatively, the image can be projected simultaneously on the monitor by attaching a camera; still further improvement may be by interface of a CPU to click and store selected images as well.

Image Analysers and Morphometry

In these techniques, microscopes are attached to video monitors and computers with dedicated software systems. Microscopic images are converted into digital images and various cellular parameters (e.g. nuclear area, cell size, etc.) can be measured. This quantitative measurement introduces objectivity to microscopic analysis.

Telepathology

It is the examination of slides under microscope set up at a distance. This can be done by using a remote control device to move the stage of the microscope or change the microscope field or magnification called as *robotic telepathology*. Alternatively and more commonly, it can be used by scanning the images and using the high-speed internet server to transmit the images to another station termed as *static telepathology*. Telepathology is employed for consultation for another expert opinion or for primary examination.

Other Types of Microscopy

DARK GROUND ILLUMINATION (DGI)

This method is used for examination of unstained living microorganisms, e.g. *Treponema pallidum*.

Principle. The microorganisms are illuminated by an oblique ray of light which does not pass through the microorganism. The condenser is blackened in the centre and light passes through its periphery illuminating the living microorganism on a glass slide against dark background.

PHASE CONTRAST MICROSCOPY

Like DGI described above, phase contrast microscopy is also used for examination of unstained structures, most often living cells for assessing their functions at the level of organelles such as mobility, phagocytosis, etc.

Principle. Illumination of varying phase and amplitude is passed through unstained cells which assesses the difference in refractive indices of various organelles; the organelles shine differently based on whether they are dense/dark (higher refractive index) or less dark (low refractive index).

POLARISING MICROSCOPE

This method is used for demonstration of birefringence, e.g. amyloid, foreign body, hair, etc.

Principle. The light is made plane polarised. Two discs made up of prisms are placed in the path of light, one below the object known as polariser and another placed in the body tube which is known as analyser. Polariser sieves out ordinary light rays vibrating in all directions allowing light waves of one orientation to pass through. The lower disc (polariser) is rotated to make the light plane polarised. During rotation, when analyser comes perpendicular to polariser, all light rays are cancelled or extinguished. Birefringent objects rotate the light rays and therefore appear bright in a dark background.

FLUORESCENT MICROSCOPE

This method is used for demonstration of naturally-occurring fluorescent material and other non-fluorescent substances or microorganisms after staining with some fluorescent dyes, e.g. *Mycobacterium tuberculosis*, amyloid, lipids, elastic fibres, etc. Light source of low wavelength (UV light) for illumination is used, most often mercury vapour lamp or xenon gas lamp.

Principle. Fluorescent microscopy is based on the principle that illumination of a substance with a low wavelength (UV region, i.e. invisible spectrum) emits light at a higher wavelength (visible spectrum), thus localising the substance with fluorescence in the visible range. Fluorescent dyes are used depending upon the type of material to be visualised, e.g. fluorescein isothiocyanate (FITC), thioflavin, etc.

ELECTRON MICROSCOPE (EM)

EM is used for study of ultrastructural details of the tissues and cells. For electron microscopy, tissue is fixed in 4% glutaraldehyde at 4°C for 4 hours. Ultrathin microsections with thickness of 100 nm are cut with diamond knives.

Principle. By using an electron beam of light, the resolving power of the microscope is increased to 50,000 to 100,000 times and very small structures can be visualised. In contrast to light microscopy, resolution of electron microscopy is 0.2 nm or less.

There are two types of electron microscopy:
1. Transmission electron microscopy (TEM)
2. Scanning electron microscopy (SEM)

Transmission Electron Microscopy (TEM)

TEM helps visualise cell's cytoplasm and organelles. For this purpose, ultrathin sections are required. TEM interprets atomic rather than molecular properties of the tissue and gives two dimensional image of the tissue.

Scanning Electron Microscopy (SEM)

SEM helps in the study of cell surface. In this three-dimensional image is produced. The image is produced on cathode ray oscillograph which can also be amplified. SEM can also be used for fluorescent antibody techniques.

Routine Histopathology Techniques and Staining

Objectives
- ➢ To learn fixation of tissues and principles of common fixatives used in a tissue laboratory.
- ➢ To be familiar with equipments and procedure of routine histopathology processing of tissues in the laboratory.
- ➢ To learn the technique of routine H & E staining of tissues.

Histology is the science of examination of normal tissues at microscopic level while histopathology is examination of tissues for presence or absence of changes in their structure due to disease processes. Both are done by examining thin sections of tissues which are coloured differently by different dyes and stains. Total or chosen representative part of tissue not more than 4 mm thick is placed in steel or plastic capsules or cassettes and is subjected to the following sequential steps (tissue processing):
- ◆ Fixation
- ◆ Dehydration ⎤
- ◆ Clearing   ⎬ *Processing*
- ◆ Impregnation ⎦
- ◆ Embedding and blocking
- ◆ Section cutting (Microtomy)
- ◆ Routine staining (H & E)

Fixation

Any tissue removed from the body starts decomposing immediately because of loss of blood supply and oxygen, accumulation of products of metabolism, action of autolytic enzymes and putrefaction by bacteria. This process of decomposition is prevented by fixation. Fixation is the method of preserving cells and tissues in life-like conditions as far as possible. During fixation, tissues are fixed in complete physical and partly in chemical state. Most fixatives act by denaturation or precipitation of cell proteins or by making soluble components of cell insoluble. Fixative produces the following *effects:*
- i. Prevents putrefaction and autolysis.
- ii. Hardens the tissue which helps in section cutting.
- iii. Makes cell insensitive to hypertonic or hypotonic solutions.
- iv. Acts as a mordant.
- v. Induces optical contrast for good morphologic examination.

An ideal fixative has the following properties:
- i. It should be cheap and easily available.
- ii. It should be stable and safe to handle.
- iii. It should be rapid in action.
- iv. It should cause minimal loss of tissue.
- v. It should not bind to the reactive groups in tissue which are meant for dyes.
- vi. It should give even penetration.
- vii. It should retain normal colour of the tissue.
- viii. It should not impart its own colour to the tissue.

TYPES OF FIXATIVES

Fixatives may be simple or compound:
- ◆ *Simple fixative* consists of one substance (e.g. formalin).
- ◆ *Compound fixative* has two or more substances (e.g. Bouin's, Zenker's).

Fixatives can also be divided into following 3 groups:

♦ *Microanatomical fixatives* which preserve the anatomy of the tissue.

♦ *Cytological fixatives* which may be cytoplasmic or nuclear and preserve respective intracellular constituents.

♦ *Histochemical fixatives* employed for demonstration of histochemical constituents and enzymes.

Commonly used fixatives are as under:
1. Formalin
2. Glutaraldehyde
3. Picric acid (e.g. Bouin's fluid)
4. Alcohol (e.g. Carnoy's fixative)
5. Osmium tetraoxide

1. Formalin

This is the most commonly used fixative in routine practise. Formalin is commercially available as saturated solution of formaldehyde gas in water, 40% by weight/volume (w/v). For all practical purposes, this 40% solution is considered as 100% formalin. For routine fixation, 10% formalin is used which is prepared by dissolving 10 ml of commercially available formalin in 90 ml of water. Duration of fixation depends upon the size and thickness of the tissue, type of tissue and its density. It takes 6-8 hours for fixation of a thin piece of tissue 4 mm thick at room temperature. The amount of fixative should be 15 to 20 times the volume of the specimen. Formalin acts by polymerisation of cellular proteins by forming methylene bridges between protein molecules.

Merits of formalin
i. Rapidly penetrates the tissues.
ii. Normal colour of tissue is retained.
iii. It is cheap and easily available.
iv. It is the best fixative for neurological tissue.

Demerits of formalin
i. Causes excessive hardening of tissues.
ii. Causes irritation of skin, mucous membranes and conjunctiva.
iii. Leads to formation of formalin pigment in tissues having excessive blood at an acidic pH which can be removed by treatment of section with alcoholic picric acid.

2. Glutaraldehyde

This is used as a fixative in electron microscopy. Glutaraldehyde is used as 4% solution at 4°C for 4 hours for fixation of tissues.

Disadvantages of glutaraldehyde
i. It is expensive.
ii. It penetrates the tissues slowly.

3. Bouin's Fluid (Picric acid)

This is used as fixative for renal and testicular needle biopsies. Bouin's fluid stains the tissues yellow. It is also a good fixative for demonstration of glycogen. It is prepared as under:

Saturated aqueous picric acid	-	375 ml
40% formaldehyde	-	125 ml
Glacial acetic acid	-	25 ml

Yellow colour in the tissue due to picric acid can be removed by washing in 50-70% ethanol.

Disadvantages
i. Makes the tissue harder and brittle.
ii. Causes lysis of RBCs.

4. Carnoy's Fixative (Alcohol)

Alcohol is mainly used for fixation of cytologic smears and endometrial curettings. It acts by denaturation of cell proteins. Both methyl and ethyl alcohol can be used. Methyl alcohol is used as 100% solution for 20-30 minutes. Ethyl alcohol is used either as 95% solution or as Carnoy's fixative for tissues which contains the following:

Ethyl alcohol (absolute)	-	300 ml
Chloroform	-	150 ml
Glacial acetic acid	-	50 ml

Carnoy's is a good fixative for glycogen and dissolves fat.

5. Osmium Tetraoxide

This is used as a fixative for CNS tissues and for electron microscopy. Osmium tetraoxide is best fixative for lipids. It is used as a 2% solution. It imparts black colour to tissues.

Dehydration

This is a process in which water from the tissues and cells is removed so that this space so created is subsequently taken up by wax. Dehydration is carried out by passing the tissues through a series of ascending grades of alcohol: 70%, 80%, 95% and absolute alcohol. If ethyl alcohol is not available, other alternatives such as methyl alcohol, isopropyl alcohol or acetone can be used.

Clearing

This is the process in which alcohol from the tissues and cells is removed (dealcoholisation) and is replaced by a fluid in which wax is soluble. It also makes the tissue transparent. Xylene is the most commonly used clearing agent. Toluene, benzene (which is carcinogenic), chloroform (which is poisonous) and cedar wood oil (which is expensive and very viscous) can also be used as clearing agents.

Impregnation

This is the process in which empty spaces in the tissues and cells after removal of clearing agent are taken up by molten paraffin wax. This hardens the tissue which helps in section cutting. Impregnation is done in molten paraffin wax which has the melting point ranging from 54-62°C.

Tissue Processors

Processes of dehydration, clearing and impregnation are carried out in a composite equipment which is known as *automated tissue processor*. Automated tissue processor can be an open (hydraulic) system or a closed (vacuum) type.

OPEN (HYDRAULIC) TISSUE PROCESSOR

It has 12 stations—10 stations are glass/steel jars and 2 stations have thermostatically controlled wax bath. These jars are used as follow:

◆ For *fixation* in formalin: 1 jar.
◆ For *dehydration* in ascending grades of alcohol: 6 jars, one each of 70%, 80%, 90% and 3 for 100%.
◆ For *clearing* in xylene: 3 jars.
◆ For *impregnation* in molten paraffin wax: 2 wax baths.

Tissue moves automatically by hydraulic mechanism from one jar to the next after fixed time schedule as set in the program (Fig. 2.1). Generally, 1.5 hours duration is given at each station and whole process takes about 18 hours

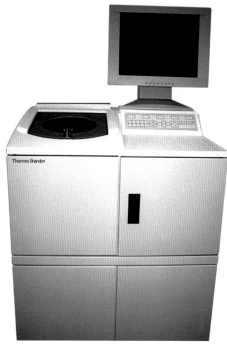

FIGURE 2.2 ◆ Vacuum tissue processor, Model Excelsior (Photograph courtesy of Thermo Shandon, UK through Towa Optics Pvt. Ltd., Delhi).

(overnight). For rapid processing, modern systems have programmes for short run in which entire tissue processing is completed in maximum of 2.5 hours; tissue stays at each station for 10-20 minutes. Nowadays, modifications are available in which vacuum system can be incorporated in open (hydraulic) type tissue processor.

CLOSED (VACUUM) TISSUE PROCESSOR

In the closed type of tissue processor, tissue cassettes are placed in a single container while different processing fluids are moved in and out sequentially according to electronically programmed cycle (Fig. 2.2). The closed or vacuum processor has the advantage that there is no hazard of contamination of the laboratory by toxic fumes unlike in open system. In addition, heat and vacuum shorten the processing time. Thus, closed tissue processors can also be applied for short schedules or rapid processing of small biopsies.

Currently, microwave technology-based tissue processors are also available which perform rapid processing of tissues.

Embedding and Blocking

Embedding of tissue is done in molten wax. Wax blocks can be conventionally prepared using metallic L (Leuckhart's) moulds; nowadays plastic moulds of different colours for

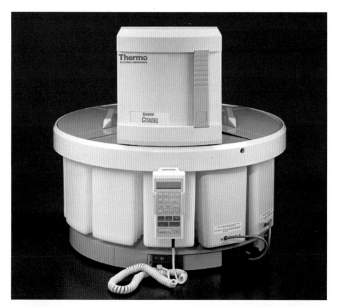

FIGURE 2.1 ◆ Automatic tissue processor (Photograph courtesy of Thermo Shandon, UK through Towa Optics India Pvt. Ltd., Delhi).

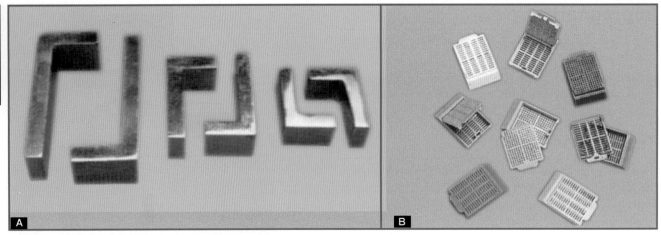

FIGURE 2.3 ◆ **A,** L (Leuckhart's) metal moulds. **B,** Plastic block moulds in different colours.

blocking are also available (Fig. 2.3). Same plastic moulds with detachable plastic covers can be used for the twin purpose of tissue capsule as well as moulds for blocking. The moulds are placed over a smooth surfaced glass tile. Molten wax is poured into the cavity in the moulds. The processed tissue pieces are put into wax with number tag and examining surface facing downward. Wax is allowed to solidify. After solidification, if L-moulds are used they are removed, while plastic mould remains with the wax block. In either case, each block contains a tissue piece carrying an identification label.

Embedding and blocking can also be performed in a special equipment called *embedding centre*. It has a wax reservoir, heated area for steel moulds, wax dispenser, and separate hot and cold plates for embedding and blocking (Fig. 2.4).

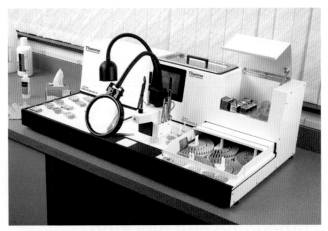

FIGURE 2.4 ◆ Tissue embedding centre, Model Histocentre (Photograph courtesy of Thermo Shandon, UK through Towa Optics (India) Pvt. Ltd., Delhi).

Section Cutting (Microtomy)

Microtome is an equipment for cutting sections and the technique of section cutting is called microtomy. There are 5 types of microtomes:
1. Rotary
2. Sliding
3. Freezing
4. Rocking
5. Base-sledge

1. *Rotary Microtome*

This is the most commonly used microtome. In this, microtome knife is fixed while the tissue block is movable (Fig. 2.5). The knife used is of stainless steel and is wedge-shaped (Fig. 2.6,A). The knife is sharpened by a process known as *honing* and *stropping*. Honing is done manually on a stone or on an electrically operated automatic hone. After honing, stropping is done which is polishing of its edge over a horse leather strop. The process of sharpening of microtome knife can also be done by automatic knife sharpener (Fig. 2.7). Nowadays, disposable blades for microtomy are also available which may be *high profile* with more width or *low profile* with narrow width (Fig. 2.6,B,C).

2. *Sliding Microtome*

In this, the tissue block is fixed while the knife is movable. These microtomes are used as freezing microtomes.

3. *Freezing Microtome*

This is discussed separately in Exercise 3.

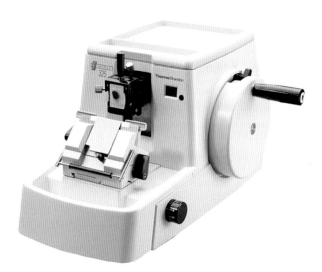

FIGURE 2.5 ◆ Rotary microtome, Model Finesse 325 (Photograph courtesy of Thermo Shandon, UK through Towa Optics India Pvt. Ltd., Delhi).

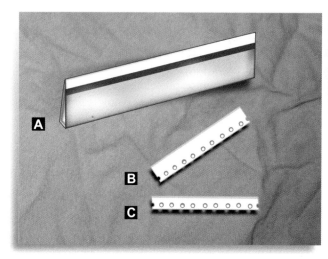

FIGURE 2.6 ◆ **A**, Plain wedge knife for rotary microtome. **B**, **C**, Disposable blades for microtomy—high profile type and low profile type respectively.

4. *Rocking Microtome*

This is a simple microtome. The knife is immovable while the tissue block is held in a spring-bearing rocking arm. It is not used nowadays.

5. *Base-Sledge Microtome*

This type of microtome is used for very hard tissues or large blocks, e.g. pieces of brain and heart.

PROCEDURE FOR MICROTOMY

Put the paraffin block having tissue in it in the rotary microtome. Cut the section by operating the microtome manually after adjusting the thickness at 3-4 μm. Sections are picked from the knife with the help of a forceps or camel hairbrush. Sections are made to float in a tissue floatation bath which is kept at a temperature of 45-50°C, i.e. 10° below the melting point of wax (Fig. 2.8). This removes folds in the

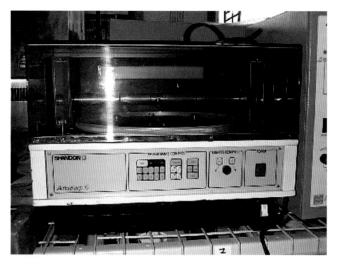

FIGURE 2.7 ◆ Automatic knife sharpener, Model Shandon Autosharp 5 (Photograph courtesy of Thermo Shandon, UK through Towa Optics India Pvt. Ltd., Delhi).

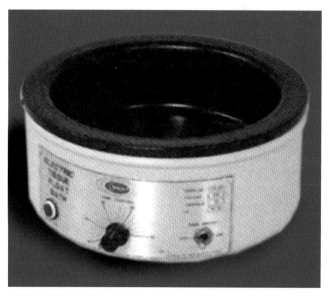

FIGURE 2.8 ◆ Tissue floatation bath (Photograph courtesy of Yorco Sales Pvt. Ltd, Delhi).

section. From tissue floatation bath, sections are picked on a clean glass slide. The glass slide is placed in an oven maintained at a temperature of 56°C for 20-30 minutes for proper drying and better adhesion. Coating adhesives for sections can be used before picking up sections; these include egg albumin, gelatin, poly-L-lysine, etc. The section is now ready for staining.

Routine Staining (H & E)

Routine staining is done with haematoxylin and eosin (H & E).

HAEMATOXYLIN

Haematoxylin is essentially a nuclear stain. This is a natural dye which is obtained from logwood of tree, *Haematoxylon campechianum*. This tree is commercially grown in Jamaica and Mexico. The natural extract from the stem of this tree is haematoxylin which is an inactive product. This product is oxidised to an active ingredient, haematein. This process of oxidation is known as *ripening* which can be done naturally in sunlight and air, or chemically by addition of oxidant like sodium iodate, $KMnO_4$ or mercuric oxide. A *mordant* is added to it (e.g. potash alum) which helps in penetrating the stain particles into the tissue.

Based on the mordant used, there are 3 main types of haematoxylins—alum haematoxylins (most commonly used), iron haematoxylins and tungsten haematoxylins. Many of the haematoxylins are alcohol soluble (e.g. Ehrlich's, Delafield's, Harris's) while others are water soluble (e.g. Mayer's, Carazzi's, Gill's).

EOSIN

Eosin is commonly used as a cytoplasmic stain. Most widely used is eosin Y dye which is both water and alcohol soluble. Commonly, it is used as 0.5-1% solution in distilled water

to which a crystal of thymol is added to inhibit growth of fungi.

Procedure for Staining

Sections are first deparaffinised (removal of wax) by placing the slide in a jar of xylene for 10-15 minutes. As haematoxylin is a water-based dye, the sections before staining are rehydrated which is done by passing the sections in a series of descending grades of alcohol and finally bringing the section to water.

- Place the slide in haematoxylin stain for 8-10 minutes.
- Rinse in water.
- *Differentiation* (i.e. selective removal of excess dye from the section) is done by putting the slide in a solution of 1% acid alcohol for 10 seconds.
- Rinse in water.
- *Blueing* (i.e. bringing of required blue colour to the section) is done by putting the section in Scott's tap water (containing sodium bicarbonate and magnesium sulphate) or saturated solution of lithium carbonate for 2-10 minutes.
- Counterstain with 1% aqueous solution of eosin for 30 seconds to 1 minute.
- One dip in tap water.
- Before mounting, the sections have to be dehydrated which is done by passing the sections in a series of ascending grades of alcohol and finally cleared in xylene, 2-3 dips in each solution.
- Mount in DPX (dextrene polystyrene xylene) or Canada balsam.

Currently, modern laboratories employ automated programmable autostainers.

Results

Nuclei	:	Blue
Cytoplasm	:	Pink
Muscle, collagen,		
RBCs, keratin,	:	Pink
colloid protein		

Exercise

3

Frozen Section and its Staining

Objectives
➤ To learn the technique and applications of frozen section.
➤ To perform staining for frozen section.

Frozen Section

When a fresh tissue is rapidly frozen, the matter within the tissue turns into ice; in this state the tissue is firm, the ice acting as an embedding medium. Therefore, sections are produced without the use of dehydrating solution, clearing agent or wax embedding. This procedure can be carried out in operation theatre complex near the operating table.

APPLICATIONS

i. It is a rapid intra-operative diagnostic procedure for pathology consultation while the patient is still under anaesthesia.
ii. It is used for determining whether the resection limits of surgical margin are free of tumour or not while the patient is still under anaesthesia.
iii. This is also used for demonstration of some special substances in the cells and tissues, e.g. fat, enzymes.

MERITS

i. This is a quick diagnostic procedure having a much shorter *turn-around-time* (i.e. time from receipt of tissue to the issue of a final report). Usually, the time needed from the receipt of tissue specimen to the study of stained sections is about 10 minutes while in routine paraffin-sectioning at least two days are required.
ii. Every type of staining can be done.
iii. There is minimal shrinkage of tissues as compared to paraffin sections.
iv. Lipids and enzymes which are lost in routine paraffin sections can be demonstrated.

DEMERITS

i. It is difficult to cut serial sections.
ii. It is not possible to maintain tissue blocks for future use.
iii. Sections cut are thicker.
iv. Structural details tend to be distorted due to lack of embedding medium.

METHODS FOR FROZEN SECTIONS

There are two methods for obtaining frozen sections:
1. Freezing microtome using CO_2 gas
2. Refrigerated microtome (cryostat).

For frozen section, best results are produced from fresh unfixed tissue and freezing the tissue as rapidly as possible.

Freezing Microtome using CO_2 Gas

In this method, freezing microtome is used which is a sliding type of microtome.

Setting of microtome and section cutting. The microtome is screwed firmly to the edge of a table by means of a stout screw. A CO_2 gas cylinder is placed near the microtome. The cylinder is then connected to the microtome by means of a special tubing. The connecting tube should not have any bends or cracks. Adjust the gauze of the microtome to a required thickness of sections. The knife is inserted in its place. Pour a few drops of water on the stage and place the selected piece of tissue on it. Short bursts of CO_2 are applied to freeze the tissue and water till the surface of the tissue is completely covered with ice. Alternatively, solid CO_2 (dry ice, cardice) can be used for freezing tissue blocks. Sections are then cut by swinging movement of knife forward and backward with a regular

(13)

rhythm. The cut sections come over the knife. From the knife, sections are picked with a camel-brush and transferred to a petri dish containing water. The sections are then placed over a glass slide with the help of a dropper. Remove the folds in the sections by tilting the slides. The slide is then passed over flame for a few seconds for fixing the sections over the slide. Section is now ready for staining with a desired stain.

Advantages

 i. It is cheap.
 ii. It requires less space.
 iii. Equipment is portable.

Disadvantages

 i. Sections cut are thick.
 ii. CO_2 gas may run out in between the procedures.
 iii. The connecting tube may be blocked due to solidified CO_2.

Refrigerated Microtome (Cryostat)

In cryostat, a rotary microtome with an antiroll plate housed in a thermostatically-controlled refrigerated cabinet is used while the rotary movement is operated from outside the cryostat. A temperature up to –30°C can be achieved (Fig. 3.1).

Setting of microtome and section cutting. Switch on the cryostat along with the knife inserted in position several hours before the procedure for attaining the operating temperature (generally –20°C or lower). A small piece of fresh unfixed tissue (4 mm) is placed on object disc of the deep freeze shelf of the cryostat for 1-2 minutes. The tissue is rapidly frozen. Now the object disc having frozen tissue is inserted into microtome object clamp. Place antiroll plate in its position. By manual movement, sections are cut at desired thickness. The antiroll plate prevents folding of sections. The section is picked from the knife directly on to the clean glass slide. A glass slide is lowered on to the knife 1 mm from section. The section comes automatically on the glass slide because of difference in temperature between the section and the slide. The section is ready for staining. The cryostat is defrosted and cleaned on weekends.

Advantages

 i. Sections cut are thin.
 ii. There is better control of temperature.
 iii. Equipment is portable.

Disadvantage

Equipment is expensive.

Staining of Frozen Sections

Sections obtained by freezing microtomy by either of the methods are stained by one of the rapid method as under:

RAPID H & E STAINING

♦ Place the section in haematoxylin for one minute.
♦ Rinse in tap water.
♦ Differentiate in 1% acid alcohol by giving one rapid dip.
♦ Rinse in water.
♦ Quick blueing is done by passing the section over ammonia vapours or rapid dip in a blueing solution.
♦ Rinse in tap water.
♦ Counterstain with 1% aqueous eosin for 3-6 seconds.
♦ Rinse in tap water.
♦ Dehydrate by passing the section through 95% alcohol and absolute alcohol, one dip in each solution.
♦ Clearing is done by passing the section through xylene, one dip.
♦ Mount in DPX.
♦ Examine under the microscope.

TOLUIDINE BLUE STAINING

♦ Place the section in toluidine blue solution 0.5% for ½ to 1 minute.
♦ Rinse in water.
♦ Mount in water or glycerine (i.e. aqueous mountant) with coverslip.
♦ Examine under the microscope.

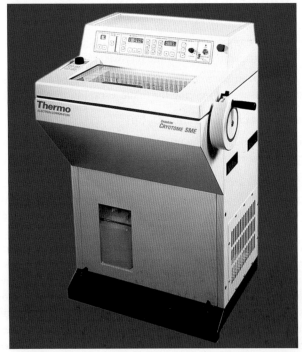

FIGURE 3.1 ♦ Cryostat, Model Cryotome (Photograph courtesy of Thermo Shandon, UK through Towa Optics India Pvt. Ltd., Delhi).

Special Stains and Immunohistochemistry

Objectives

➢ To learn broad principles of common special stains in surgical pathology and interpretation of their results.
➢ To learn the principle of immunohistochemical (IHC) staining and applications of common IHC stains.

Special (or histochemical) stains and immunohistochemical (IHC) stains are ancillary staining techniques used on paraffin-embedded sections to improve the morphologic diagnosis made on routine H & E staining.

Special Stains

Special stains, also called histochemical stains, are applied for demonstration of certain specific substances/constituents of the cells/tissues. The staining depends upon physical, chemical or differential solubility of the stain with the tissues. The principles of some of the staining procedures are well known while those of others are unknown. Some of the common special stains in use in the laboratory are as under (Fig. 4.1):

SUDAN BLACK/OIL RED O

These stains are used for demonstration of fat.

Principle. Sudan black and oil red O stains are based on physical combination of the stain with fat. It involves differential solubility of stain in fat because these stains are more soluble in fat than the solvent in which these are prepared. The stain leaves the solvent and goes into the fat.

Procedure for oil red O staining

◆ Cut frozen section.
◆ Rinse in 60% isopropyl alcohol.

◆ Put in oil red O solution for 5-10 minutes.
◆ Rinse in 60% isopropyl alcohol.
◆ Wash in water.
◆ Counterstain with haematoxylin for 1-2 minutes.
◆ Wash with water and blue.
◆ Rinse in water.
◆ Mount in glycerin or any other aqueous mountant.

Result

With oil red O

Fat	:	Bright red
Nuclei	:	Blue

With Sudan black

Fat	:	Black
Nuclei	:	Red

VAN GIESON

This stain is used for staining of collagen fibres.

Principle. It is based on the differential staining of collagen and other tissues (e.g. muscle) depending upon the porosity of tissue and the size of the dye molecule. Collagen with larger pore size takes up the larger molecule red dye (acid fuchsin) in an acidic medium, while non-porous muscle stains with much smaller molecule dye (picric acid).

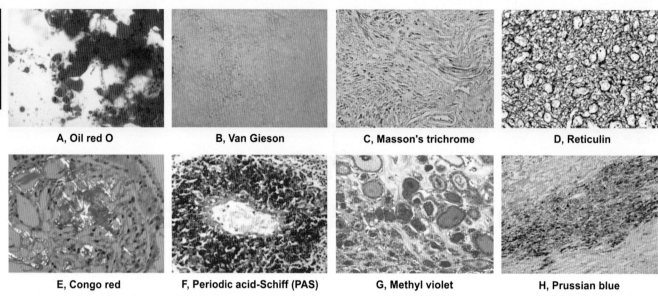

| A, Oil red O | B, Van Gieson | C, Masson's trichrome | D, Reticulin |
| E, Congo red | F, Periodic acid-Schiff (PAS) | G, Methyl violet | H, Prussian blue |

FIGURE 4.1 ◆ Common special stains. **A**, Oil red O for fat. **B**, Van Gieson for collagen. **C**, Masson's trichrome for muscle. **D**, Reticulin for reticulin fibre. **E**, Congo red for amyloid. **F**, Periodic acid-Schiff (PAS) for glycogen. **G**, Methyl violet for metachromasia. **H**, Prussian blue for iron.

Result

Collagen	:	Red
Nuclei	:	Blue
Other tissues	:	Yellow
(including muscle and RBC's)		

MASSON'S TRICHROME

This stain is used for staining of muscle.

Principle. The principle is the same as for van Gieson outlined above.

Result

Muscle	:	Red
Nuclei	:	Blue-black
Collagen	:	Blue-green

RETICULIN

This is used for demonstration of reticulin fibres.

Principle. Reticulin stain employs silver impregnation method. There is local reduction and selective precipitation of silver salt which get impregnated on the tissue.

Result

Reticulin fibres	:	Black
Nuclei	:	Colourless
Collagen	:	Brown

CONGO RED

This stain is used for demonstration of amyloid, an extracellular fibrillar proteinaceous substance.

Principle. Congo red dye has selective affinity for amyloid and attaches through non-polar hydrogen bonds. It gives green birefringence when viewed by polarised light.

Result

Amyloid elastic fibres : Red

Only amyloid gives green birefringence in polarised light.

PERIODIC ACID-SCHIFF (PAS)

PAS stain is used for demonstration of glycogen and mucopolysaccharides.

Principle. Tissues/cells containing 1,2 glycol group are converted into dialdehyde with the help of an oxidising agent which then reacts with Schiff's reagent to give magenta colour. Schiff's reagent is colourless.

Result

PAS positive substances	:	Magenta
Nuclei	:	Blue

PAS positive substances are glycogen, fungi, basement membrane, neutral mucin and hyaline cast.

METHYL VIOLET

This is a metachromatic stain, i.e. the tissues are stained in a colour which is different from the colour of the stain itself. It is used for demonstration of amyloid in tissue.

Principle. This depends upon the type of dye (stain) used and character of the tissue which unites with the dye. Tissues containing SO_4, PO_4 or $COOH$ groups react with basic dyes and cause their polymerisation, which in turn leads to production of colour that is different from the original dye.

Result

Metachromatic positive tissue	:	Red to violet
Other tissues	:	Blue

Other metachromatic stains used are crystal violet, toluidine blue.

PRUSSIAN BLUE/PERL'S REACTION

This is used for demonstration of iron.

Principle. Ferric ions present in the tissue combine with potassium ferrocyanide forming ferric-ferrocyanide.

Result

Iron	:	Blue
Cytoplasm and nuclei	:	Red to pink

Immunohistochemical Stains

Immunohistochemistry (IHC) is the application of immunologic techniques to the cellular pathology.

Principle. The technique of IHC is used to detect the status and localisation of particular antigen in the cells (membrane, cytoplasm or nucleus) by use of specific antibodies which are then visualised by chromogen (using DAB which gives brown colour). This then helps in determining cell lineage specifically, or is used to confirm a specific infection.

TECHNIQUE OF IHC

Immunoperoxidase technique employing labelled antibody method to *formalin-fixed paraffin sections* is now widely used. Currently, two most commonly used procedures in IHC are as under:

i) Peroxidase-antiperoxidase (PAP) method in which PAP reagent is pre-formed stable immune-complex which is linked to the primary antibody by a bridging antibody.

ii) Avidin-biotin conjugate (ABC) immunoenzymatic technique in which biotinylated secondary antibody serves to link the primary antibody to a large preformed complex of avidin, biotin and peroxidase.

Most commonly used chromogen is diaminobenzidine tetrahydrochloride or DAB.

INTERPRETATION

It is important to remember that *different antigens are localised at different sites in cells* (membrane, cytoplasm or nucleus) and accordingly positive brown staining is seen and interpreted at those sites, e.g. membranous staining for leucocyte common

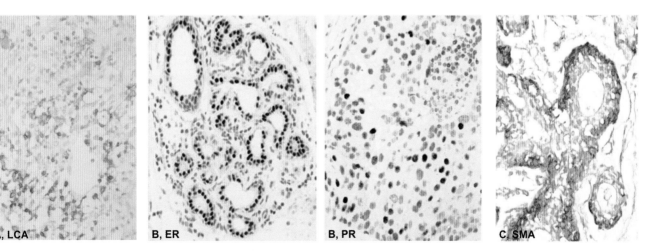

FIGURE 4.2 ◆ Examples of IHC stains. **A,** Membranous staining for LCA. **B,** Nuclear staining for ER/PR in breast carcinoma. **C,** Cytoplasmic staining for smooth muscle antigen (SMA) in myoepithelium in breast acinus.

antigen (LCA), nuclear staining for oestrogen-progesterone receptors (ER-PR), cytoplasmic staining for smooth muscle actin (SMA), etc. (Fig. 4.2).

APPLICATIONS OF IHC

Use of IHC has added objectivity, specificity and reproducibility to the surgical pathologist's diagnosis. IHC stains are used for the following purposes, in order of diagnostic utility:

1. **Tumours of uncertain histogenesis.** A panel of antibodies is chosen to resolve diagnostic problem cases. The selection of antibodies is made on the basis of clinical history, morphologic features and differential diagnosis considered on routine staining, and also based on results of other relevant investigations.

2. **Prognostic markers in cancer.** These include: proto-oncogenes (e.g. HER-2/neu overexpression in carcinoma breast), tumour suppressor genes or antioncogenes (e.g. *Rb* gene, *p53*), growth factor receptors (e.g. epidermal growth factor receptor or EGFR), and tumour cell proliferation markers (e.g. Ki67, proliferation cell nuclear antigen PCNA).

3. **Prediction of response to therapy.** IHC is widely used to predict therapeutic response in two important tumours—carcinoma of the breast and prostate. The results of oestrogen-receptors and progesterone-receptors (ER-PR) in breast cancer have significant prognostic correlation, though the results of androgen-receptor studies in prostatic cancer have limited prognostic value.

4. **Infections.** IHC stains are applied to confirm infectious agent in tissues by use of specific antibodies against microbial DNA or RNA, e.g. detection of viruses (HBV, CMV, HPV, herpesviruses), bacteria (e.g. *Helicobacter pylori*), and parasites (*Pneumocystis carinii*), etc.

However, IHC stains cannot be applied to distinguish between neoplastic and non-neoplastic lesions, or between benign and malignant tumours. These distinctions have to be done by traditional methods in surgical pathology.

Surgical Pathology Request Form

Objectives

➢ To learn to send a proper and complete requisition for surgical pathology examination of biopsy/excised organ.
➢ To fill out a sample of Surgical Pathology Request Form.

The receipt of the biopsy/excised organ in the surgical pathology laboratory is followed by a series of complex steps in the laboratory before the surgical pathologist issues histopathology report which has a great bearing in the management of patient by the clinician. The time spent between tissue accession in the laboratory and issuance of report is called *turnaround time (TAT)*. These days, there is justified need and urgency for reducing the TAT owing to shorter hospital stay of the patient.

Although the skill and expertise of histopathologist entrusted with the job of "sign-outs" (or reporting) is of importance, the very nature of histopathology as a speciality is such that it has its limitations and potentials, and thus the final pathology report depends heavily on the input received from the requisitioning clinician. There are several ways of communication between the surgical pathologist and the surgeon but one which has stood the test of time and also for proper record-keeping in pathology department for future reference, is the *Surgical Pathology Request Form* that accompanies the specimen. In view of other patient-related priorities of the main surgeon at the time of surgery or biopsy, unfortunately the job of filling out this request form is invariably assigned to a juniormost person in the surgical team who may or may not be fully conversant with the entire details of the patient. Many a times, an inadequate data on the request form results in avoidable delay or incomplete report, or a report based on misinterpretation of microscopic findings by the pathologist. Thus, there is certainly need for future and present resident doctors in clinical departments sending biopsies to be familiar with the essential clinical data to be

provided to the pathologist and treat these request forms differently than the requests for routine haematology, biochemistry or clinical pathology tests.

Design of the Request Form

The Surgical Pathology Request Form must be designed by the pathology service department in such a way that it has a place for patient identity and separate columns for various aspects of clinical data. The latter includes as brief history, findings of physical and local examination, operative findings, results of other relevant investigations including radiological findings, clinical/differential diagnosis and cross-reference of a previous procedure (e.g. FNA or biopsy) if done and examined earlier. In the author's department, this form has also a place informing the clinician how to prepare 10% formalin, ratio of formalin and the specimen, and re-emphasising the need by the pathologist for clinical data to be filled out while sending request for histopathologic examination.

In more modern set ups, the entire information of clinical data is available to the pathologist through hospital and laboratory network and hence paperless working.

Sample Request Form

Figure 5.1 shows a completely and appropriately filled out sample request form that accompanied a requisition for histopathologic examination of a specimen of "modified radical mastectomy (MRM) with axillary clearance" in a case who had earlier undergone FNA in the same department.

GOVERNMENT MEDICAL COLLEGE HOSPITAL
SECTOR-32, CHANDIGARH

DEPARTMENT OF PATHOLOGY

Name	RR
Age/Sex	58/F
CR No.	120703824
Ward/OPD	General Surgery
Date: 12/07/12	Income: 20,000/-

Referred by   Dr AK Dalal

Site of biopsy   Right breast

Material sent   MRM (right) with axillary clearance

Clinical Data   Locally advanced breast cancer (LABC) right.
6 × 5 cm central tumour, Peau de orange over
tumour, nipple retracted. Left breast normal.

Biopsy No.   S-4410/12

Radiological and any other investigations   B/L mammography: Asymmetric area of increased density in superolateral quadrant
(right breast) suspicious of malignancy.
Bone scan: Degenerative changes in the spine but no metastasis.

Provisional diagnosis   Ca breast (right) with metastasis in axillary lymph node

Previous cytology/histopathology no, if any   A-1315/12 FNA right breast showed infiltrating duct carcinoma.
FNA right axillary lymph node showed metastasis

Date   12/07/2012   Signature....................

For use in the Department of Pathology

Received	Sectioned	
Processed	Stained	
Blocked	Reported	Technician

Directions for sending tissue for Histopathological Examination:

A.   (i)   Tissue after removal should be transferred to 10% formalin immediately.

      (ii)   Ratio of tissue to formalin should be 1 to 15 for proper fixation.

      (iii)   Prepare formalin (10%) as follows:

               Formalin   10 ml

               Tap water   90 ml

B.   If clinical summary is not given, the report is likely to be withheld or delayed.

C.   Clearly state if any special information is desired from laboratory.

SURGICAL PATHOLOGY REQUEST

FIGURE 5.1 ◆ A sample of Surgical Pathology Request Form for dispatch of a specimen of modified radical mastectomy (MRM)
with axillary clearance.

During their learning period, the students of pathology must be exhorted to undertake the exercise of writing a Surgical Pathology Request Form on different specimens in a manner similar to teaching them prescription writing in another department. This way, it will be possible to re-emphasise the justifiable need by the pathologist for a completed surgical request form to the future resident doctors who would be sending such requests.

Section Two

GENERAL PATHOLOGY

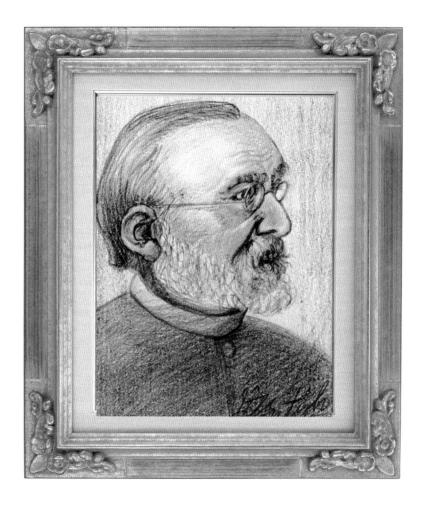

RUDOLF VIRCHOW (1821–1902)
'Father of Modern Pathology'

German physician, who described cellular basis of disease and introduced histopathology as a diagnostic branch. Important discoveries going by his name include: Virchow cells (lepra cell), Virchow node (enlarged left supraclavicular lymph node in cancer of the stomach), Virchow space in brain tissue, and Virchow's triad in pathogenesis of thrombosis.

Section Contents

Degenerations

Objectives
> To learn common forms of degenerations with examples—hydropic change (e.g. vacuolar nephropathy), hyaline change (e.g. leiomyoma), myxoid degeneration (e.g. ganglion).
> To describe salient gross and microscopic features of these conditions.

The term degeneration has been used conventionally to denote morphologic expression of reversible form of cell injury. These include earliest form of cell injury (e.g. hydropic change kidney), deposition of pink proteinaceous hyaline material at intracellular or extracellular location (e.g. in uterine leio-myoma), and accumulation of mucoid material in epithelial tissues or myxoid material in connective tissues (e.g. in ganglion cyst).

Vacuolar Nephropathy

Vacuolar nephropathy is the initial or reversible change seen grossly as "cloudy change" and microscopically as well-defined "hydropic vacuoles" due to accumulation of water within the cytoplasm of the convoluted tubules in the kidney. Most commonly, it is due to impaired regulation of sodium and potassium at the level of cell membrane resulting in intracellular accumulation of sodium (and water) and escape of potassium. Common causes are acute and subacute cell injury from various causes such as bacterial toxins, chemicals, poisoning, burns, high fever, intravenous administration of hypertonic glucose or saline, etc.

G/A The kidneys are slightly enlarged due to swelling and pale due to compression of blood vessels. The cut surface has cloudy, opaque appearance and bulges out.

M/E
  i. The epithelial cells of proximal convoluted tubules show small clear well-defined vacuoles in their cytoplasm.

These vacuoles are watery in character (hydropic change) and do not stain for fat or glycogen; they represent distended endoplasmic reticulum.
  ii. The microvasculature in the renal interstitium is compressed due to swollen tubular epithelial cells (Fig. 6.1).

Hyaline Change in Leiomyoma

The word hyaline simply refers to morphologic appearance of the material that has glassy, pink, homogeneous appearance when routinely stained with haematoxylin and eosin. Hyaline change (or hyalinisation) represents an end-stage of many diverse and unrelated lesions. It may be intracellular or extracellular. Hyaline degeneration in leiomyoma, a benign smooth muscle tumour, is an example of extracellular hyaline in the connective tissue.

G/A Uterine leiomyomas, depending upon location, may be subserosal, intramural or submucosal. Leiomyoma is a circumscribed, firm to hard tumour. Cut surface presents a whorled appearance. Hyaline change in leiomyoma is common and appears glassy and homogeneous (Fig. 6.2).

M/E
  i. There is a mixture of smooth muscle fibres and fibrous tissue in varying proportions. Some of the muscle fibres may be cut longitudinally and some transversely.
  ii. Smooth muscle fibres admixed with fibrous tissue are arranged in a whorled pattern at many places.

(23)

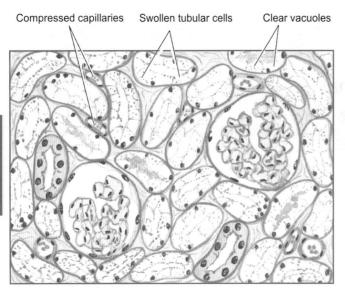

Compressed capillaries   Swollen tubular cells   Clear vacuoles

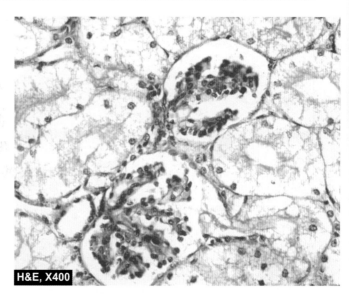

H&E, X400

FIGURE 6.1 ◆ Vacuolar nephropathy. The tubular epithelial cells are distended with cytoplasmic clear vacuoles while the interstitial vasculature is compressed. The nuclei of affected tubules are pale.

iii. The cytoplasm of smooth muscle fibres is more pink and their nuclei are short, plump and fusiform while the cytoplasm of fibroblasts is light pink in colour and nuclei are longer, slender and have pointed ends.

iv. Areas of hyaline change appear as pink, homogeneous and acellular lying in the centre of the whorls or between them (Fig. 6.3).

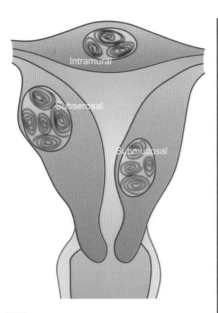

Intramural
Subserosal
Submucosal

A

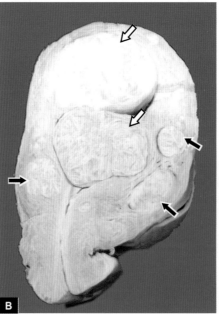

B

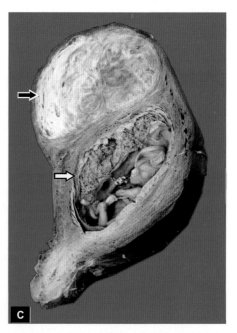

C

FIGURE 6.2 ◆ Leiomyomas uterus. **A**, Diagrammatic appearance of common locations and characteristic whorled appearance on cut section. **B**, Sectioned surface of the uterus shows multiple circumscribed, firm nodular masses of variable sizes—submucosal (white arrows) and intramural (black arrows) in location having characteristic whorling. **C**, The opened up uterine cavity shows an intrauterine gestation sac with placenta (white arrow) and a single circumscribed, enlarged, firm nodular mass in intramural location (black arrow) having grey-white whorled pattern.

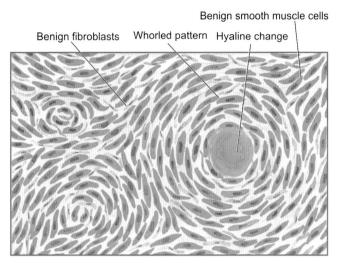
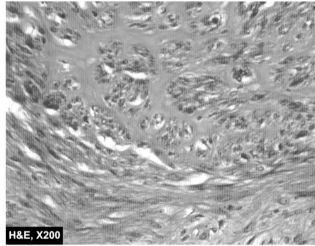

Benign fibroblasts Whorled pattern Hyaline change

Benign smooth muscle cells

H&E, X200

FIGURE 6.3 ◆ Leiomyomas. Microscopy shows whorls of smooth muscle cells which are spindle-shaped, having abundant cytoplasm and oval nuclei and mixed with fibrous tissue. The hyaline material appears homogeneous, pink and glassy.

Myxoid Degeneration in Ganglion

While mucus is the normal watery secretion of mucous glands (epithelial mucin) or by certain connective tissue cells, especially in the foetus (connective tissue mucin), myxoid or mucoid degeneration refers to exaggerated form of the process and may involve both these types of mucin. In the early stages of a ganglion of the wrist, connective tissue mucin develops in the synovial membrane in connection with the tendon sheath.

G/A The lesion appears most commonly as a cyst containing soft mucoid material.

M/E
  i. The cyst of ganglion is composed of fibrous wall devoid of any specialised lining.
  ii. Centre of the cyst contains a mass of acellular basophilic myxoid material (Fig. 6.4).
  iii. Connective tissue mucin stains positively with colloidal iron and alcian blue.

Myxoid change   Cyst wall

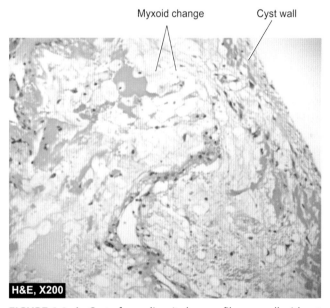

H&E, X200

FIGURE 6.4 ◆ Cyst of ganglion. It shows a fibrous wall without any distinct lining. The wall shows areas of basophilic myxoid material.

Intracellular Accumulations

Objectives
➢ To learn common forms of intracellular accumulations with examples—fat (e.g. fatty change liver), melanin (e.g. naevus), anthracotic pigment (e.g. anthracotic pigment in lung), lipofuscin (e.g. brown atrophy heart).
➢ To describe salient gross and microscopic features of these conditions.

Intracellular accumulations of substances in abnormal amounts may occur within the cytoplasm of cells under various conditions that may produce cell injury. These substances may be constituents of normal metabolism produced in excess (e.g. fatty change), normal endogenous pigments in excess (e.g. melanin), abnormal pigment produced endogenously (e.g. lipofuscin), or pigments entering the body exogenously (e.g. anthracosis).

Fatty Change Liver

Fatty change (steatosis) is seen most commonly in the liver since it is the major organ involved in fat metabolism. The causes include alcohol abuse (most common cause in industrialised world), protein malnutrition, obesity, diabetes mellitus, anoxia, and various toxins (carbon tetrachloride, chloroform, ether, etc.).

G/A The liver is enlarged and yellow with tense, glistening capsule and rounded margins. The cut surface bulges slightly and is pale-yellow and greasy to touch (Fig. 7.1).

M/E
 i. Fat in the cytoplasm of the hepatocytes is seen as clear area which may vary from minute droplets in the cytoplasm of a few hepatocytes *(microvesicular)* to distention of the entire cytoplasm of most cells by coalesced droplets *(macrovesicular)* pushing the nucleus to periphery of the cell (Fig. 7.2).

ii. When steatosis is mild, centrilobular hepatocytes are mainly affected, while the progressive accumulation of fat involves the entire lobule.

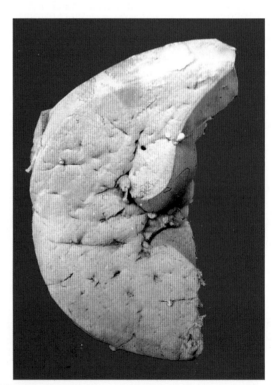

FIGURE 7.1 ◆ Fatty liver. Sectioned slice of the liver shows pale yellow parenchyma with rounded borders.

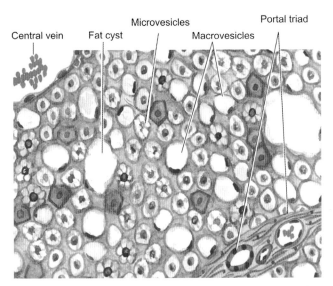
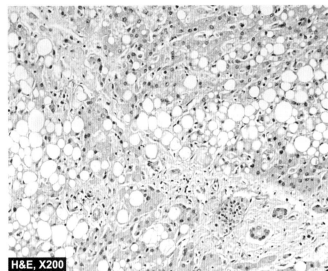

Central vein   Fat cyst   Microvesicles   Macrovesicles   Portal triad

H&E, X200

FIGURE 7.2 ◆ Fatty liver. Many of the hepatocytes are distended with large fat vacuoles pushing the nuclei to the periphery (macrovesicles), while others show multiple small vacuoles in the cytoplasm (microvesicles).

iii. Occasionally, the adjacent cells containing fat rupture and produce fatty cysts.

iv. Infrequently, lipogranulomas may appear consisting of collection of macrophages, lymphocytes and multi-nucleate giant cells.

v. Special stains such as Sudan III, Sudan IV, Sudan Black and Oil Red O can be employed to demonstrate fat in the tissue.

Melanin Pigment in Compound Naevus

Common moles or naevi (more appropriately termed nevocellular naevi) are the common benign neoplasms of the skin arising from melanocytes. There are numerous clinical and histologic types of nevocellular naevi and have variable clinical appearance.

G/A A mole clinically and grossly appears as a small tan dot 0.1-0.2 cm in diameter initially but subsequently enlarges to a uniform coloured tan to brown area which may be flat or slightly elevated and having regular, circular or oval outline.

M/E

i. The lesion is composed of melanocytes forming aggregates or nests at the dermo-epidermal junction (junctional naevus) which subsequently migrate to the underlying dermis (compound naevus). The older lesions may be entirely confined to dermis (dermal naevus).

ii. The melanocytes forming naevi are round to oval cells and have round or oval nuclei. The cytoplasm of naevus cells is homogeneous and contains abundant granular brown-black melanin pigment (Fig. 7.3).

iii. The pigment is more marked in the naevus cells in the lower epidermis and upper dermis but the cells in the mid-dermis and lower dermis hardly contain any pigment.

Anthracotic Pigment in Lung

The common, benign and asymptomatic deposition of carbon dust in the lungs of most urban dwellers due to atmospheric pollution and cigarette smoke is termed anthracosis of the lung. Anthracosis is thus not a lung disease in true sense. However, coal-miners may inhale very large amount of particulate carbon and develop a severe form of anthracosis called coal-miners' pneumoconiosis.

G/A The lungs as well as the involved hilar lymph nodes are black in colour. The cut section shows blackish mottling due to aggregates of anthracotic pigment.

M/E

i. Anthracotic pigment, black in colour, is deposited in the macrophages around respiratory bronchioles, beneath the pleura, and in the hilar lymph nodes.

ii. While anthracosis is not associated with any significant loss of pulmonary function, coal-workers' pneumo-coniosis is characterised by coal macule and coal nodule

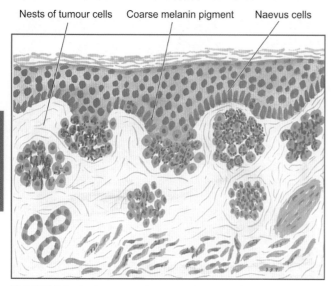

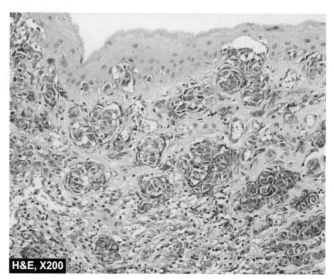

H&E, X200

FIGURE 7.3 ◆ Compound naevus showing clusters or lobules of benign naevus cells in the dermis as well as in lower epidermis. These cells contain coarse, granular, brown black melanin pigment.

consisting of carbon-laden macrophages admixed with some amount of collagen (Fig. 7.4).

Brown Atrophy Heart

Brown atrophy of the heart is the term used for intracellular accumulation of yellowish-brown lipid pigment called lipofuscin (*lipo* = fat, *fuscus* = brown) in the myocardial fibres. This pigment is also known as lipochrome or wear and tear or ageing pigment.

G/A The change is seen in the heart of ageing patients or patients with severe malnutrition and cancer cachexia. The heart is small in weight and light brown in colour.

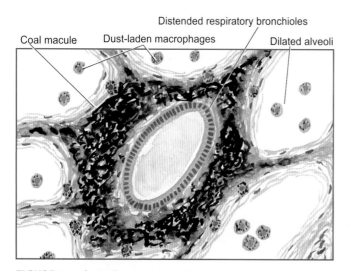

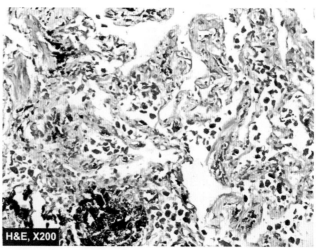

H&E, X200

FIGURE 7.4 ◆ Anthracosis lung. There is abundant coarse black carbon pigment in the septal walls and around the respiratory bronchiole.

Perinuclear lipofuscin granules

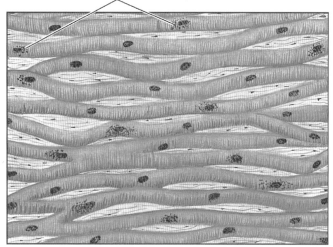

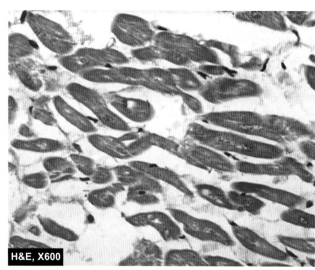

H&E, X600

FIGURE 7.5 ◆ Brown atrophy of the heart. The lipofuscin pigment granules are seen in the cytoplasm of the myocardial fibres, especially around the nuclei.

M/E

i. The myocardial fibres contain golden-brown, finely granular, intracytoplasmic pigment, often in perinuclear location.

ii. The myocardial fibres show changes of atrophy (Fig. 7.5).

iii. Lipofuscin can be stained by fat stains but differs from other lipids in being fluorescent and acid fast.

Amyloidosis

Objectives
➢ To learn common examples of deposition of amyloid in tissues (e.g. kidney, spleen, liver).
➢ To describe salient gross and microscopic features of these conditions.

Amyloidosis is extracellular deposition of fibrillar protein-aceous amyloid material in different organs. On routine staining, it appears pink and homogeneous; it shows positive staining with Congo Red (congophilia) which on polarising microscopy depicts characteristic apple-green birefringence.

Amyloidosis Kidney

Amyloidosis of the kidney is most common and most serious because of its ill-effects on renal function. The deposits in the kidneys are found in most cases of secondary amyloidosis and in about one-third cases of primary amyloidosis.

G/A The kidneys may appear normal, enlarged or terminally contracted due to ischaemic effect of narrowing of vascular lumina. The cut surface is pale, waxy and translucent (Fig. 8.1).

M/E
  i. The amyloid is seen as amorphous, eosinophilic, hyaline extracellular material. It is deposited mainly in the *glomeruli*, initially on the glomerular basement membrane but later extends to produce luminal narrowing and distortion of the glomerular capillary tuft.
 ii. The amyloid deposits in the *tubules* begin close to the tubular epithelial basement membrane. Subsequently, the deposits may produce degenerative changes in the tubular epithelial cells and amyloid casts in the tubular lumina.

 iii. The walls of small *arteries and arterioles* in the interstitium of the kidney are narrowed due to amyloid deposit (Fig. 8.2).
 iv. *Congo red staining* imparts pink or red colour to the amyloid when seen in ordinary light but demonstrates green birefringence when viewed under polarising microscopy (Fig. 8.3, A, B).

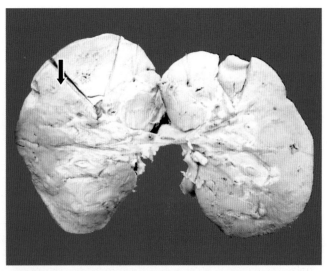

FIGURE 8.1 ◆ Amyloidosis of kidney. The kidney is small and pale in colour. Sectioned surface shows loss of corticomedullary distinction (arrow) and pale, waxy translucency.

(30)

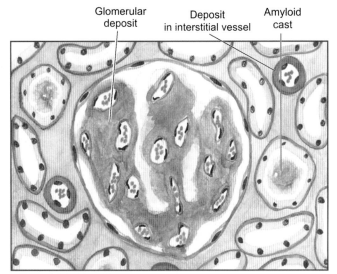

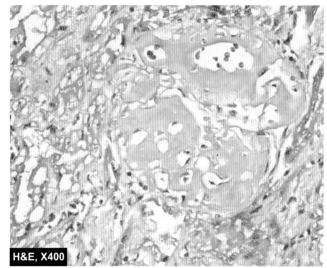

H&E, X400

FIGURE 8.2 ◆ Amyloidosis of kidney. The amyloid deposits are seen mainly in the glomerular capillary tuft. The deposits are also present in peritubular connective tissue producing atrophic tubules and amyloid casts in the tubular lumina, and in the arterial wall in the interstitium producing luminal narrowing.

Amyloidosis Spleen

Splenic amyloid may have two patterns—one associated primarily with deposition in the stroma of the red pulp (lardaceous spleen) and the second within the stroma of the white pulp (sago spleen).

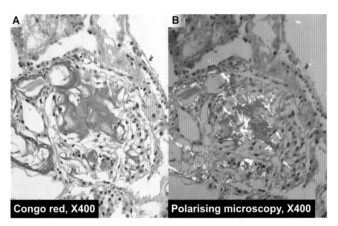

Congo red, X400　Polarising microscopy, X400

FIGURE 8.3 ◆ Amyloidosis kidney, Congo red stain. **A**, The amyloid deposits are seen mainly in the glomerular capillary tuft stained red-pink (Congophilia). **B**, Viewing the same under polarising microscopy, the congophilic areas show apple-green birefringence.

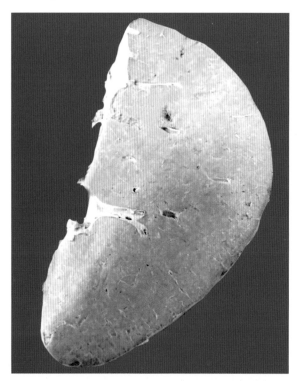

FIGURE 8.4 ◆ Lardaceous amyloidosis of the spleen. The sectioned surface shows presence of pale, waxy translucency in a map-like pattern.

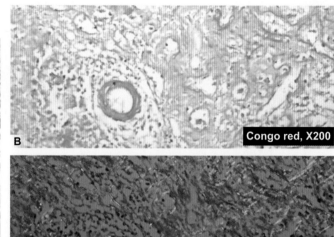

Atrophied white pulp

Pink acellular material

Expanded red pulp

A

H&E, X200

B

Congo red, X200

C

Polarising microscopy, X200

FIGURE 8.5 ◆ Amyloidosis spleen. **A,** The pink acellular amyloid material is seen in the red pulp causing atrophy of while pulp. **B,** Congo red staining shows Congophilia as seen by red-pink colour. **C,** When viewed under polarising microscopy the corresponding area shows apple-green birefringence.

G/A The spleen may be normal-sized or may cause moderate to marked splenomegaly. The cut surface of the spleen shows one of the two patterns of deposition—*lardaceous spleen* characterised by diffuse map-like areas of pale, waxy translucency (Fig. 8.4) or, alternatively, *sago spleen* seen as multiple pale foci corresponding to the regions of splenic follicles.

M/E
 i. In *lardaceous spleen,* the amyloid deposits are seen in the walls of splenic sinuses and the region of the red pulp.
 ii. In *sago spleen*, the amyloid deposits begin in the walls of the arterioles of the white pulp and eventually replacing the splenic follicles (Fig. 8.5, A).
 iii. *Congo red staining* gives pink or red colour to amyloid by light microscopy and when viewed in polarising light shows green birefringence (Fig. 8.5, B, C).

Amyloidosis Liver

Involvement of the liver is seen in about half the cases of systemic amyloidosis.

G/A Amyloidosis may not be apparent or may cause moderate to marked enlargement. The cut surface is pale, waxy and translucent.

M/E
 i. The amyloid deposits begins in the space of Disse obliterating the space that lies between the hepatocytes and sinusoidal endothelial cells.
 ii. Later, the deposits compress the cords of hepatocytes resulting in atrophy and shrinkage of liver cells and replace the cords of hepatocytes by amyloid (Fig. 8.6, A).
 iii. Congo red staining demonstrates pink red colour to amyloid by light microscopy and shows green birefringence when viewed under polarising microscopy (Fig. 8.6, B,C).

Central vein   Amyloid deposit   Atrophied hepatocytes   Portal triad

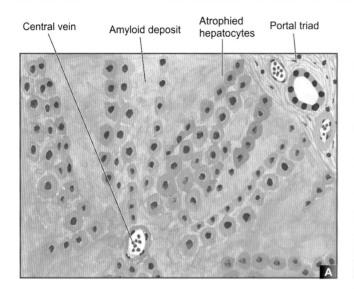

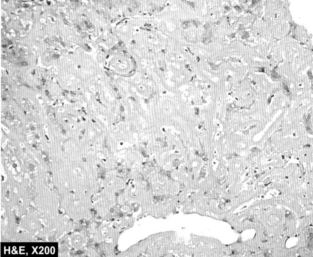

H&E, X200

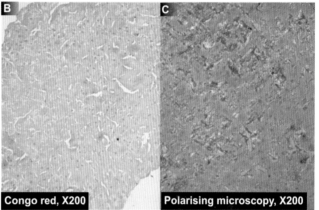

Congo red, X200   Polarising microscopy, X200

FIGURE 8.6 ◆ Amyloidosis of the liver. **A**, The deposition is extensive in the space of Disse causing compression and pressure atrophy of hepatocytes. **B**, Congo Red staining shows congophilia which under polarising microscopy shows apple-green birefringence **(C)**.

Necrosis

Objectives
➢ To learn common forms of necrosis with common examples—coagulative necrosis (e.g. infarct kidney), liquefactive necrosis (e.g. infarct brain), caseous necrosis (e.g. tuberculous lymphadenitis), and fat necrosis (e.g. acute pancreatitis).
➢ To describe salient gross and microscopic features of these conditions.

Necrosis is defined as morphologic expression of irreversible cell death. Depending upon etiologic agent producing it and pathogenetic mechanisms, major forms of necrosis can be distinguished. These are: coagulative necrosis due to cessation of blood supply (e.g. infarct kidney), liquefactive necrosis due to degradation of tissue by hydrolytic enzymes (e.g. infarct brain), caseous necrosis due to infection with tubercle bacilli (e.g. tuberculosis lymph node) and fat necrosis due to enzymatic degradation of fatty tissues and pancreas (e.g. acute pancreatitis).

Coagulative Necrosis (Infarct) Kidney

Coagulative necrosis is the most common type of necrosis caused by irreversible focal cell injury, most often from sudden cessation of blood supply or ischaemia (infarction). The characteristic examples of coagulative necrosis are seen in infarcts of the kidney, heart and spleen, resulting from thromboemboli.

G/A Renal infarcts are often multiple and may be bilateral. Characteristically, they are pale or anaemic and wedge-shaped with base resting under the capsule and apex pointing towards the medulla. Generally, a narrow rim of renal tissue under the capsule is spared because it draws its blood supply from the capsular vessels. The cut surface of renal infarct in the initial 2 to 3 days is red and congested but by 4th day the centre

becomes pale yellow. At the end of one week, the infarct is typically anaemic and depressed below the surface of the kidney (Fig. 9.1).

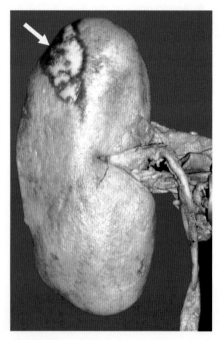

FIGURE 9.1 ◆ Infarct kidney. The wedge-shaped infarct is slightly depressed on the surface. The apex lies internally and wide base is on the surface. The central area is pale while the margin is haemorrhagic.

(34)

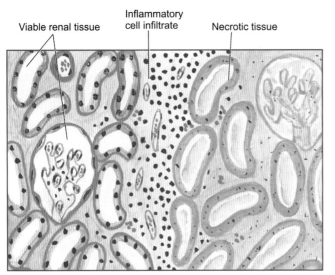

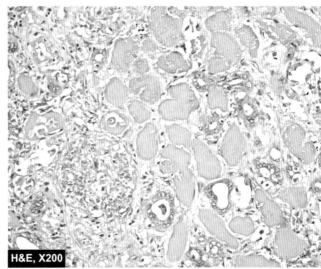

H&E, X200

FIGURE 9.2 ◆ Coagulative necrosis in infarct kidney. The affected area on right shows cells with intensely eosinophilic cytoplasm of tubular cells but the outlines of tubules are still maintained. The nuclei show granular debris. The interface between viable and non-viable area shows non-specific chronic inflammation and proliferating vessels.

M/E

  i. The hallmark of coagulative necrosis kidney is that architectural outlines of glomeruli and tubules may be preserved though all cellular details are lost.

  ii. The margin of infarct shows inflammatory reaction, initially by polymorphonuclear cells but later macrophages, lymphocytes and fibrous tissue predominate (Fig. 9.2).

Liquefactive Necrosis (Infarct) Brain

Liquefactive necrosis results commonly due to bacterial infections which constitute powerful stimuli for release of hydrolytic enzymes causing liquefaction. The common example is infarct of the brain.

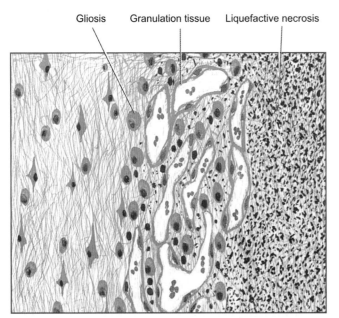

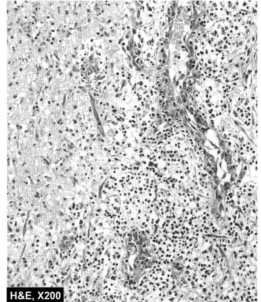

H&E, X200

FIGURE 9.3 ◆ Liquefactive necrosis brain. The necrosed area on right side of the field shows a cystic space containing cell debris, while the surrounding zone shows granulation tissue and gliosis.

G/A The affected area of the brain is soft with liquefied centre containing necrotic debris. Later, a cyst wall is formed.

M/E

i. The cystic space contains necrotic cell debris and macrophages containing phagocytosed material.

ii. The cyst wall is formed by proliferating capillaries, inflammatory cells and proliferating glial cells (gliosis) (Fig. 9.3).

Caseous Necrosis (Tuberculosis) Lymph Node

Caseous necrosis is a distinctive form of necrosis encountered in the foci of tuberculous infections. It combines the features of both coagulative and liquefactive necrosis. Tuberculous lymphadenitis is a common example of caseous necrosis.

G/A The lymph nodes are matted together. The cut surface shows characteristic map-like areas of yellowish, granular, soft necrotic material resembling dry cheese (Fig. 9.4).

M/E

i. The necrotic foci are composed of structureless, eosinophilic and granular debris which may contain foci of dystrophic calcification.

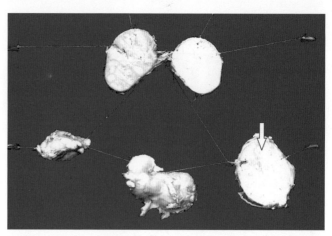

FIGURE 9.4 ◆ Caseous necrosis in tuberculous lymphadenitis. Multiple lymph nodes are matted together and surrounded by fat. Sectioned surface shows merging capsules of adjacent nodes and large areas of yellowish caseation necrosis (arrow).

ii. The area surrounding caseous necrosis shows characteristic granulomatous inflammatory reaction consisting of slipper-shaped epithelioid cells with interspersed giant cells of Langhans' type and peripheral mantle of lymphocytes (Fig. 9.5).

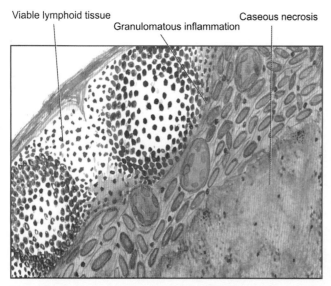

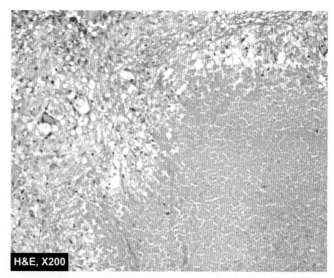

FIGURE 9.5 ◆ Tuberculous lymphadenitis. Area of caseation necrosis is surrounded by epithelioid cells having characteristic slipper-shaped nuclei, with interspersed Langhans' giant cells, and peripherally surrounded by lymphocytes.

Enzymatic Fat Necrosis Pancreas

Enzymatic fat necrosis of pancreas is the term used for focal areas of destruction of fat in the peritoneal cavity resulting from liberation of activated pancreatic lipases. This occurs in the fatal condition of acute pancreatitis.

G/A Fat necrosis appears as yellowish-white firm deposits. Formation of calcium soaps imparts the necrosed foci firmer and chalky-white appearance.

M/E

  i. The necrosed fat cells have cloudy shadowy appearance.
 ii. There are foci of calcium soaps identified in the tissue sections as amorphous, granular and basophilic material.
iii. There is surrounding zone of inflammatory reaction (Fig. 9.6).

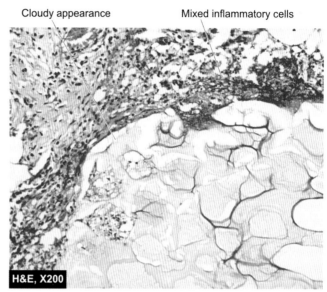

Cloudy appearance   Mixed inflammatory cells

H&E, X200

FIGURE 9.6 ◆ Fat necrosis in acute pancreatitis. There is cloudy appearance of adipocytes and coarse basophilic granular debris, peripherally surrounded by inflammatory granulation tissue.

Gangrene and Pathologic Calcification

Objectives

➤ To learn types of gangrene with common examples (e.g. wet gangrene bowel, dry gangrene foot) and types of pathologic calcification (e.g. dystrophic calcification in Monckeberg's arteriosclerosis).

➤ To describe salient gross and microscopic features of these conditions.

Gangrene is a form of ischaemic necrosis in which there is superadded bacterial infection. Depending upon type of pathogenetic mechanism and organs involved, there are two main forms of gangrene—*dry gangrene* due to obstruction in arterial blood supply (e.g. dry gangrene foot) and *wet gangrene* due to obstruction in drainage of venous blood or arterial obstruction (e.g. gangrene bowel).

Deposition of calcium salts at sites other than bones is called pathologic calcification. It is of 2 main types—*dystrophic calcification* in which the deposition occurs in degenerated (e.g. Monckeberg's arteriosclerosis) or necrotic tissues (e.g. in caseous necrosis as described on page 36) with normal blood calcium levels, and *metastatic calcification* in which the deposition occurs in normal tissues and is associated with raised blood calcium levels.

Wet Gangrene Bowel

Wet gangrene occurs in tissues and organs which contain fluid, e.g. bowel, lung, etc.

G/A The affected zone of the small bowel is suffused with blood causing haemorrhagic infarction which may be due to thromboembolic occlusion of the superior mesenteric artery commonly, or less often from thrombosis of the

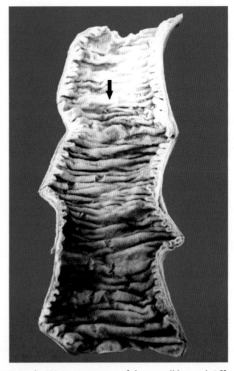

FIGURE 10.1 ◆ Wet gangrene of the small bowel. Affected part is soft, swollen and dark. Line of demarcation between gangrenous segment and the viable bowel is not clear cut (arrow).

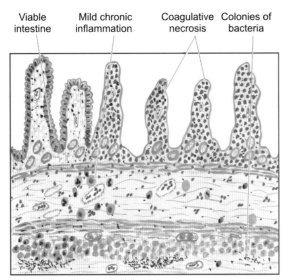

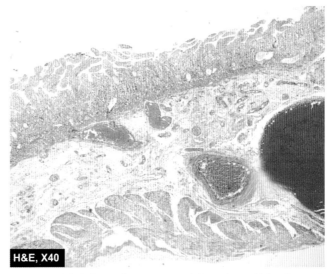

H&E, X40

FIGURE 10.2 ◆ Gangrene small bowel. The affected area shows non-viable infarcted segment and thrombosed blood vessels. The junction of normal with gangrenous segment is indistinct and there is inflammatory reaction.

mesenteric veins. In *arterial thromboembolic occlusion*, the line of demarcation between gangrenous bowel and normal bowel is usually sharp while *venous occlusion* may lead to a more diffuse appearance. The affected zone is dilated and the external surface may be dark purple, green and black. The mucosa shows haemorrhages and necrosis (Fig. 10.1).

M/E

i. There is coagulative and/or liquefactive necrosis affecting the entire thickness of the affected segment of the bowel and exudate on the serosa.

ii. Bacterial colonies may be identified in different layers of the affected bowel.

iii. The blood vessels in the bowel wall may show thrombi.

iv. The line of demarcation between the viable and gangrenous segment shows acute inflammatory cells (Fig. 10.2).

Dry Gangrene Foot

The typical form of dry gangrene is seen in most distal part of the foot when the arteries to the foot are obliterated, most often from arteriosclerosis in old age.

G/A The affected part of the foot is dry, shrunken and dark black resembling the foot of mummy. A line of separation is seen at the junction of viable tissue with gangrenous part (Fig. 10.3).

M/E

i. There is coagulative necrosis of the affected tissue identified by outlines of cells without nuclear and cytoplasmic details.

ii. In addition, there is blurring and smudging of outlines of cells with disintegration and breaking up.

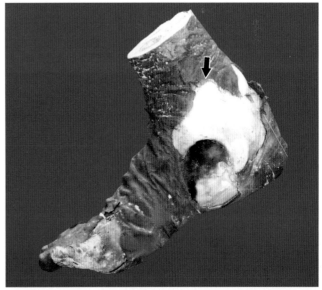

FIGURE 10.3 ◆ Dry gangrene of foot. The affected part is dry, shrunken and dark black. There is a well-delineated line of demarcation between the unaffected and affected area (arrow).

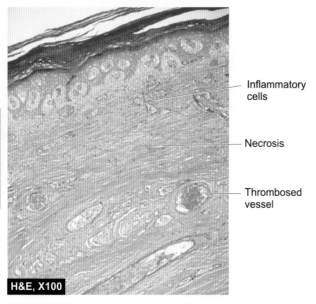

H&E, X100

FIGURE 10.4 ◆ Dry gangrene foot. There is coagulative necrosis of soft tissues while the margin with viable tissue shows non-specific chronic inflammation.

Inflammatory cells

Necrosis

Thrombosed vessel

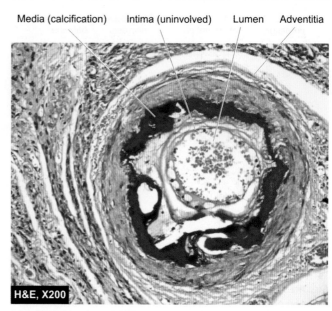

Media (calcification) Intima (uninvolved) Lumen Adventitia

H&E, X200

FIGURE 10.5 ◆ Monckeberg's arteriosclerosis (Medial calcific sclerosis). There is calcification in the degenerated tunica media and no inflammation.

iii. The line of separation shows inflammatory granulation tissue (Fig. 10.4).

Monckeberg's Arteriosclerosis

Monckeberg's arteriosclerosis or medial calcific sclerosis is dystrophic calcification in the degenerated media of large and medium-sized muscular arteries, especially of extremities and of the genital tract in the elderly (e.g. in uterine myometrium).

G/A Medial calcification produces pipestem-like rigidity of affected artery without significant luminal narrowing. However, coexistent changes of atherosclerosis may be present.

M/E

i. Smooth muscle of media is replaced by acellular hyalinised fibrous tissue.

ii. Foci of dystrophic calcification are seen in the media as basophilic coarse granules (Fig. 10.5).

iii. Inflammation is conspicuously absent.

Derangements of Body Fluids

Objectives
➢ To learn important forms of derangements of body fluids with examples—pulmonary oedema, chronic venous congestion (e.g. CVC lung, CVC liver, CVC spleen).
➢ To describe salient gross and microscopic features of these conditions.

Derangements of body fluids are of 2 types:
◆ Due to alterations in normal water, electrolytes and proteins within the body (e.g. oedema).
◆ Hemodynamic derangements, either due to altered volume of blood (e.g. venous congestion of different organs), or due to circulatory obstruction (e.g. thrombus formation in vessels and infarcts of various organs). The latter group is discussed in the next exercise separately.

Pulmonary Oedema

Pulmonary oedema is a common clinical and pathologic condition resulting from haemodynamic disturbances or from direct increase in capillary permeability.

G/A The lungs are voluminous, heavy, firm, wet and show marked pitting on pressure. Initially, fluid accumulates in the basal region of the lower lobes. Cut surface of lungs permits

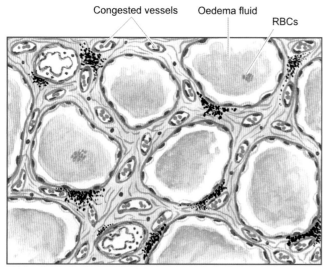
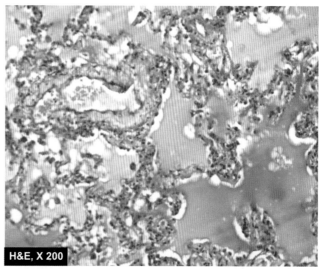

FIGURE 11.1 ◆ Pulmonary oedema. The alveolar capillaries are congested. The alveolar spaces as well as interstitium contain eosinophilic, granular, homogeneous and pink proteinaceous oedema fluid alongwith some RBCs and inflammatory cells.

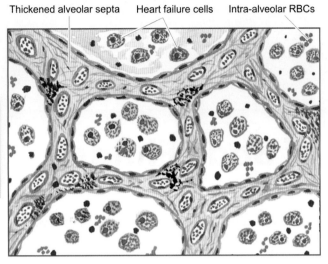

Thickened alveolar septa   Heart failure cells   Intra-alveolar RBCs

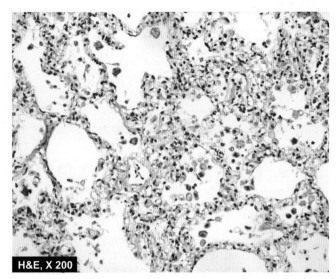

H&E, X 200

FIGURE 11.2 ◆ CVC lung. The alveolar septa are widened and thickened due to congestion, oedema and mild fibrosis. The alveolar lumina contain heart failure cells (alveolar macrophages containing haemosiderin pigment).

escape of frothy blood-tinged fluid due to mixture of air and oedema fluid.

M/E
  i.   Initially, alveolar septa are widened due to accumulation of oedema fluid.
  ii. Later, the proteinaceous fluid appears in the alveolar spaces and appears as pink granular material and may have some admixed RBCs and macrophages (Fig. 11.1).

CVC Lung

Chronic venous congestion (CVC) of lungs and consequent pulmonary oedema occur in elevated left atrial pressure which raises the pulmonary venous pressure, e.g. in mitral stenosis in rheumatic heart disease.

G/A Both lungs are dark brown in colour, heavy and firm. Cut surface shows brown colouration referred to as *brown induration*.

M/E
  i.   Vessels in the alveolar septa are dilated and congested.
  ii. Rupture of dilated and congested capillaries may result in minute intra-alveolar haemorrhages.
  iii. The characteristic finding is the presence of large number of alveolar macrophages filled with yellow-brown haemosiderin pigment, so called *heart failure cells* in the alveoli (Fig. 11.2).

  iv. Pulmonary oedema is a common accompaniment of venous congestion of the lungs.

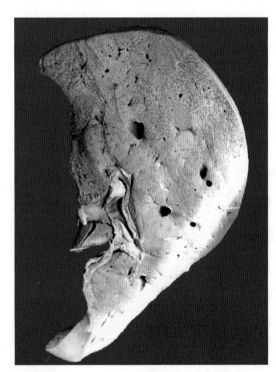

FIGURE 11.3 ◆ Nutmeg liver. The cut surface shows mottled appearance—alternate pattern of dark congestion and pale fatty change.

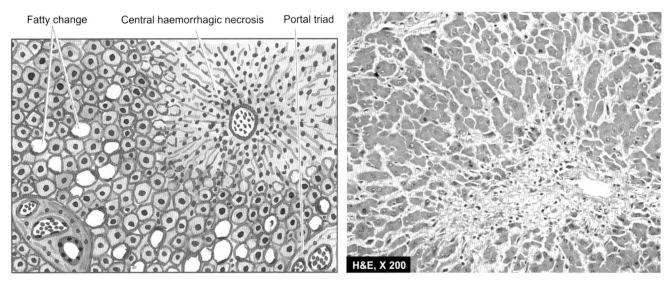

Fatty change   Central haemorrhagic necrosis   Portal triad

H&E, X 200

FIGURE 11.4 ◆ CVC liver. The centrilobular zone shows marked degeneration and necrosis of hepatocytes accompanied by haemorrhage while the peripheral zone shows mild fatty change of liver cells.

CVC Liver

The liver is particularly vulnerable to chronic passive congestion in right heart failure.

G/A The liver is enlarged and tender. The cut surface shows characteristic alternate dark areas representing congested centre of each lobule, and light areas being the fatty peripheral part, so called *nutmeg liver* (Fig. 11.3).

M/E
  i. The central vein and the sinusoids in the centrilobular region are distended with blood.
  ii. The hepatocytes in the centrilobular region undergo degeneration and atrophy, probably as a result of anoxia.
  iii. Eventually, the centrilobular zone shows central haemorrhagic necrosis (Fig. 11.4).
  iv. The peripheral hepatocytes are either normal or may show fatty change.

CVC Spleen

Chronic venous congestion (CVC) of the spleen may result from systemic causes (e.g. in right heart failure) or local causes (e.g. in cirrhosis of liver).

G/A The spleen becomes enlarged, firm and tense. The weight of the organ is increased (250 gm or more). The capsule may get thickened and fibrous. The cut surface shows fibrosis and

is meaty in appearance with indistinct malpighian corpuscles (Fig. 11.5).

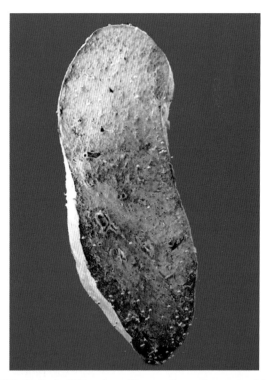

FIGURE 11.5 ◆ CVC spleen (Congestive splenomegaly). The spleen is enlarged and heavy. Cut surface shows grey-tan parenchyma.

Thickened capsule   Congested sinusoids   Gamna-Gandy body

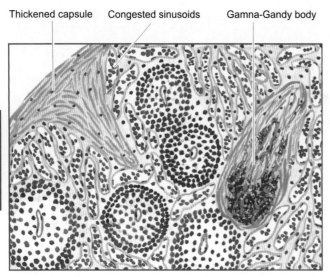 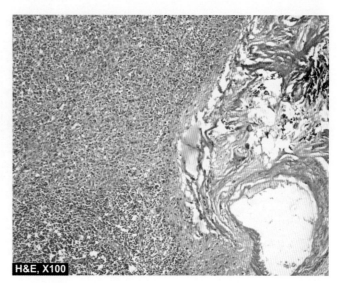

H&E, X100

FIGURE 11.6 ◆ Histological appearance of CVC spleen. The sinuses are dilated and congested. There is increased fibrosis in the red pulp, capsule and the trabeculae. A Gamna-Gandy body is also seen.

M/E

i. The red pulp shows marked congestion and dilatation of sinusoids with areas of recent and old haemorrhages.

ii. The haemorrhages may get organised and show diffuse fibrosis together with iron pigment and calcium deposits, so called siderotic nodules or Gamna-Gandy bodies (Fig. 11.6).

iii. In the late stages, there is hyperplasia of pigment-laden macrophages and thickening of fibrous framework of the organ, termed fibrocongestive splenomegaly.

Obstructive Circulatory Disturbances

Objectives

➤ To learn important forms of circulatory disturbances due to obstruction in circulation with examples—thrombus artery and, types of infarcts in different organs.

➤ To describe salient gross and microscopic features of these conditions.

As discussed in previous exercise, haemodynamic derangements may occur due to either altered volume of blood (e.g. venous congestion of different organs), or due to circulatory obstruction (e.g. thrombus formation in vessels and infarcts of various organs). The latter group is discussed here.

Thrombus Artery

Thrombi may occur anywhere in the arteries but one of the most common sites is in the coronary arteries.

G/A Coronary arterial thrombi are generally firmly attached to the vessel wall (mural) and occlude the lumen (occlusive). The arterial thrombus invariably overlies an atherosclerotic lesion. A slit-like lumen may be formed on contraction of freshly-formed thrombus restoring some flow. Arterial thrombus is grey-white and friable. The cut surface shows laminations called the lines of Zahn.

Arterial wall   Lines of Zahn   Residual lumen   Thrombus

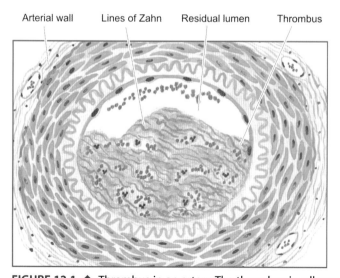 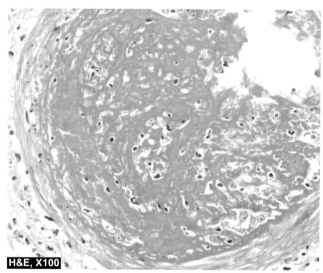

H&E, X100

FIGURE 12.1 ◆ Thrombus in an artery. The thrombus is adherent to the arterial wall and is seen occluding most of the lumen. It shows lines of Zahn composed of granular-looking platelets and fibrin meshwork with entangled red cells and leucocytes.

M/E

i. The internal elastic lamina is degenerated and disrupted at the site of attachment of thrombus to the vessel wall.

ii. The residual lumen of the original artery is slit-like and shows flowing blood (Fig. 12.1).

iii. The structure of thrombus shows lines of Zahn composed of layers of light-staining fibrin strands and platelets enmeshed in dark-staining red cells.

iv. The underlying atheromatous plaque may be seen.

v. Organised thrombus shows ingrowth of granulation tissue at the base having spindle cells and capillary channels.

Pale Infarct Spleen

Splenic infarction is one of the common types resulting from occlusion of the splenic artery or its branches.

G/A Infarcts of spleen are often multiple and pale or anaemic. They are usually wedge-shaped with their base lying on the splenic capsule and apex pointing inwards (Fig. 12.2).

M/E

i. There is coagulative necrosis of the cells in the affected area, i.e. outlines of cells and structures are identified but without intact nuclei and cytoplasmic details.

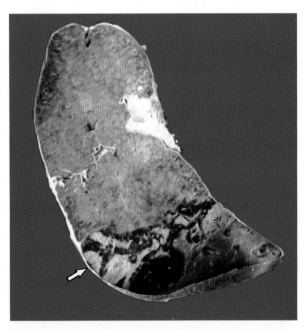

FIGURE 12.2 ◆ Pale infarct spleen. A wedge-shaped area of pale colour with base resting under the capsule is seen while the margin is congested tan (arrow).

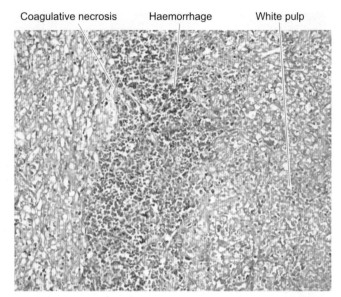

Coagulative necrosis   Haemorrhage   White pulp

FIGURE 12.3 ◆ Pale infarct spleen showing outlines of cells in infarcted area on left.

ii. Margin of the infarct with the viable tissue shows zone of inflammatory reaction, initially acute and later chronic (Fig. 12.3).

Haemorrhagic Infarct Lung

Embolism of pulmonary arteries may produce pulmonary infarction, though not always.

G/A Pulmonary infarcts are variable in size and are always red or haemorrhagic because the organ has dual blood supply. The infarct appears as firm, bright red, wedge-shaped area, with the base of the wedge at the surface and covered by fibrinous pleural exudate. The infarcted area is slightly raised above the adjacent area. The cut surface is dark red (Fig. 12.4).

M/E

i. There is ischaemic necrosis of the lung parenchyma in the affected area of haemorrhage, i.e. the alveolar walls, bronchioles and vessels in the infarcted zone show outlines but loss of nuclear and cytoplasmic details (Fig. 12.5).

ii. Margin of the infarct shows inflammatory infiltrate, initially by neutrophils and later their place is taken by macrophages and haemosiderin.

iii. If the infarct is caused by an infected embolus, the infarct shows more intense neutrophilic infiltration.

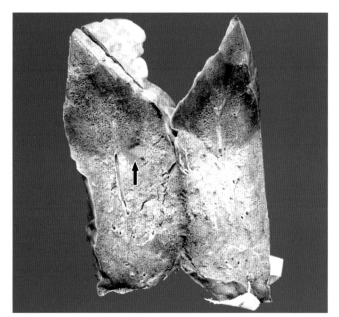

FIGURE 12.4 ◆ Haemorrhagic infarct lung. The sectioned surface shows dark tan firm area (arrow) with base on the pleura.

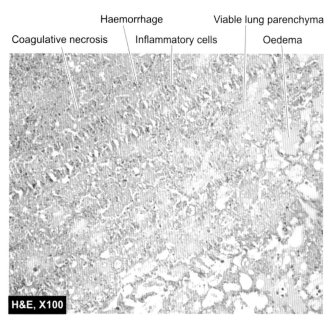

FIGURE 12.5 ◆ Haemorrhagic infarct lung. Infarcted area shows ghost alveoli filled with blood.

Types of Inflammation

Objectives

➢ To learn general types of inflammation with examples—acute inflammation (e.g. abscess lung), chronic non-specific inflammation (e.g. chronic inflammatory granulation tissue) and granulomatous inflammation (e.g. tuberculous lymphadenitis).

➢ To describe salient gross and microscopic features of these conditions.

Inflammation is local response by the host to injury from various agents. Depending upon the body's defense capacity and duration of response, it may be *acute* (e.g. abscess) or *chronic*. Chronic inflammation is further subdivided into 2 types: chronic nonspecific inflammatory reaction, and specific or chronic granulomatous reaction such as in tuberculosis, leprosy, sarcoidosis, etc.

Abscess Lung

Abscess is the formation of cavity as a result of extensive tissue necrosis following pyogenic bacterial infection accompanied by intense neutrophilic infiltration. Abscess of the lung may occur due to inhalation, embolic phenomena, and pneumonia.

G/A Abscess is more common in the right lung and may occur in upper or lower lobe. Size of the cavity may vary from small to fairly large. The wall is ragged and necrotic but advanced lesions may show fibrous and smooth wall (Fig. 13.1). The inhalation abscess may communicate with the bronchus.

M/E

i. The wall of the abscess shows dense infiltration by polymorphonuclear leucocytes and varying number of macrophages.

ii. More chronic cases show fibroblasts at the periphery.

iii. Alveolar walls in the affected area are destroyed.

iv. Lumen of the abscess contains pus consisting of purulent exudate, some red cells, fragments of tissue debris and fibrin (Fig. 13.2).

Chronic Inflammatory Granulation Tissue

Granulation tissue is the granular and pink appearance of the tissue in a healing ulcer and in secondary union of wounds.

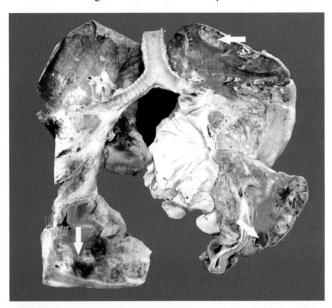

FIGURE 13.1 ◆ Lung abscess. The pleura is thickened. Cut surface of the lung shows multiple cavities 1-4 cm in diameter, having irregular and ragged inner walls (arrow). The lumina contain necrotic debris. The surrounding lung parenchyma is consolidated.

Neutrophils   Necrosis   Bacterial colony

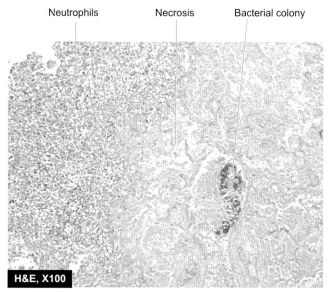

H&E, X100

FIGURE 13.2 ◆ Lung abscess. The photomicrograph shows abscess formed by necrosed alveoli and dense acute and chronic inflammatory cells.

G/A Floor of the lesion contains pink granulations composed of the vascular connective tissue, while the edges are sloping and bluish-white.

M/E

i. Surface of the ulcer contains mixture of blood, fibrin and inflammatory exudate.
ii. The zone underneath contains granulation tissue composed of proliferating fibroblasts, newly-formed small blood vessels and varying number of inflammatory cells which are initially polymorphs but in the later stages macrophages and lymphocytes predominate.

iii. The epithelium grows from the edge of the wound as spurs.
iv. Granulation tissue matures from below upwards and late stage shows dense collagen, scanty vascularity and fewer inflammatory cells (Fig. 13.3).

Tuberculous Lymphadenitis

Tuberculosis of the lymph nodes is always secondary to tuberculosis elsewhere.

G/A The lymph nodes are enlarged and are matted together due to periadenitis. The cut surface in the tuberculous areas is yellow, cheesy, opaque and caseous while elsewhere is grey brown (Fig. 13.4,A).

M/E

i. The caseous areas show nuclear debris due to fragmented coagulated cells (Fig. 13.4,B).
ii. The periphery of caseous foci shows granulomatous inflammation consisting of epithelioid cells (identified by large size, epithelium-like appearance, abundant pale cytoplasm and oval vesicular nuclei), surrounded by lymphocytes and some plasma cells. Epithelioid cells may fuse to form giant cells in the granuloma and may have nuclear arrangement at the periphery of the cell (Langhans' giant cell) or the nuclei may be distributed haphazardly (foreign body giant cell) (Fig. 13.5).

Plasma cells   Lymphocytes   Fibroblasts
Neovascularisation   Macrophages   Ulcer   Neutrophils

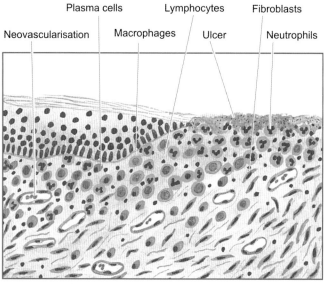

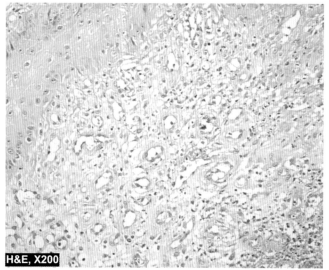

H&E, X200

FIGURE 13.3 ◆ Active granulation tissue has inflammatory cell infiltrate, newly formed blood vessels and young fibrous tissue in loose matrix.

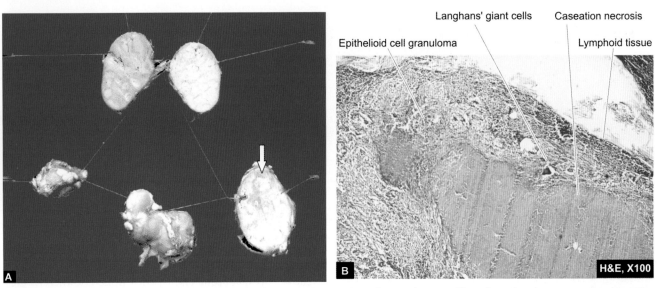

FIGURE 13.4 ◆ Caseating granulomatous lymphadenitis. **A,** Cut section of matted mass of lymph nodes shows merging capsules and large areas of caseation necrosis (arrow). **B,** Caseating epithelioid cell granulomas with some Langhans' giant cells in the cortex of lymph node.

iii. Depending upon the age of granuloma, fibroblasts may surround the granulomas.

iv. It is not uncommon to find areas of dystrophic calcification appearing as bluish granularity in the caseous areas (Fig. 13.6).

v. Ziehl-Neelsen staining may demonstrate presence of acid-fast bacilli.

vi. Normal nodal architecture may be seen at the periphery only.

FIGURE 13.5 ◆ Tuberculous lymphadenitis. Characteristic sliper-shaped epithelioid cells, minute caseation necrosis and Langhans' giant cells.

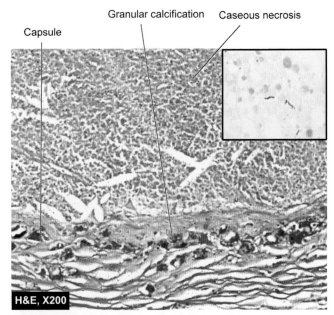

FIGURE 13.6 ◆ Tuberculous lymphadenitis. Large areas of caseation necrosis with dystrophic calcification, surrounded by epithelioid cells. Inbox shows AFB.

Granulomatous Inflammation—Tuberculosis

Objectives
➤ To learn tuberculous granulomatous inflammation with common examples—fibrocaseous tuberculosis lung, tuberculosis intestine, military tuberculosis lung and spleen.
➤ To describe salient gross and microscopic features of these conditions.

As discussed in previous exercise, granulomatous inflammation is a form of specific chronic inflammatory reaction that occurs in response to poorly digestible agents. Infection with organism, *Mycobacterium tuberculosis*, is singular most important example characterised by caseating granulomatous inflammatory reaction in different organs such as lungs, lymph nodes, and many other organs.

Fibrocaseous Tuberculosis Lung

The breakdown of caseous tissue in the lung in chronic cases results in cavitary fibrocaseous tuberculosis.

G/A The cavity is seen most commonly at the apex and is fairly large and may communicate through the bronchial wall (open tuberculosis). In progressive form of the disease, however, cavities may be formed in the lower lobe too. Wall of the cavity is smooth (unlike ragged lining of the pyogenic abscess), fibrous and may be traversed by bronchi and blood vessels (Fig. 14.1).

M/E
i. Basic lesion is the *tubercle*, consisting of epithelioid cells, lymphocytes and giant cells, and central area of caseation necrosis. The tubercles coalesce to form confluent areas.
ii. Periphery of the lesion shows proliferating fibroblasts and fibrosis (Fig. 14.2).

iii. The arterioles may show endarteritis obliterans closing the lumen.
iv. The surrounding alveoli may contain cellular exudate.

Tuberculosis Intestine

Intestinal tuberculosis occurs in 3 forms: primary, secondary and hyperplastic. Secondary tuberculosis of small intestine is most common.

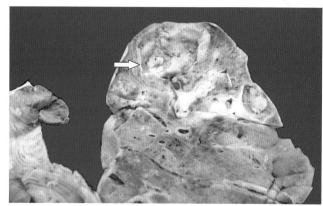

FIGURE 14.1 ◆ Chronic fibrocaseous tuberculosis lung. Sectioned surface of the lung shows a cavity in the apex of the lung (arrow). The cavity is lined by yellowish caseous necrotic material. The lung tissue around the cavity is consolidated.

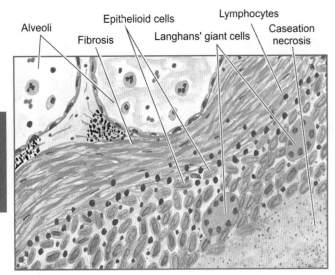

Alveoli · Fibrosis · Epithelioid cells · Langhans' giant cells · Lymphocytes · Caseation necrosis

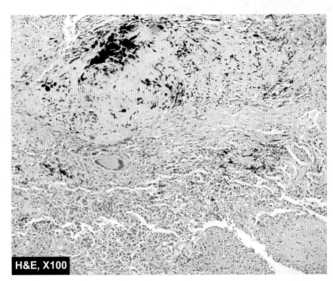

H&E, X100

FIGURE 14.2 ◆ Fibrocaseous tuberculosis lung. The cavity shows caseation necrosis while the wall shows epithelioid cells admixed with lymphocytes and some Langhans' giant cells and surrounded at the periphery by fibrosclerosis.

G/A The intestine shows large ulcers which are transverse to the long axis of the bowel. These ulcers may be coated with caseous material. Advanced cases show transverse fibrous strictures and intestinal obstruction (Fig. 14.3).

M/E

 i. Presence of caseating tubercles in all the layers of intestine (Fig. 14.4).
 ii. Ulceration of mucosa with slough on the surface.
 iii. Variable fibrosis in the muscular layer.

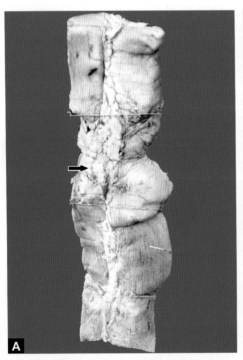

A

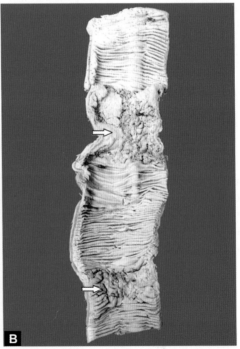

B

FIGURE 14.3 ◆ Intestinal tuberculosis. **A,** The external surface shows strictures and cut section of lymph node showing caseation necrosis (black arrow). **B,** The lumen shows transverse ulcers and strictures (transverse to the long axis of intestine) (arrows). The intestinal wall in the strictrous areas is thickened and grey-white and mucosa over it is ulcerated.

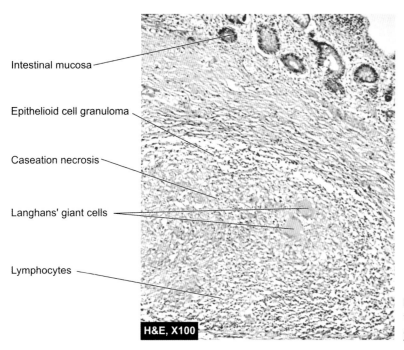

Intestinal mucosa

Epithelioid cell granuloma

Caseation necrosis

Langhans' giant cells

Lymphocytes

H&E, X100

FIGURE 14.4 ◆ Tuberculosis small intestine. The wall of intestine shows caseating epithelioid cell granulomas.

Miliary Tuberculosis Lung

If the caseous pulmonary tuberculous lesion discharges its contents into a blood vessel or lymphatic, it results in lympho-haematogenous dissemination of tuberculosis which may be confined to the lungs or may involve other organs.

G/A The lungs show intense congestion and minute millet seed-sized (1 to a few mm in diameter) yellowish-white firm lesions in which caseous centre may not be visible grossly (Fig. 14.5).

M/E
  i. The tubercles (as described above) are seen in the fibrous stromal framework of the lung and contain minute areas of caseation necrosis in the centre.
 ii. The intervening lung alveoli are either empty or may contain cellular exudate (Fig. 14.6).

Miliary Tuberculosis Spleen

Lympho-haematogenous spread of chronic pulmonary tuberculosis may result in acute miliary tuberculosis of the spleen.

G/A The miliary tubercles are scattered throughout the liver. They appear as yellowish-white firm lesions of a few millimeters in diameter (Fig. 14.7).

M/E
  i. Tubercles with minute areas of central caseation necrosis are seen scattered in the splenic parenchyma.
 ii. The neighbouring splenic parenchyma may show congestion (Fig. 14.8).

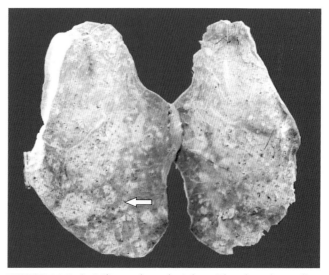

FIGURE 14.5 ◆ Miliary tuberculosis lung. The pleural as well as sectioned surface shows presence of minute (about pinhead sized) yellowish nodules with central necrosis called miliary tubercles (arrow).

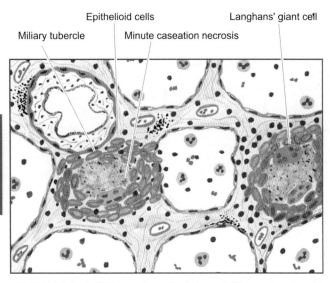

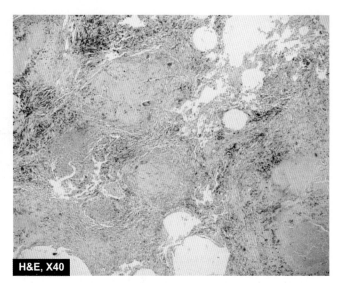

FIGURE 14.6 ◆ Miliary tuberculosis lung. Miliary tubercle with minute area of caseation necrosis surrounded by epithelioid cells, mantle of lymphocytes and peripheral fibroblasts.

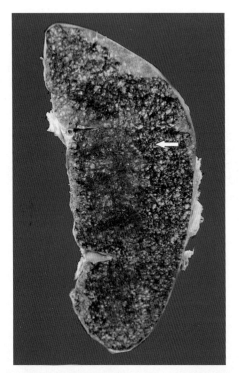

FIGURE 14.7 ◆ Miliary tuberculosis spleen. The capsule as well as sectioned surface shows presence of minute (about pinhead sized) yellowish nodules with central necrosis called tubercles (arrow).

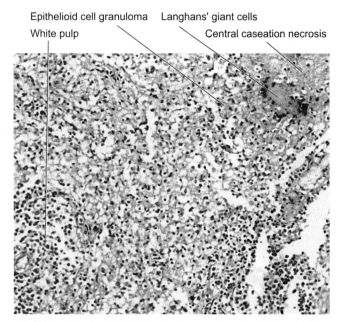

FIGURE 14.8 ◆ Miliary tuberculosis spleen. Small caseating granuloma is seen in the splenic parenchymal tissue.

Exercise
15

Other Granulomatous Inflammations

Objectives
➤ To learn common examples of granulomatous inflammation other than tuberculosis—leprosy (lepromatous and tuberculoid) and sarcoidosis.
➤ To describe salient gross and microscopic features of these conditions.

Although tubeculosis is the most common example of granulomatous inflammation (Exercise 14), granuloma formation may occur in many other conditions. A few other examples studied in this exercise are those of two polar forms of leprosy (lepromatous and tuberculoid) and sarcoidosis.

Lepromatous Leprosy

Leprosy or Hansen's disease caused by *Mycobacterium leprae* affects the skin and peripheral nerves. The causative organism is less acid-fast than the tubercle bacillus. The polar form of lepromatous leprosy lacks cell-mediated immunity.

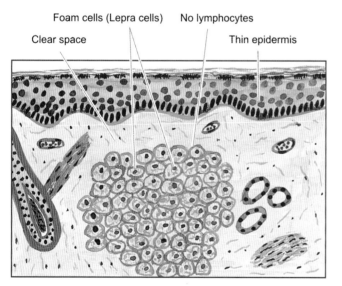

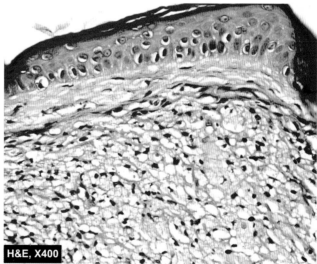

H&E, X400

FIGURE 15.1 ◆ Lepromatous leprosy (LL). There is a clear subepidermal zone and underlying collection of foamy macrophages or lepra cells.

G/A The lepromatous lesions are characterised by development of nodules or masses formed in the skin, particularly on the face, hands and feet.

M/E

i. The dermis contains large aggregates of lipid-laden foamy macrophages known as *lepra cells.*

ii. The dermal infiltrate of lepra cells characteristically does not encroach upon the basal layer of epidermis leaving uninvolved *(clear zone)* subepidermal dermis.

iii. The overlying epidermis is *thin and flat* (Fig. 15.1).

iv. With Fite-Faraco stain, lepra cells are crowded with acid-fast lepra bacilli *(multibacillary leprosy)*(Fig. 15.2).

Tuberculoid Leprosy

Tuberculoid leprosy is the other polar form that represents high resistance (i.e. good cell-mediated immune response).

G/A The skin lesions have hyperpigmented margins and pale centre. Neuronal involvement predominates in tuberculoid leprosy and small nerves may be destroyed.

M/E

i. The dermis shows granulomas which closely resemble *hard tubercles,* i.e. they consist of epithelioid cells, Langhans' giant cells and a few lymphocytes at the periphery but generally little or no caseation necrosis.

ii. The granulomas erode the basal layer of the epidermis, i.e. there is *no clear zone.*

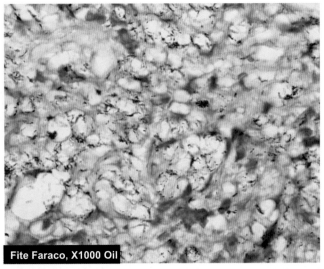

Fite Faraco, X1000 Oil

FIGURE 15.2 ◆ Lepra bacilli in LL. Numerous globi and cigarettes-in-pack appearance of lepra bacilli inside foamy macrophages.

iii. Lesions of tuberculoid leprosy have predilection for *dermal nerves* which may be destroyed and infiltrated by epithelioid cells and lymphocytes (Fig. 15.3).

iv. With Fite-Faraco stain, lepra bacilli are almost never found *(paucibacillary leprosy).*

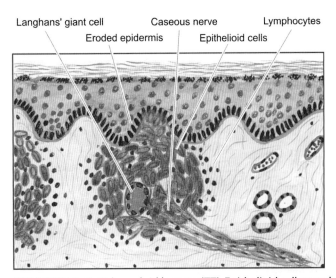

Langhans' giant cell   Caseous nerve   Lymphocytes
Eroded epidermis   Epithelioid cells

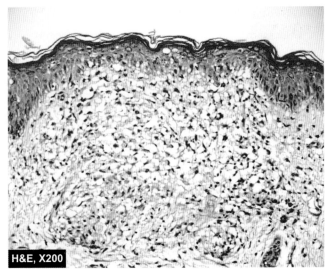

H&E, X200

FIGURE 15.3 ◆ Tuberculoid leprosy (TT). Epithelioid cell granulomas eroding the basal layer of epidermis.

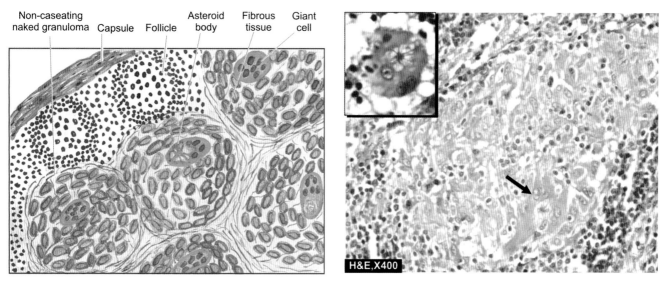

Non-caseating naked granuloma   Capsule   Follicle   Asteroid body   Fibrous tissue   Giant cell

H&E, X400

FIGURE 15.4 ◆ Sarcoidosis in lymph node. Characteristically, there are non-caseating epithelioid cell granulomas which have paucity of lymphocytes. A giant cell with inclusions is also seen in the photomicrograph (arrow) as also as inbox.

Sarcoidosis Lung

Sarcoidosis is a systemic disease of unknown etiology. The lesions are generalized and may affect various organs and tissues but the brunt of the disease is borne by the lungs and lymph nodes.

M/E

i. There are non-caseating epithelioid cell granulomas having Langhans' and foreign body giant cells.

ii. Typically, sarcoid granulomas are devoid of lymphocytes, i.e. they are "naked" granulomas (Fig. 15.4)

iii. Old granulomas may show condensation of fibrosis at the periphery.

iv. Sometimes, giant cells may show various types of cytoplasmic inclusions, e.g. asteroid bodies, Schaumann's bodies, and conchoid bodies (Fig. 15.4, inbox).

Fungal Infections

Objectives

➢ To learn pathology of common fungal infections in tissues—oral candidiasis, madura foot, aspergillosis lung, rhinosporidiosis nose.

➢ To describe salient gross and microscopic features of these conditions.

Many of the fungal infections in human beings are opportunistic, i.e. they occur under conditions with impaired host immune mechanisms. A few important representative examples discussed in this exercise are oral candidiasis, madura foot, aspergillosis lung and rhinosporidiosis nose.

Oral Candidiasis

Candidiasis is an opportunistic infection caused commonly by *Candida albcans*. Candida in human beings is a normal commensal in mucocutaneous surfaces but becomes pathogenic in impaired immunity.

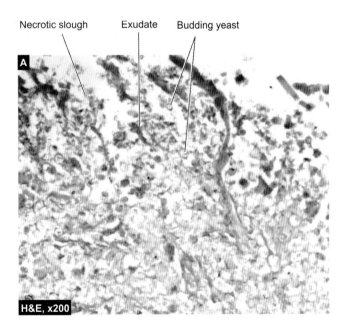
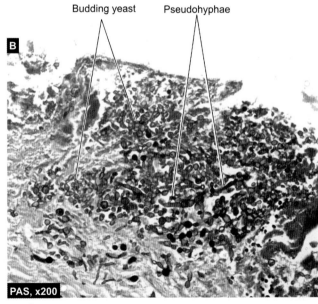

FIGURE 16.1 ◆ Ulcer containing budding yeast form and non-branching pseudohyphal form of candida **(A)** best identified in PAS stain **(B)**.

G/A Clinically, candida produces superficial infection of the skin and mucous membranes or may invade the deeper tissues. Oral thrush, as it is commonly called in oral cavity, is creamy white pseudomembrane formed on the tongue, soft palate and buccal mucosa.

M/E

i. Candidiasis may produce ulcers at the affected site.

ii. The organisms appear as budding spores or as non-branching pseudohyphal form (Fig. 16.1,A).

iii. The organisms are positive with periodic acid Schiff (PAS) stain (Fig.16.1,B).

Madura Foot

Eumycetoma is a chronic suppurative infection caused by true fungi, most commonly by *Madurella mycetomatis* or *Madurella grisea*. Foot is the most common location of the lesion.

G/A The affected site in chronic lesions produces swelling and black granules from discharging sinuses.

M/E

i. The lesion shows the sinus tract discharging purulent material and grains.

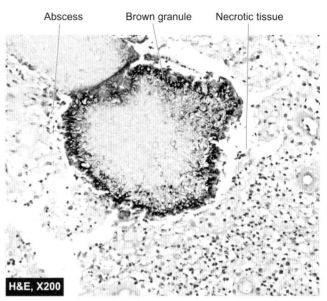

FIGURE 16.2 ◆ Madura foot. Brown granule lying in necrotic tissue of the discharging sinus.

ii. The grains of brown colonies of the fungus are seen in the purulent foci (Fig. 16.2).

iii. The surrounding tissue shows mononuclear inflammatory cell reaction and fibrosis.

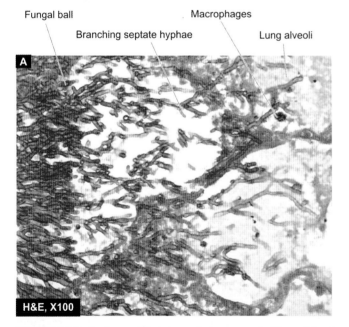

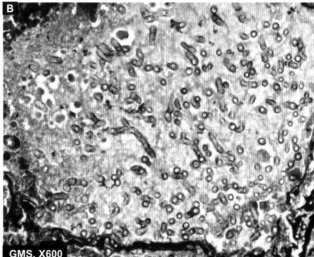

FIGURE 16.3 ◆ Aspergillosis lung. **A**, Acute-angled branching hyphae lying in necrotic debris and acute inflammatory exudates in lung abscess **B**, The organisms are identified by fungal stain, Gomori's methenamine silver (GMS).

Aspergillosis Lung

Aspergillosis is the most common opportunistic fungal infection, usually involving the lungs. The most common human pathogen is *Aspergillus fumigatus*. It occurs in 3 forms—allergic bronchopulmonary aspergillosis, aspergilloma and invasive aspergillosis.

G/A Aspergilloma occurs in pulmonary cavities or in bronchiectasis as fungal ball.

M/E

   i. Structure of an abscess cavity is seen showing chronic inflammatory cells in the wall and necrotic centre (Fig. 16.3,A).

   ii. There is a mass of tangled hyphae lying within a cavity with fibrous wall.

   ii. The organism has characteristic septate hyphae (2-7 μm in diameter) and has multiple dichotomous branching at acute angles, best seen in special stain, Gomori's methenamine silver (GMS) (Fig. 16.3,B).

Rhinosporidiosis Nose

Rhinosporidiosis of the nose is caused by the fungus, *Rhinosporidium seeberi*.

G/A Rhinosporidiosis occurs in a nasal polyp typically. The polypoid mass is gelatinous with smooth and shining surface.

M/E

   i. Structure of nasal polyp of inflammatory or allergic type is seen, i.e. subepithelial loose oedematous connective tissue containing mucous glands and varying number of inflammatory cells like lymphocytes, plasma cells and eosinophils. The surface of the polyp is covered by respiratory epithelium which may show squamous metaplasia.

   ii. Large number of organisms of the size of erythrocytes with chitinous wall are seen in the thick-walled sporangia. Spores are also seen in the submucosa and on the surface of the mucosa (Fig. 16.4).

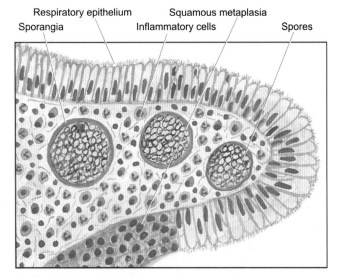

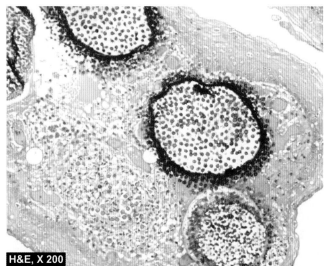

H&E, X 200

FIGURE 16.4 ◆ Rhinosporidiosis in a nasal polyp. The spores are present in sporangia under the nasal mucosa as well as are intermingled in the inflammatory cell infiltrate.

Actinomycosis and Parasitic Infections

Objectives
➢ To learn pathology in actinomycosis and some common examples of tissue parasites—cysticercosis, hydatid cyst.
➢ To describe salient gross and microscopic features of these conditions.

Actinomycosis, unlike its name (mycosis meaning fungus), is a chronic suppurative bacterial infection caused by aerobic bacteria, *Actinomyces israelii*.

Parasitic infections and infestations are quite common and may cause disease due to their presence in the lumen of intestine, infiltration in the blood, or their presence inside the tissues. Here, we discuss a few examples of parasites which infect tissues, e.g. cysticercosis and hydatid cyst.

Actinomycosis Skin

Actinomycosis, a chronic suppurative disease caused by anaerobic bacteria, *Actinomyces israelii*, is of 4 types: cervicofacial, thoracic, abdominal and pelvic. However, head and neck region is the most common location of the lesion.

G/A There is a firm swelling in the region of the lower jaw initially, but later sinuses and abscesses are formed. The pus contains characteristic yellow *sulphur granules* (Fig. 17.1).

M/E
i.   The inflammatory reaction is a granuloma with central suppuration. Centre of the lesion shows abscess and at the periphery are seen chronic inflammatory cells, giant cells and fibroblasts.
ii. The bacterial colony, sulphur granule, characterised by basophilic radiating filaments with hyaline, eosinophilic, club-like ends is seen in the centre of suppuration (Fig. 17.2).

Cysticercosis Soft Tissue

Cysticercus cellulosae is caused by the larval stage of pork tapeworm, *Taenia solium*. The most common sites in the body are skeletal muscle, brain (Fig. 17.3), skin and heart.

G/A The lesions may be solitary or multiple and appear as round to oval white cyst, about 1 cm in diameter (Fig. 17.3). The cyst contains milky fluid.

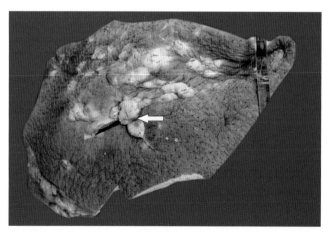

FIGURE 17.1 ◆ Skin surface shows multiple draining sinuses with blackish grains (arrow). These sinuses extend into underlying tissues as well.

(61)

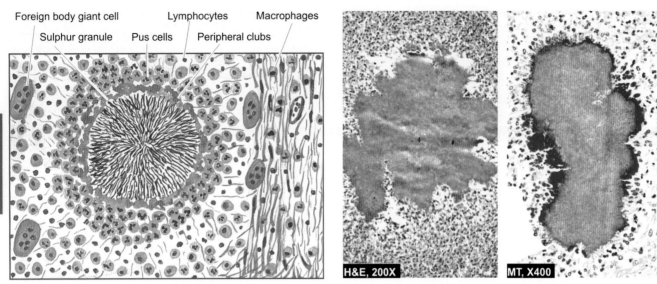

Foreign body giant cell   Lymphocytes   Macrophages
Sulphur granule   Pus cells   Peripheral clubs

H&E, 200X   MT, X400

FIGURE 17.2 ◆ Actinomycosis. Microscopic appearance of sulphur granule lying inside an abscess. The margin of the colony shows hyaline filaments highlighted by Masson's trichrome (MT) stain (right photomicrograph).

M/E

i. The cysticercus cellulosae lying in the cyst shows continuity of epithelium on surface and that lining the body canal. Sometimes the parasite is degenerated or even calcified.

ii. The dead and degenerated forms incite intense tissue reaction. The cyst wall is lined by palisades of histiocytes. It is surrounded by inflammatory cell reaction consisting of mixed infiltrate including prominence of eosinophils (Fig. 17.4).

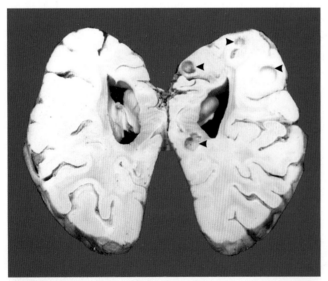

FIGURE 17.3 ◆ Neurocysticercosis. The sliced surface of the cerebral hemispheres of the brain shows many whitish nodules and cysts, about 1 cm in diameter (arrowheads).

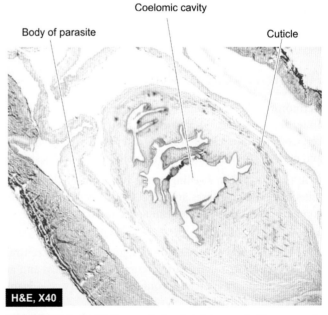

Coelomic cavity
Body of parasite   Cuticle

H&E, X40

FIGURE 17.4 ◆ Cysticercosis in skeletal muscle. The worm is seen in the cyst while the cyst wall below contains palisad layer of histiocytes.

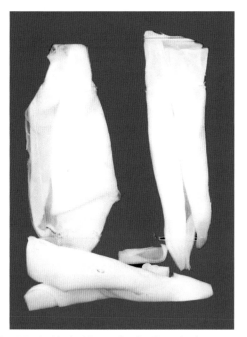

FIGURE 17.5 ◆ Hydatid cyst in the liver. It shows a cyst wall composed of curled up whitish membranous layer resembling the membrane of a hard-boiled egg.

Hydatid Cyst Liver

Hydatid disease occurs as a result of infection by the larval stage of the tapeworm, *Echinococcus granulosus*. The liver is a common site for development of hydatid cyst.

G/A The cyst may vary in size and may attain the size over 10 cm in diameter. The cyst wall has laminated membrane and the lumen contains clear fluid (Fig. 17.5).

M/E The cyst wall is composed of 3 distinguishable layers (Fig. 17.6):

i. Outer *Pericyst* is the inflammatory reaction by the host consisting of mononuclear cells, eosinophils, some giant cells and surrounded peripherally by fibroblasts.

ii. *Ectocyst* is the characteristic intermediate layer composed of acellular, chitinous laminated, hyaline material.

iii. *Endocyst* is the inner germinal layer bearing the daughter cysts and scolices bearing row of hooklets (Fig. 17.6, inbox).

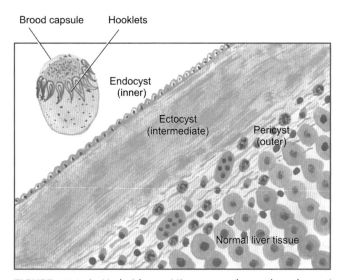

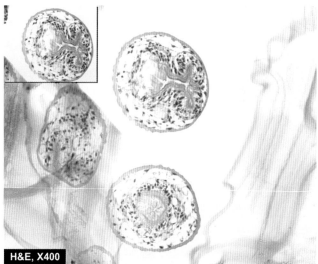

FIGURE 17.6 ◆ Hydatid cyst. Microscopy shows three layers in the wall of hydatid cyst—endocyst, ectocyst and pericyst. Inbox (right figure) shows a scolex with a row of hooklets.

Exercise
18

Adaptive Disorders of Growth

Objectives
➢ To learn adaptive disorders of growth with common examples (e.g. testicular atrophy, cardiac hypertrophy, reactive hyperplasia lymph nodes, squamous metapalsia cervix).
➢ To describe salient gross and microscopic features of these conditions.

Cellular adaptations are the adjustments which cells make in response to various stresses. These include decreasing or increasing the cell size (atrophy and hypertrophy), or increasing their number (hyperplasia), or changing the pathway of differentiation of cells (metaplasia and dysplasia).

A few common examples of these are discussed below except dysplasia which is discussed in Exercise 40.

Testicular Atrophy

Atrophy means reduction in number and size of cells which were once normal. Testicular atrophy may occur from various causes; senility is one common cause of atrophy.

G/A In testicular atrophy, the testis is small in size, firm and fibrotic.

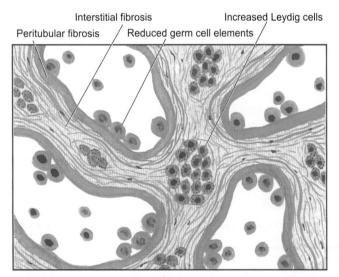
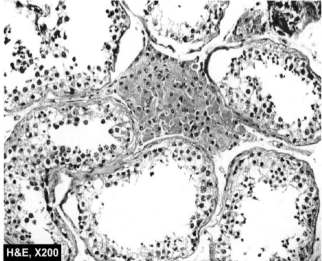

FIGURE 18.1 ◆ Testicular atrophy. Some of the seminiferous tubules show hyalinisation while others show peritubular fibrosis. The spermatogenic elements are reduced in number. The interstitium shows prominence of Leydig cells.

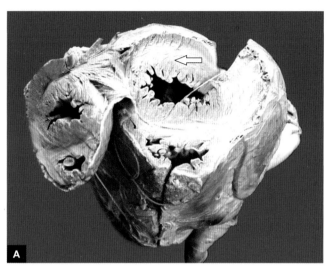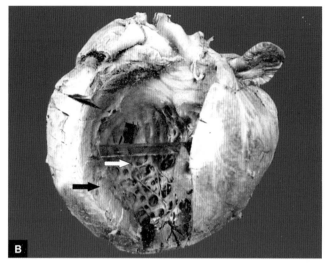

FIGURE 18.2 ◆ **A,** Concentric cardiac hypertrophy. The weight of the heart is increased. A slice of the heart is cut off at the apex revealing lumina and walls of both the ventricles. The left ventricular wall is thickened concentrically around the chamber (arrow) while the left ventricular lumen is obliterated. **B,** Eccentric cardiac hypertrophy. The weight of the heart is increased. The free left ventricular wall is thickened (black arrow) while the left ventricular lumen is dilated (white arrow). The right ventricular lumen and wall are unaffected.

M/E

  i. *Seminiferous tubules:* There is progressive depletion of germ cell elements. The tubular basement membrane is thickened and there is peritubular fibrosis. Some tubules may show hyalinisation.

  ii. *Interstitial stroma:* There is increase in interstitial fibrovascular stroma in which Leydig cells are prominent, seen singly or as clusters (Fig. 18.1).

Cardiac Hypertrophy

Hypertrophy is an increase in the size of parenchymal cells resulting in enlargement of the organ. Hypertrophy of the cardiac muscle occurs commonly due to aortic stenosis and systemic hypertension.

G/A The heart is enlarged and heavy and may weigh as much as 700-800 g as compared to average normal weight of 350 g. Cross-section of the heart at the apex shows left ventricular hypertrophy. Thickness of the left ventricular wall is over 2 cm compared to normal up to 1.5 cm. Cardiac hypertrophy without dilatation of the chamber is termed *concentric* and when associated with dilatation is termed *eccentric* (Fig. 18.2).

M/E

  i. There is an increase in the size of individual muscle fibres with prominent nuclei.

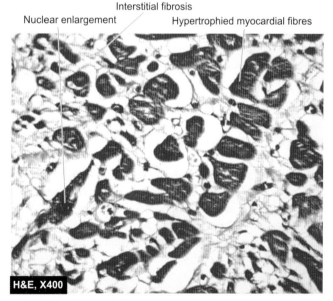

FIGURE 18.3 ◆ Cardiac hypertrophy. Individual myocardial fibres are thick and have prominent vesicular nuclei.

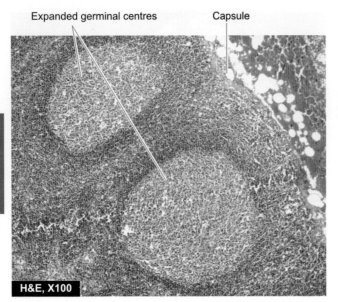

Expanded germinal centres   Capsule

H&E, X100

FIGURE 18.4 ◆ Reactive hyperplasia lymph node, follicular type.

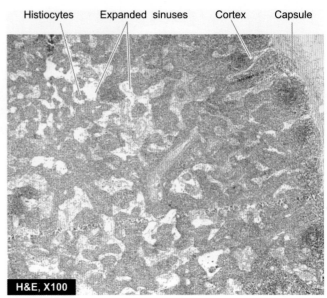

Histiocytes   Expanded sinuses   Cortex   Capsule

H&E, X100

FIGURE 18.5 ◆ Reactive hyperplasia lymph node, sinus histiocytosis type.

ii. Foci of degenerative changes and necrosis in the hypertrophied myocardium may be seen (Fig. 18.3).

Reactive Hyperplasia Lymph Node

Hyperplasia means an increase in the number of the cells of a part. Lymphoid tissue readily undergoes reactive hyperplasia in response to local irritation.

G/A The affected lymph nodes are enlarged, firm and non-tender.

M/E Reactive hyperplasia of lymph nodes in chronic nonspecific lymphadenitis shows one of the following three patterns:
  i. *Follicular hyperplasia* is most common and is characterised by enlargement and prominence of germinal centres of lymphoid follicles (Fig. 18.4).
  ii. *Paracortical lymphoid hyperplasia* is due to hyperplasia and enlargement of paracortex so that lymphoid follicles are effaced.

iii. *Sinus histiocytosis* refers to distention and engorgement of the sinusoids of the lymph node with histiocytes and endothelial cells (Fig. 18.5).

Squamous Metaplasia Cervix

Squamous metaplasia is defined as a reversible change of one type of epithelium to the squamous type which is a less well-specialised epithelium.

G/A Squamous metaplasia of the cervix is commonly encountered in prolapsed uterus. The cervix is pearly white and isthmus is elongated.

M/E
  i. Columnar lined mucosa as well as cervical glands show foci of squamous cell change.
  ii. Surface of the cervix may show keratinisation and hyperkeratosis.
  iii. There is generally some degree of subepithelial chronic inflammatory cell infiltrate (Fig. 18.6).

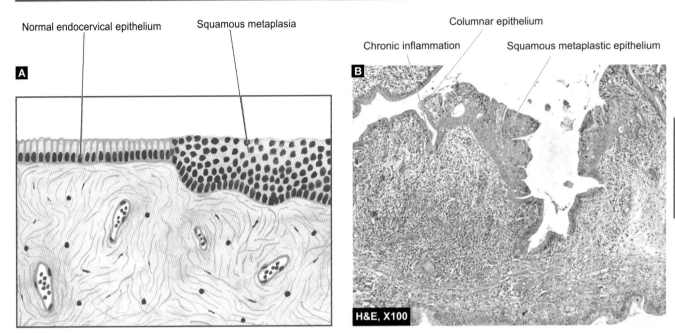

Normal endocervical epithelium   Squamous metaplasia

Columnar epithelium

Chronic inflammation   Squamous metaplastic epithelium

A

B

H&E, X100

FIGURE 18.6 ◆ **A,** Schematic diagram showing change in uterine cervix from normal mucus-secreting endocervical epithelium to squamous metaplastic epithelium. **B,** Squamous metaplasia cervix. Part of some of the glands are lined by columnar epithelium while other parts show change to squamous lining.

Primary Epithelial Tumours

Objectives
➢ To learn pathology of common primary epithelial benign and malignant tumours with examples (e.g. squamous cell papilloma, squamous cell carcinoma, malignant melanoma, basal cell carcinoma).
➢ To describe salient gross and microscopic features of these tumours.

Neoplasms or tumours may be *benign* when slow growing and localised, and *malignant* when they proliferate rapidly and spread to the other sites. Common term used for the malignant tumours is *cancer*.

Tumours arising from epithelium of various sites are named by the prefix of cell of origin, followed by—oma. For example, the term for benign epithelial tumour of squamous epithelium of skin and mucosa is squamous cell papilloma. Malignant epithelial tumours are called carcinomas, e.g. malignant tumour of squamous epithelium is termed squamous cell carcinoma. Similarly, malignant epithelial tumour of melanin-pigment epithelium is called malignant melanoma, and of basal layer of epidermis is called basal cell carcinoma. These examples are discussed in this exercise.

Squamous Cell Papilloma

Squamous cell papilloma is a common benign epithelial tumour of the skin and mucosa.

G/A Surface of the tumour shows finger-like processes (Fig. 19.1).

M/E
  i. The epidermis is thickened but orderly and is thrown into finger-like processes or papillae.
  ii. The central core of the papillae is composed of loose fibrovascular tissue (Fig. 19.2).

Squamous Cell Carcinoma

Squamous cell (or epidermoid) carcinoma occurs most commonly in the skin, oral cavity, oesophagus, uterine cervix, penis and at the edge of chronic ulcers.

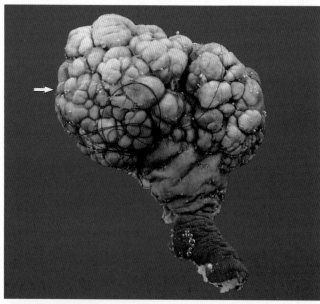

FIGURE 19.1 ◆ Squamous cell papilloma skin. The skin surface shows a papillary growth on the surface (arrow) having a pedicle. It is elevated above the adjoining normal skin without any invasion.

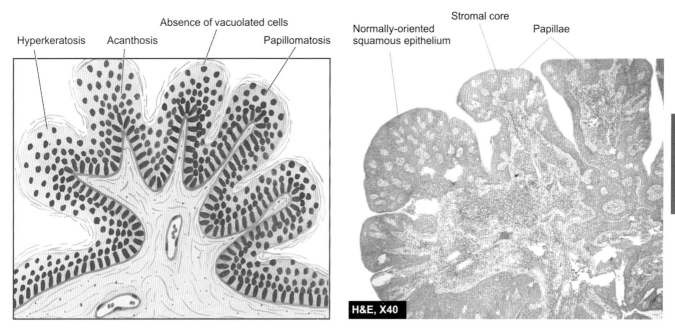

FIGURE 19.2 ◆ Squamous cell papilloma. Finger-like projections are covered by normally-oriented squamous epithelium while the stromal core contains fibrovascular tissue.

G/A The tumour is either in the form of nodular and ulcerative growth, or fungating and polypoid mass without ulceration. The margin of the growth is elevated and indurated. Cut section of the growth shows grey-white endophytic as well as exophytic tumour (Fig. 19.3).

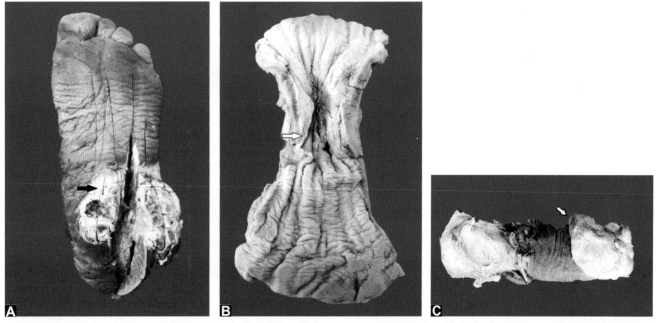

FIGURE 19.3 ◆ Squamous cell carcinoma. **A,** The skin surface on the sole of the foot shows a fungating and ulcerated growth (arrow). **B,** Carcinoma oesophagus showing narrowing of the lumen and thickening of the wall (arrow). **C,** Carcinoma penis showing fungating growth on the coronal sulcus (arrow).

Keratin pearls

Whorls of malignant squamous cells

Downward proliferation

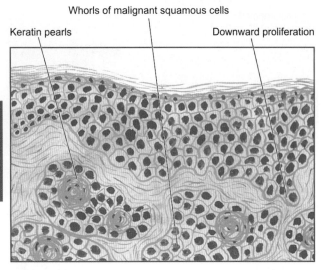

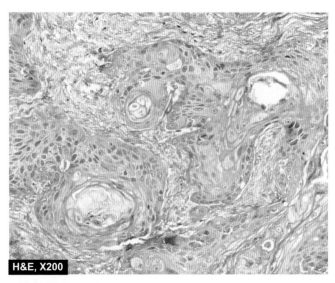

H&E, X200

FIGURE 19.4 ◆ Squamous cell carcinoma, well-differentiated. The dermis is invaded by downward proliferating epidermal masses of cells which show atypical features. A few horn pearls with central laminated keratin are present. There is marked inflammatory reaction in the dermis between the masses of tumour cells.

M/E

i. There is downward as well as outwards proliferation of squamous epithelium with increased number of layers which show loss of orderly maturation.

ii. These masses of tumour cells invade through the basement membrane into subepithelium or dermis.

iii. In better-differentiated tumours, the tumour cells are arranged in concentric layers or whorls and contain concentric layers of keratin material in the centre of the cell whorls (Fig. 19.4).

iv. The tumour cells show variable degree of differentiation and anaplasia and accordingly labeled as well-differentiated, moderately-differentiated, and poorly-differentiated.

v. The masses of tumour cells are separated by lymphocytes.

Malignant Melanoma

Malignant melanoma or melanocarcinoma is the malignant counterpart of naevus and is the most rapidly spreading malignant tumour of the skin, mucosa and other melanin containing sites.

G/A Malignant melanoma may appear as flat, macular or slightly elevated, nodular lesion. The lesion exhibits variation in pigmentation appearing in shades of black, brown, grey, blue or red. The borders are irregular (Fig. 19.5).

M/E

i. The tumour has marked junctional activity at the epidermo-dermal junction and grows horizontally as well as downwards into the dermis.

ii. The invading tumour cells are arranged in a variety of patterns—solid masses, sheets, islands, nests, etc.

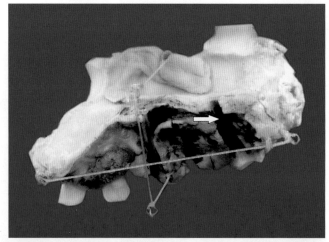

FIGURE 19.5 ◆ Malignant melanoma oral cavity. In this hemi-maxillectomy specimen, whitish oral mucosa shows an elevated blackish area with ulceration. Cut surface shows blackish tumour with irregular outlines (arrow).

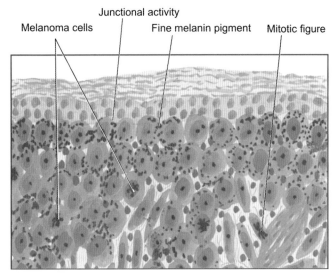
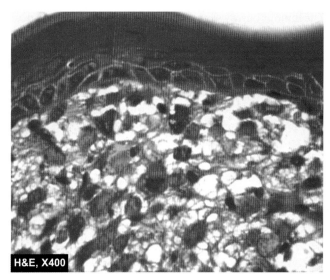

H&E, X400

FIGURE 19.6 ◆ Malignant melanoma. There is marked junctional activity at the dermal-epidermal junction. Tumour cells resembling epithelioid cells with pleomorphic nuclei and prominent nucleoli are seen as solid masses in the dermis. Many of the tumour cells contain fine granular melanin pigment.

iii. The individual tumour cell are usually larger than the naevus cells, contain large vesicular nuclei with peripherally condensed chromatin and having prominent eosinophilic nucleoli. The cytoplasm is amphophilic (Fig. 19.6).

iv. Melanin pigment is present in the cytoplasm in the form of uniform fine granules (unlike coarse pigment granules at the periphery of the lesion in benign naevus).

Basal Cell Carcinoma

Basal cell carcinoma or rodent ulcer is a locally invasive slow-growing tumour of the skin of face in the middle-aged that rarely metastasises.

G/A The tumour is commonly a nodular growth with central ulceration (nodulo-ulcerative). The margins of the tumour are pearly white and rolled while the base shows ulceration.

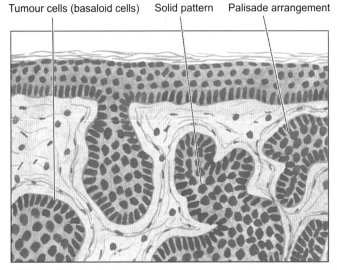
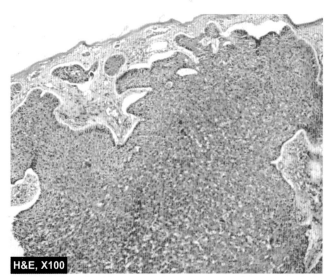

H&E, X100

FIGURE 19.7 ◆ Solid basal cell carcinoma. The dermis is invaded by irregular masses of basaloid cells with characteristic peripheral palisaded appearance.

The tumour burrows into the underlying tissues like a rodent and destroys them.

M/E

i. The tumour cells resemble normal basal cell layer of the skin and grow downwards from the epidermis in a variety of patterns—solid masses, nests, islands, strands, keratotic masses, adenoid, etc.

ii. All patterns of tumour cells have one common characteristic feature—the cells forming the periphery of tumour have parallel alignment or show palisading (basaloid cells).

iii. The tumour cells are basophilic with hyperchromatic nuclei (Fig. 19.7).

iv. Stroma shrinks away from epithelial tumour nests, creating clefts which help in differentiating it from the adnexal tumours.

Mesenchymal and Metastatic Tumours

Objectives
➤ To learn pathology of common primary mesenchymal benign and malignant tumours with examples (e.g. lipoma, pleomorphic sarcoma) and metastatic carcinoma and sarcoma (e.g. metastatic carcinoma lymph node, metastatic sarcoma lung).
➤ To describe salient gross and microscopic features of these tumours.

Just like epithelial tumours, benign mesenchymal tumours are also suffixed as—oma with prefix of cell of origin (e.g. lipoma) while malignant mesenchymal tumours are called sarcomas with prefix of cell of origin (e.g. liposarcoma).

All malignant tumours have 2 common features—anaplasia and invasion or spread. Invasiveness of cancers may be by direct local spread, or to other sites such as by lymphatics to lymph nodes (most carcinomas) and by haemotogenous spread (most sarcomas) to distant sites. Examples of metastases discussed below are metastatic carcinoma in lymph nodes and metastatic sarcoma in lung.

Lipoma

Lipoma is a common benign tumour occurring in the subcutaneous tissues.

G/A The tumour is small, encapsulated, round to oval. The cut surface is soft, lobulated, yellowish and greasy (Fig. 20.1).

M/E
  i. A thin fibrous capsule surrounds the periphery.
  ii. The tumour is composed of lobules of mature adipose cells separated by thin fibrovascular septa (Fig. 20.2).

Pleomorphic Rhabdomyosarcoma

Malignant tumour of skeletal muscle origin is called rhabdomyosarcoma. There are 4 histologic types—embryonal, botyroid, alveolar and pleomorphic. The pleomorphic rhabdomyosarcoma occurs in older adults (past 4th decade), commonly in the extremities, and is a highly malignant tumour.

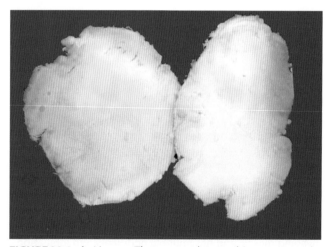

FIGURE 20.1 ◆ Lipoma. The tumour shows a thin outer capsule. Cut surface is soft, lobulated, yellowish and greasy.

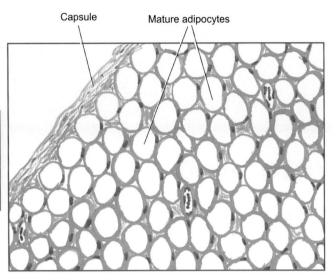

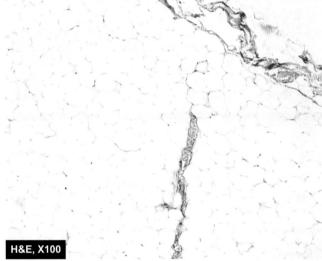

H&E, X100

FIGURE 20.2 ◆ Lipoma. The tumour composed of mature fat cells is enclosed by thin fibrous capsule.

G/A The tumour forms a well-circumscribed, soft, whitish mass with areas of haemorrhages and necrosis (Fig. 20.3).

M/E

i. The tumour cells are arranged in interlacing bundles and fascicles.

ii. The tumour is composed of highly anaplastic cells having bizarre appearance and many multinucleate giant cells (Fig. 20.4).

iii. The tumour cells may have variety of shapes—racquet shape, tadpole appearance, large strap cells, ribbon shape, etc.

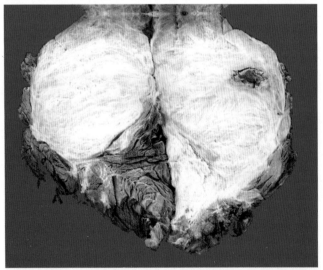

FIGURE 20.3 ◆ Pleomorphic rhabdomyosarcoma. Sectioned surface shows an irregular and unencapsulated tumour invading muscle and has multiple nodularity and lobulations. Cut surface is grey-white fleshy with areas of haemorrhage and necrosis.

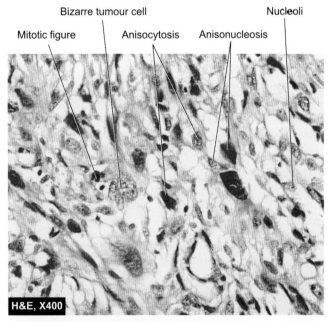

H&E, X400

FIGURE 20.4 ◆ Pleomorphic rhabdomyosarcoma. Marked pleomorphism, anisonucleosis, hyperchromatic nuclei, prominent nucleoli, mitotic figures and bizarre tumour cells.

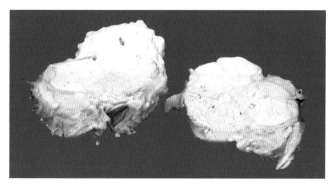

FIGURE 20.5 ◆ Metastatic carcinoma in lymph nodes. Matted mass of lymph nodes is surrounded by fat. Cut surface shows large irregular areas of grey-white colour replacing grey-brown nodal tissue.

iv. In some cases, cross striations may be demonstrable in the cytoplasm of the tumour cells in routine staining or by special stain, PTAH.

Metastatic Carcinoma Lymph Node

The regional lymph nodes may show metastatic deposits, most commonly from carcinomas but sometimes sarcomas may also metastasise to the regional lymph nodes.

G/A The affected lymph nodes are enlarged and matted. Cut surface shows homogeneous, grey-white deposits with areas of necrosis (Fig. 20.5).

M/E The features of metastatic carcinoma reproduce the picture of primary tumour. In a metastatic carcinoma from infiltrating duct carcinoma of the breast, the features are as under:
  i. Initially, the tumour is seen in the subcapsular sinus but advanced cases show replacement of the nodal architecture by masses of malignant cells.
  ii. The tumour is seen as solid nests, cords and poorly-formed glandular structures.
  iii. The tumour cells show varying degree of anaplasia and mitotic activity.
  iv. Part of cortex and capsule of the lymph node are intact (Fig. 20.6).

Metastatic Sarcoma Lung

Sarcomas commonly metastasise through haematogenous route to lungs, liver, bones, kidneys, etc. Some carcinomas, however, too spread by haematogenous route.

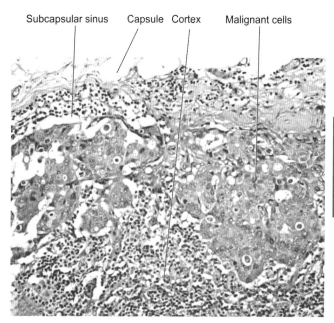

Subcapsular sinus   Capsule   Cortex   Malignant cells

FIGURE 20.6 ◆ Metastatic carcinoma in lymph node. Lymphatic spread beginning by lodgement of tumour cells in subcapsular sinus via afferent lymphatics entering at the convex surface of the lymph node.

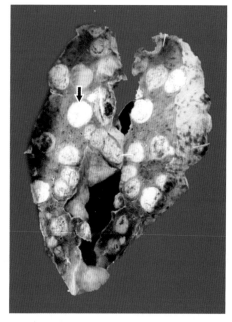

FIGURE 20.7 ◆ Metastatic sarcoma lung. Cut surface of the lung shows replacement of spongy parenchyma by multiple, variable-sized, circumscribed nodular masses (arrow). These masses are grey-white in colour and some show areas of haemorrhage and necrosis.

Lung parenchyma   Sarcoma cells   Mitotic figure

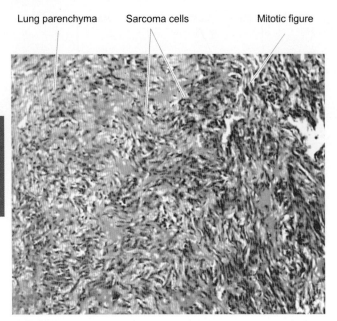

FIGURE 20.8 ◆ Metastatic sarcoma lung. Large masses of highly pleomorphic mesenchymal cells have replaced lung tissue on right.

G/A In lung, the metastatic nodules are scattered throughout all lobes. The tumour nodules are circumscribed, soft and fleshy (Fig. 20.7).

M/E The metastatic tumour reproduces the picture of primary sarcoma. In metastatic deposits from malignant fibrous histiocytoma, the features are as under:

   i. Tumour cells are arranged as whorls, fascicles and bundles.

   ii. The tumour cells are highly pleomorphic and are oval to spindle-shaped.

  iii. Multinucleate tumour giant cells are seen.

  iv. The background may show myxoid material and areas of necrosis.

   v. There is generally rich vascularity (Fig. 20.8).

Section Three

SYSTEMIC PATHOLOGY

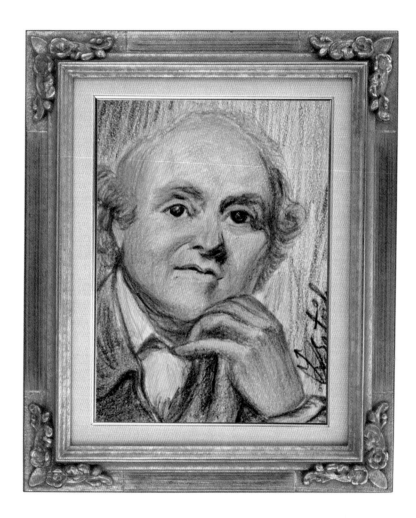

JOHN HUNTER (1728–1793)
'Founder of Medical Museum Techniques'

Scottish surgeon regarded as the greatest surgeon-anatomist of all times.
He established unique collection of pathological specimens that later resulted in
Hunterian Museum of the Royal College of Surgeons, London.
He described syphilitic chancre (Hunterian chancre) and adductor
canal (Hunterian canal). His brother William Hunter was famous anatomist of his time.

Section Contents

Atherosclerosis and Vascular Tumours

Objectives
➢ To learn pathology of atheroma of the aorta and common examples of tumours of blood vessels (e.g. capillary haemangioma skin, cavernous haemangioma liver) and lymphatics (e.g. lymphangioma tongue).
➢ To describe salient gross and microscopic features of these conditions.

Atherosclerosis is a form of thickening and hardening of medium and large sized muscular arteries due to fibrofatty plaques on the intima.

Majority of benign tumours of blood vessels and lymphatics are malformations or hamartomas which occur on the skin and mucosal surfaces and less often in the deeper tissues. A few common examples are described below.

Atheroma Aorta

A fully-developed atherosclerotic lesion is called atheromatous plaque or atheroma. It is located most commonly in the aorta (Fig. 21.1) and major branches of the aorta including coronaries.

G/A The atheromatous plaque in the coronary is eccentrically located bulging into the lumen from one side. The plaque lesion is white to yellowish-white and may have ulcerated surface. Cut section shows firm *fibrous cap* and central yellowish-white soft porridge-like *core*. Frequently, there is grittiness owing to calcification in the lesion.

M/E The appearance of plaque varies depending upon the age of lesion. However, the following features are invariably present:
  i. The superficial luminal part of *fibrous cap* is covered by endothelium and is composed of smooth muscle cells, dense connective tissue and extracellular matrix.

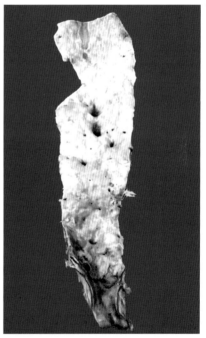

FIGURE 21.1 ◆ Fully-developed atheroma. The opened up aorta shows arterial branches coming out. The intimal surface shows yellowish-white lesions, slightly raised above the surface. A few have ulcerated surface. Many of these lesions are located near the ostial openings on the intima, thus partly occluding them.

(79)

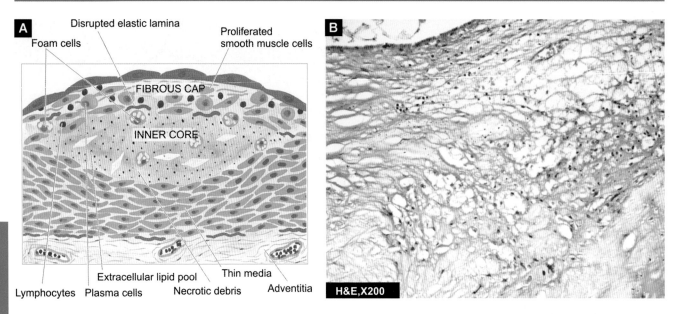

FIGURE 21.2 ◆ A, Diagrammatic view of the histologic appearance of a fully-developed atheroma. **B,** Atheromatous plaque showing fibrous cap and central core.

ii. The cellular area under the fibrous cap is composed of macrophages, foam cells and lymphocytes.

iii. The deeper central soft *core* consists of extracellular lipid material, cholesterol clefts, necrotic debris and lipid-laden foam cells (Fig. 21.2).

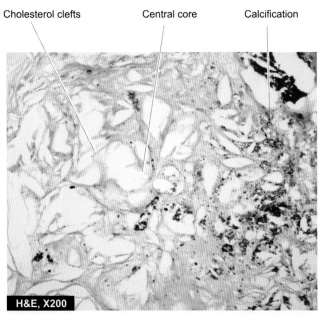

FIGURE 21.3 ◆ Complicated plaque lesion. There is critical narrowing of the coronary due to atheromatous plaque having dystrophic calcification.

iv. Calcium salts are deposited in the vicinity of necrotic area and in the lipid pool deep in the thickened intima (Fig. 21.3).

Capillary Haemangioma Skin

Haemangiomas are common lesions on the skin in infancy and childhood.

G/A Haemangioma is a small or large, flat or slightly elevated, red to purple, soft and lobulated lesion varying in size from a few millimeters to a few centimeters in diameter.

M/E The lesion is well-defined but in the form of unencapsulated lobules.

i. The lobules are composed of capillary-sized, thin-walled, blood-filled vessels.

ii. The vessels are lined by single layer of plump endothelial cells surrounded by a layer of pericytes.

iii. Some stromal connective tissue separates lobules of blood vessels (Fig. 21.4).

Cavernous Haemangioma Liver

Cavernous haemangioma is a single or multiple, discrete or diffuse, soft and spongy mass.

G/A Cavernous haemangioma varies from 1 to 2 cm in diameter and is located in the organ in the form of red to blue, soft and spongy mass.

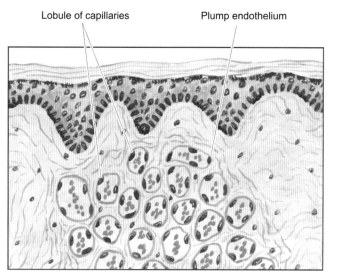

Lobule of capillaries   Plump endothelium

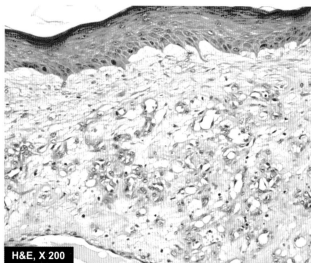

H&E, X 200

FIGURE 21.4 ◆ Capillary haemangioma of the skin. Lobules of capillary-sized vessels lined by plump endothelial cells and containing blood are lying in the dermis.

M/E

i. The lesion is composed of thin-walled cavernous vascular spaces, filled partly or completely with blood.

ii. The vascular spaces are lined by flattened endothelial cells.

iii. The intervening stroma consists of scanty connective tissue (Fig. 21.5).

Lymphangioma Tongue

Lymphangiomas are lymphatic counterparts of haemangioma and may be capillary or cavernous type, the latter being more common.

G/A Lymphangioma is a spongy mass which infiltrates the adjacent soft tissue diffusely.

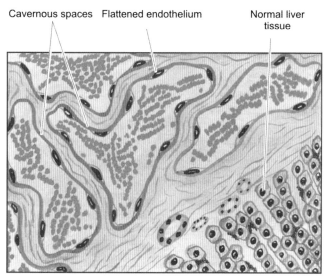

Cavernous spaces   Flattened endothelium   Normal liver tissue

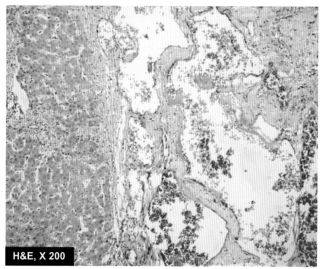

H&E, X 200

FIGURE 21.5 ◆ Cavernous haemangioma of the liver. Large cavernous spaces containing blood are seen in the liver tissue. Scanty connective tissue stroma is seen between the cavernous spaces.

Lymphoid follicle | Muscle bundles | Cavernous spaces | Stratified squamous mucosa | Lymph

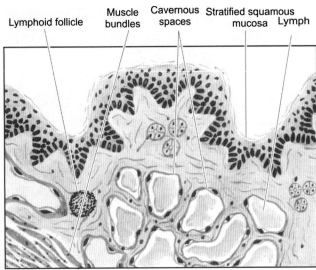
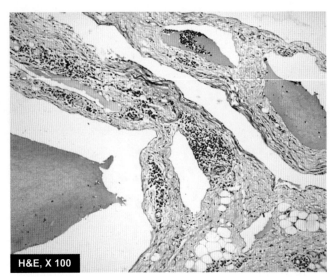

H&E, X 100

FIGURE 21.6 ◆ Cavernous lymphangioma of the tongue. Large cystic spaces lined by the flattened endothelial cells and containing lymph are present. Stroma shows scattered collection of lymphocytes.

M/E

i. There are large dilated lymphatic spaces containing homogeneous pink lymph fluid.

ii. These spaces are lined by flattened endothelial cells.

iii. The intervening stromal tissue consists of connective tissue and lymphoid infiltrate, sometimes lymphoid follicles.

iv. Skeletal muscle bundles are present in the intervening stroma showing infiltration of the lesion into the muscle (Fig. 21.6).

Diseases of the Heart

Objectives
➤ To learn pathology of common examples of diseases of layers of the heart (e.g. bacterial endocarditis, myocardial infarction, chronic ischaemic heart disease, fibrinopurulent pericarditis).
➤ To describe salient gross and microscopic features of these conditions.

In this exercise, we will learn a few common and important examples of diseases affecting various tissues of the heart— endocardium (e.g. bacterial endocarditis), myocardial ischaemia (e.g. healed myocardial infarct, chronic ischaemic heart disease or chronic IHD) and pericardium (e.g. fibrinopurulent percarditis).

Bacterial Endocarditis

Bacterial endocarditis (BE) is a serious bacterial infection of the valvular and mural endocardium, more often on pre-

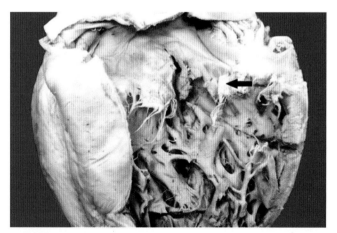

FIGURE 22.1 ◆ Vegetations on valves in bacterial endocarditis. The chambers and valves of the left heart are opened up. The mitral valve on its atrial (superior) surface show irregular, soft, elevated, greyish areas of varying size (arrow).

diseased heart, and is characterised by typical infected and friable vegetations. The disease exists in 2 forms—acute (ABE) and subacute (SABE) forms, the latter being more common.

G/A The vegetations are mainly found on the valves of left heart, most frequently on the atrial surface of mitral valve, ventricular surface of aortic valve, and combined mitral and aortic valvular involvement. The vegetations are variable in size, grey to greenish, irregular, and typically friable (Fig. 22.1). They may be flat, filiform, fungating or polypoid.

M/E The vegetations of BE consist of 3 zones:
  i. *Outer layer or cap* composed of eosinophilic material of fibrin and platelets.
  ii. Underneath is the *basophilic zone* containing colonies of bacteria in untreated cases.
  iii. The *deeper zone* consists of nonspecific inflammatory reaction in the cusp (Fig. 22.2).

Healed Myocardial Infarct

The myocardial infarct undergoes healing in about 6 weeks.

G/A The infarcted area is replaced by a thin, grey-white, hard, shrunken fibrous scar compared to adjacent uninvolved grey-brown myocardium (Fig. 22.3).

M/E
  i. There is replacement of an irregular area of the myocardium by dense fibrocollagenous tissue with foci of entrapped groups of myocardial fibres.

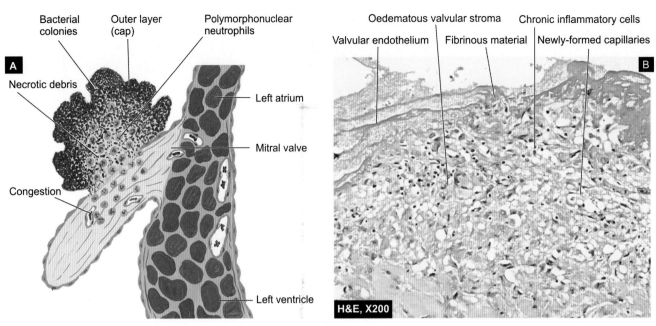

FIGURE 22.2 ◆ Infective (bacterial) endocarditis. Microscopic structure of a vegetation of BE on the surface of the mitral valve shows three layers (from within outside)—fibrin cap on luminal surface, basophilic layer of bacteria and deeper zone of inflammatory reaction with prominence of neutrophils.

ii. The neighbouring myocardial fibres may show compensatory hypertrophy.

iii. The affected area of healed infarct shows old granulation tissue seen by infiltrate of some pigmented macrophages, lymphocytes and plasma cells and a few capillary sized blood vessels (Fig. 22.4).

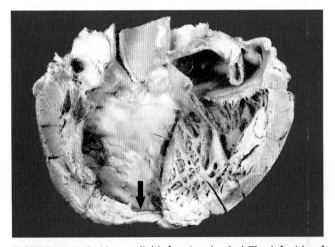

FIGURE 22.3 ◆ Myocardial infarction, healed. The left side of the heart has been opened. The left ventricular wall shows a grey-white and firm but thin area of scarring near the apex (arrow).

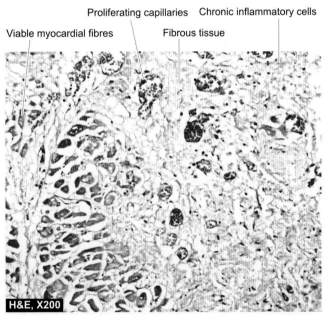

FIGURE 22.4 ◆ Myocardial infarction (old). The infarcted zone shows large area of fibrous replacement of the myocardium. The adjacent area shows old granulation tissue and myocardial hypertrophy.

Variable-sized
myocardial fibres

Hypertrophied
myocardial fibre

Periarteriolar
myocardial fibrosis

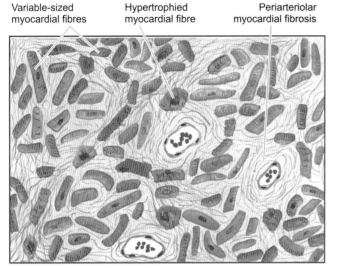

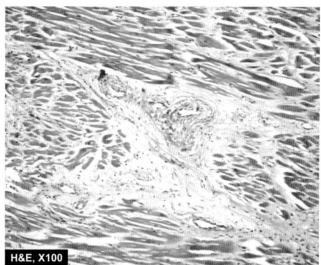

H&E, X100

FIGURE 22.5 ◆ Chronic ischaemic heart disease. There is patchy myocardial fibrosis, especially around terminal branches of coronaries in the interstitium. The adjacent single cells and groups of myocardial cells show myocytolysis and hypertrophy.

Chronic Ischaemic Heart Disease

Chronic IHD is found in elderly patients of progressive ischaemia who have had repeated episodes of angina due to coronary disease.

G/A The heart may be normal sized or hypertrophied. The left ventricular wall shows foci of grey-white fibrosis.

M/E
  i. There are scattered areas of myocardial fibrosis, especially around arterioles (terminal branches of coronaries) in the interstitial tissue of the myocardium.
 ii. The neighbouring myocardial fibres show variation in fibre size and changes of myocardial hypertrophy (Fig. 22.5).
iii. Areas of brown atrophy may be seen, i.e. presence of lipofuscin pigment in the myocardial fibres.

Fibrinopurulent Pericarditis

Purulent and fibrinopurulent pericarditis is mainly caused by pyogenic bacteria, and less often by fungi and parasites. It may occur by direct extension from neighbouring inflammation, or spread by haematogenous and lymphatic routes.

G/A The pericardial cavity and the surface contain thick creamy pus. Advanced cases may show healing by organization and hence adhesions may be seen.

M/E
  i. Pericardial surface is coated with purulent exudate.
 ii. The fibrocollagenic tissue of the pericardium contains numerous chronic inflammatory cells with predominance of neutrophils (Fig. 22.6).

Pericardium   Fibrinous material   Inflammatory cells   Myocardium

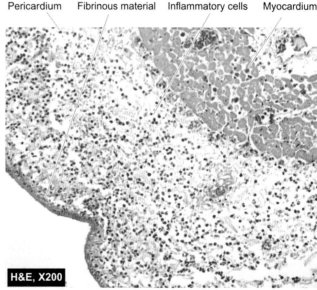

H&E, X200

FIGURE 22.6 ◆ Fibrinopurulent pericarditis. The pericardial surface shows presence of pink serofibrinous exudate while the space between the two layers of pericardium shows acute inflammatory cells admixed with exudate.

Pneumonias

Objectives
➢ To learn pathology of common types and stages of pneumonias, e.g. lobar pneumonia (acute congestion stage, red and grey hepatisation stage) and bronchopneumonia.
➢ To describe salient gross and microscopic features of these conditions.

Pulmonary tuberculosis (Exercise 14), lung abscess (Exercise 13), fungal infections (Exercise 16) and pneumonia are the most common infections of pulmonary tissues. Pneumonia (or pneumonitis) is defined as acute inflammation of the lung parenchyma distal to terminal bronchioles. Based on the anatomic part of lung involved, pneumonias are of 3 main types: *lobar pneumonia* (affecting a large portion of a lobe/lobes of one or both the lungs), *broncho- (or lobular) pneumonia* involving terminal bronchioles and alveolar tissue surrounding it, and *interstitial (or atypical) pneumonia* which is mostly of viral etiology.

Lobar Pneumonia— Acute Congestion Stage

Acute congestion stage is the initial stage of lobar pneumonia which represents the early acute inflammatory response to bacterial infection that lasts for 1 to 2 days.

PMNs and RBCs (some)

Widened septa   Oedema fluid

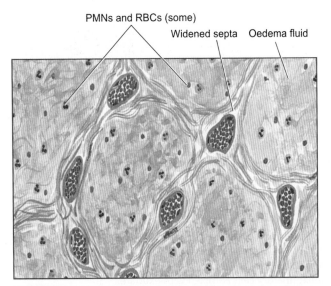

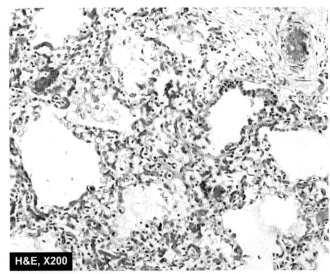

H&E, X200

FIGURE 23.1 ◆ Lobar pneumonia, acute congestion. There is congestion of septal walls while the air spaces contain pale oedema fluid and a few red cells.

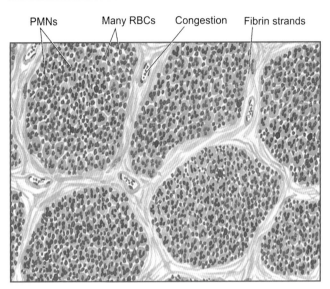

PMNs　Many RBCs　Congestion　Fibrin strands

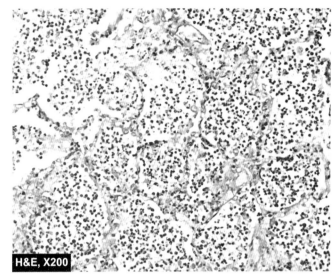

H&E, X200

FIGURE 23.2 ◆ Lobar pneumonia, red hepatisation. The alveoli are filled with cellular exudate of neutrophils and some red cells.

G/A The affected lobe is enlarged, heavy, dark red and congested. Cut surface exudes blood-stained frothy fluid.

M/E

i. There is dilatation and congestion of capillaries in the alveolar walls.

ii. The air spaces contain pale eosinophilic oedema fluid.

iii. A few red cells and neutrophils are seen in the intra-alveolar fluid (Fig. 23.1).

iv. Bacteria may be demonstrable by Gram's staining.

Lobar Pneumonia— Red Hepatisation Stage

Red hepatisation phase lasts for 2 to 4 days. The term *hepatisation* in pneumonia refers to liver-like consistency of the affected lobe on cut section.

G/A The affected lobe is red, firm and consolidated. Cut surface of the involved lobe is air-less, red-pink, dry, granular and has liver-like consistency.

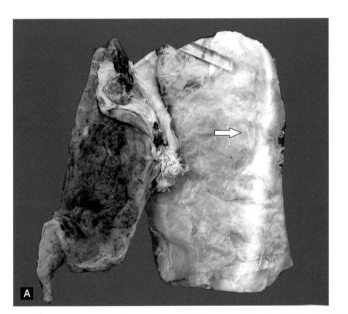

A

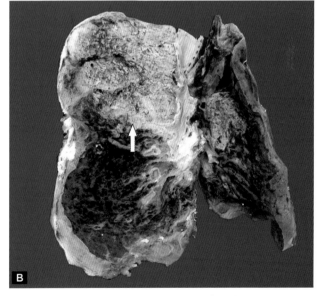

B

FIGURE 23.3 ◆ Grey hepatisation (late consolidation) (4-8 days). **A,** The pleural surface shows some serofibrinous exudate (arrow). **B,** Sectioned surface of the lung shows grey-brown, firm area of consolidation affecting a lobe (arrow) while the rest of the lung is spongy.

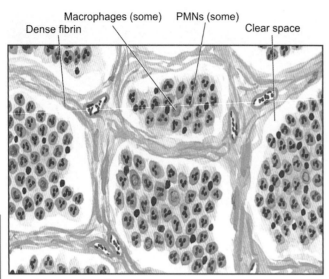

Dense fibrin   Macrophages (some)   PMNs (some)   Clear space

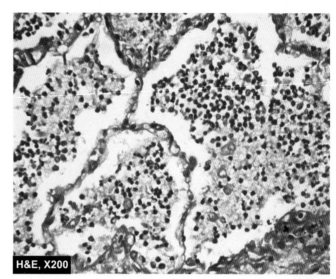

H&E, X200

FIGURE 23.4 ◆ Lobar pneumonia, grey hepatisation. The cellular exudate is separated from septal wall by a clear space. The exudate consists of neutrophils as well as macrophages.

M/E
  i. Air spaces contain strands of fibrin.
 ii. There is marked cellular exudate of neutrophils and extravasation of red cells (Fig. 23.2).
iii. Neutrophils may show ingested bacteria.

Lobar Pneumonia— Grey Hepatisation Stage

This phase lasts for 4-8 days.

G/A The affected lobe is firm and heavy. The pleural surface may show some serofibrinous exudate. Cut surface is dry, granular and grey in appearance with liver-like consistency (Fig. 23.3).

M/E
  i. The fibrin strands in the air spaces are dense.
 ii. The lumina of alveoli contain disintegrated neutrophils and many macrophages.
iii. A clear space separates septal walls from the cellular exudate (Fig. 23.4).

Bronchopneumonia

Bronchopneumonia or lobular pneumonia is infection of terminal bronchioles that extends into the surrounding alveoli resulting in patchy consolidation of the lung.

G/A Bronchopneumonia is identified by patchy areas of red or grey consolidation affecting one or more lobes, more often

bilaterally and involving lower zones of lungs more frequently. On cut surface, patchy consolidated lesions appear dry, granular, firm, red or grey in colour, 3 to 4 cm in diameter.

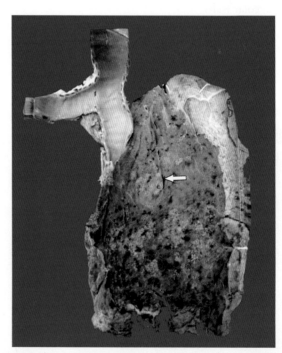

FIGURE 23.5 ◆ Bronchopneumonia. The pleural surface shows some serofibrinous deposits. Sectioned surface of the lung shows multiple, small, grey-brown, firm, patchy or granular areas of consolidation around bronchioles (arrow). These areas are seen affecting a lobe while the rest of the lung is spongy.

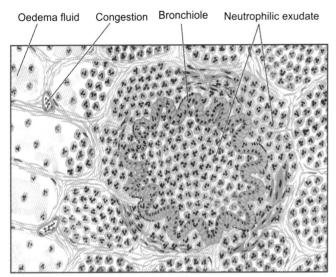
Oedema fluid   Congestion   Bronchiole   Neutrophilic exudate

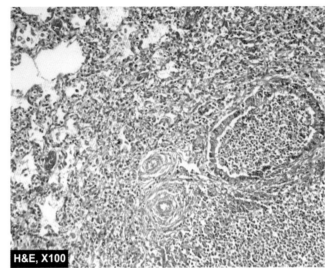
H&E, X100

FIGURE 23.6 ◆ Microscopic appearance of bronchopneumonia. The bronchioles as well as the adjacent alveoli are filled with exudate consisting chiefly of neutrophils. The alveolar septa are thickened due to congested capillaries and neutrophilic infiltrate.

These lesions are slightly elevated over the surface centred around a bronchiole, best picked up by feeling with fingers on cut section (Fig. 23.5).

M/E

i. Changes of acute bronchiolitis characterised by acute inflammatory cells in the bronchiolar walls are seen.

ii. There is suppurative exudate of neutrophils in the peribronchiolar alveoli.

iii. There is widening of alveolar septa by congested capillaries and leucocytic infiltration.

iv. Alveoli away from the involved area contain oedema fluid (Fig. 23.6).

Chronic Obstructive Pulmonary Diseases and Lung Cancer

Objectives

➢ To learn pathology of a few examples of obstructive lung diseases (e.g. emphysema, bronchiectasis) and lung cancer (e.g. squamous cell carcinoma and small cell carcinoma).

➢ To describe salient gross and microscopic features of these conditions.

Chronic obstructive pulmonary diseases or COPD are a group of pathologic conditions in which there is chronic, partial or complete, obstruction to the airflow at any level from the trachea to the terminal airways. COPD includes 4 main conditions: chronic bronchitis and bronchial asthma (both of which are more of medical problems), emphysema and bronchiectasis (both of which have major pathologic changes in the lungs and are hence discussed here). Besides, pathology of two major forms of bronchogenic cancer—squamous cell and small cell carcinoma, are discussed here.

Emphysema

Emphysema is permanent dilatation of air spaces distal to the terminal bronchiole resulting in destruction of the walls of dilated air spaces.

G/A The lungs show varying-sized sub-pleural bullae and blebs. These spaces are air-filled cyst-like or bubble-like structures, 1 cm or larger in diameter (Fig. 24.1).

M/E

i. There is dilatation of air spaces and destruction of septal walls of part of acinus involved.

ii. Alveolar walls are ruptured with spurs of broken septa between adjacent alveoli.

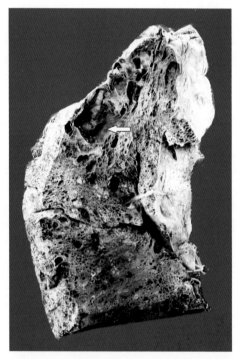

FIGURE 24.1 ◆ Bullous emphysema of the lung. The lung is expanded and has thin-walled cysts or bullae visible on the pleural surface. Sectioned surface of the lung shows many large air-filled sacs, a few centimeters in diameter (arrow), located under the pleura.

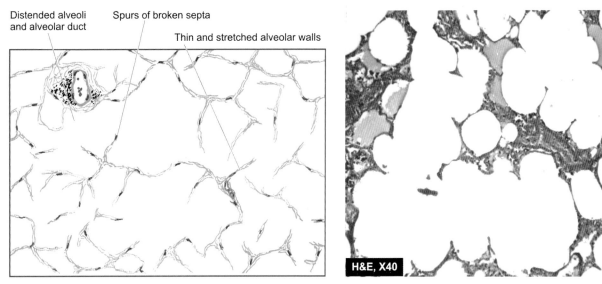

Distended alveoli and alveolar duct

Spurs of broken septa

Thin and stretched alveolar walls

H&E, X40

FIGURE 24.2 ◆ Emphysema. There is dilatation of air spaces and destruction of septal walls.

iii. Capillaries in the septal walls are thinned and stretched.

iv. Changes of bronchitis are often present (Fig. 24.2).

Bronchiectasis

Bronchiectasis is abnormal and irreversible dilatation of the bronchi and larger bronchioles.

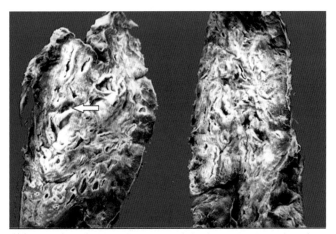

FIGURE 24.3 ◆ Bronchiectasis of the lung. Sectioned surface of the lung shows honey-combed appearance of the lung in its lower lobes where many thick-walled dilated cavities with cartilaginous wall are seen (arrow).

G/A Bilateral involvement of lower lobes of lungs is seen more frequently. The pleura is usually fibrotic and thickened. Cut surface of affected lower lobes shows characteristic honey-combed appearance due to dilated airways containing mucopus and thickening of their walls (Fig. 24.3).

M/E

i. There is infiltration of the bronchial walls by acute and chronic inflammatory cells with destruction of normal muscle and elastic tissue with replacement fibrosis.

ii. There is fibrosis of the intervening lung parenchyma and interstitial pneumonia.

iii. Bronchial epithelium may be normal, ulcerated or may show squamous metaplasia (Fig. 24.4).

Squamous Cell Carcinoma Lung

This has been the most common type of bronchogenic carcinoma world over until recently but is now most common in developing countries while in the western world non-smoking related adenocarcinoma has become most common.

G/A The tumour is often hilar or central arising from a large bronchus, may be of variable size and invades the adjacent lung parenchyma. Cut surface of the tumour shows extensive necrosis and cavitation (Fig. 24.5).

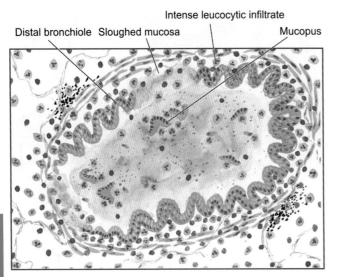
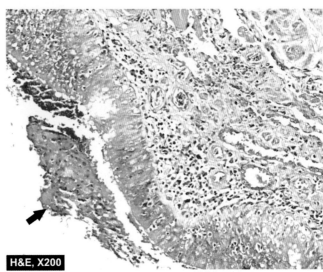

Distal bronchiole Sloughed mucosa Intense leucocytic infiltrate Mucopus

H&E, X200

FIGURE 24.4 ◆ Microscopic appearance of a dilated distal bronchiole in bronchiectasis. The bronchial wall is thickened and infiltrated by acute and chronic inflammatory cells. The mucosa is sloughed off at places with exudate of mucopus in the lumen (arrow).

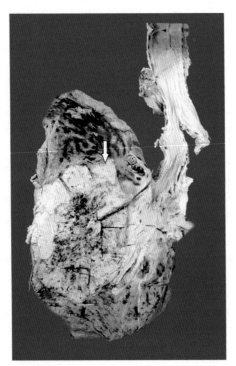

FIGURE 24.5 ◆ Squamous cell carcinoma of the lung, hilar type. Sectioned surface shows grey-white, fleshy, thickening of the bronchus at its bifurcation, partly occluding the lumen (arrow). The tumour is also seen extending irregularly into adjacent lung parenchyma and hilar lymph nodes.

M/E
  i. Varying grades of differentiation from well-differentiated with keratinisation (Fig. 24.6) to poorly-differentiated and sarcoma-like spindle cell carcinoma may be seen.
 ii. Intercellular bridges or keratinisation are often seen in better differentiated tumour.
iii. The edge of the tumour often shows squamous metaplasia, epithelial dysplasia and carcinoma in situ.

Small Cell Carcinoma Lung

Small cell carcinoma is a variant of bronchogenic carcinoma arising from argentaffin cells and is a highly malignant tumour.

G/A The tumour is frequently hilar or central in location. The tumour appears as a nodule 1-5 cm in diameter with ulcerated surface. Cut surface of the tumour is yellowish-white with areas of necrosis and haemorrhages.

M/E
  i. Tumour cells are uniform, small (slightly larger than lymphocytes) with dense round or oval nuclei having diffuse chromatin, inconspicuous nucleoli and scanty granular cytoplasm.

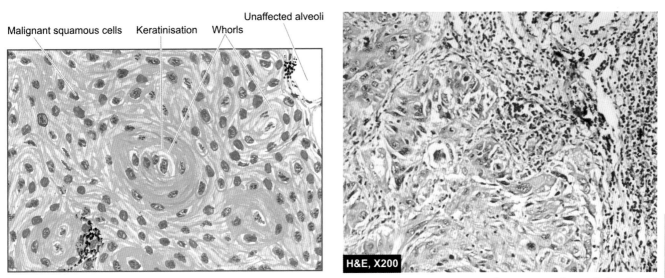

FIGURE 24.6 ◆ Squamous cell carcinoma of the lung. Islands of invading malignant squamous cells are seen. A few well-developed cell nests with keratinisation are evident.

ii. Tumour cells are arranged in cords, aggregates and ribbons, or around small blood vessels forming pseudorosettes (Fig. 24.7).

iii. The granules of the tumour cells are positive for neurosecretory marker, chromogranin (Fig. 24.7, inbox).

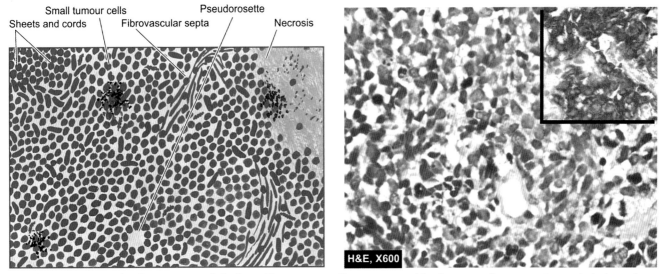

FIGURE 24.7 ◆ Small cell carcinoma of the lung. The tumour cells are arranged in sheets, cords, aggregates and at places form pseudorosettes. The individual tumour cells are small, uniform, lymphocyte-like with scanty granular cytoplasm. Inbox in right figure shows IHC staining for chromogranin as brown cystoplasmic granules.

Diseases of the Jaws, Salivary Glands and Stomach

Objectives
➤ To learn pathology of an example each of tumours of jaws (e.g. ameloblastoma) and salivary glands (e.g. pleomorphic adenoma) and examples of common diseases of the stomach (e.g. peptic ulcer and adenocarcinoma).
➤ To describe salient gross and microscopic features of these conditions.

Odontogenic tumours of the jaw derived from odontogenic apparatus are generally benign (ameloblastoma being the most common) but there are some examples of malignant countrparts.

The major and minor salivary glands can give rise to a variety of benign and malignant tumours, parotid being the most common site (85%).

The stomach is involved in a variety of conditions: inflammatory (gastritis of various types), peptic ulcers, and tumour and tumour like lesions or polyps, etc. A few common examples of these organs are discussed here.

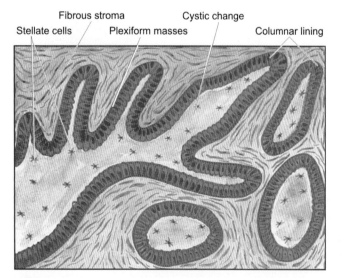

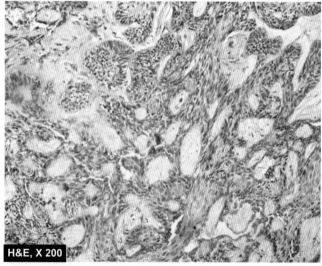

H&E, X 200

FIGURE 25.1 ◆ Ameloblastoma, follicular pattern. Epithelial follicles are seen in fibrous stroma. The follicles are composed of central area of stellate cells and peripheral layer of cuboidal or columnar cells. A few follicles show central cystic change .

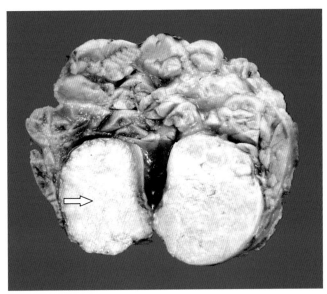

FIGURE 25.2 ◆ Pleomorphic adenoma (mixed salivary tumour) of the parotid gland. The salivary tissue is identified on section by lobules of soft tissue separated by thin septa. The cut surface of the tumour shows grey-white and light-bluish variegated semitranslucent parenchyma (arrow).

Ameloblastoma

Ameloblastoma is the common benign but locally aggressive epithelial odontogenic tumour, commonly in the mandible and maxilla.

G/A The tumour is grey-white, usually solid, sometimes cystic, replacing the affected bone.

M/E
  i. Follicular pattern is the most common, characterised by follicles of varying size and shape which are separated by fibrous tissue.
  ii. The follicles consist of central area of stellate cells and peripheral layer of cuboidal or columnar cells (Fig. 25.1).
  iii. Other less common patterns include plexiform masses, acanthomatous pattern, basal cell pattern, and granular cell pattern.

Pleomorphic Adenoma

Pleomorphic adenoma is the most common tumour in the major (60-75%) and minor (50%) salivary glands. It is the commonest tumour in the parotid gland.

G/A The tumour is circumscribed, pseudoencapsulated, rounded and multilobulated, firm mass, 2-5 cm in diameter (Fig. 25.2). The cut surface is grey-white and bluish, variegated, with soft to mucoid consistency.

M/E The pleomorphic adenoma has two components: epithelial and mesenchymal (Fig. 25.3):
  i. *Epithelial component* consists of various patterns like ducts, acini, tubules, sheets and strands of monomorphic cells of ductal or myoepithelial origin. These ductal cells

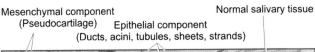

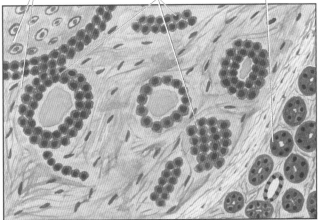

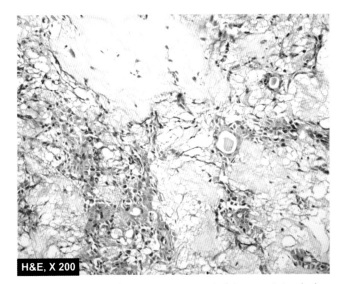

FIGURE 25.3 ◆ Pleomorphic adenoma, typical microscopic appearance. The epithelial element is composed of ducts, acini, tubules, sheets and strands of cuboidal and myoepithelial cells. These are seen randomly admixed with mesenchymal elements composed of pseudocartilage.

are cuboidal or columnar while myoepithelial cells are polygonal or spindle-shaped.

ii. *Mesenchymal component* present in loose connective tissue includes myxoid, mucoid and chondroid matrix which simulates cartilage (pseudocartilage).

Peptic Ulcer

Peptic ulcers are areas of degeneration and necrosis of mucosa of the stomach and duodenum.

G/A Gastric ulcers are found predominantly along the lesser curvature in the region of pyloric antrum, more commonly on the posterior wall. Duodenal ulcers are commonly found in first part of the duodenum, more commonly on the anterior wall. Typically, peptic ulcers of either gastric or duodenal mucosa are small (1-2.5 cm in diameter), round to oval and characteristically punched out. The mucosal folds converge towards the ulcer (Fig. 25.4).

M/E Chronic peptic ulcers have 4 histologic zones *(from within outside)* (Fig. 25.5):

i. *Necrotic zone* lies in the floor of the ulcer. The tissue elements show coagulative necrosis giving eosinophilic smudgy appearance with nuclear debris.

ii. *Superficial exudative zone* lies underneath the necrotic zone and is composed of fibrinous exudate containing

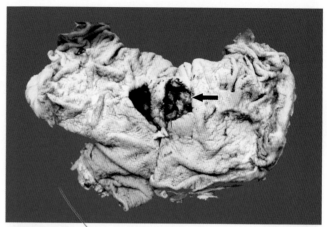

FIGURE 25.4 ◆ Benign chronic gastric ulcer. Partial gastrectomy specimen is identified by thick muscular wall and irregular mucosal folds. The luminal surface shows a punched out round to oval ulcer, about 1 cm in diameter (arrow) and penetrating in to muscularis layer.

necrotic debris and a few leucocytes, predominantly neutrophils.

iii. *Granulation tissue zone* is seen merging into the necrotic zone. It is composed of nonspecific chronic inflammatory infiltrate and proliferating capillaries.

iv. *Zone of cicatrisation* is seen outer to the layer of granulation tissue and is composed of dense fibrocollagenic scar tissue.

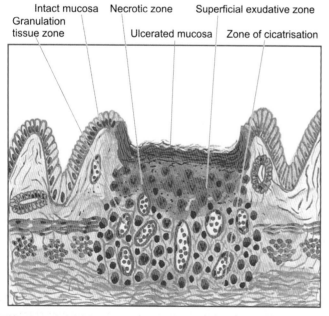

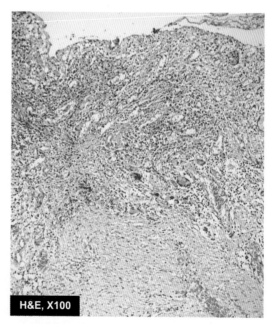

H&E, X100

FIGURE 25.5 ◆ Chronic peptic ulcer. Histologic zones of the ulcer are illustrated. The mucosal surface shows necrosis, ulceration, and inflammation.

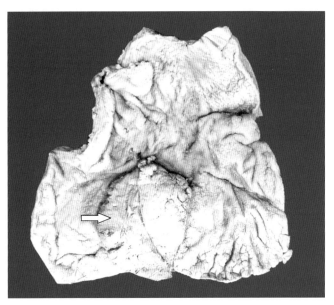

FIGURE 25.6 ◆ Ulcerative carcinoma stomach. The luminal surface of the stomach in the region of the pyloric canal shows an elevated irregular growth with ulcerated surface and raised margins (arrow).

Adenocarcinoma Stomach

Invasive gastric carcinoma extends beyond the basement membrane of mucosal layer into the muscularis propria and is seen most often in the region of pyloric canal.

G/A Most common pattern is flat, infiltrating and ulcerative growth with irregular necrotic base and raised margin (Fig. 25.6). Other gross patterns include fungating (polypoid), scirrhous (linitis plastica), colloid (mucoid) and ulcer-cancer.

M/E

i. Tubular and acinar pattern of growth is seen infiltrating the stomach wall.
ii. The tumour invades into the wall of stomach for variable depth.
iii. The tumour cells show varying degree of anaplasia but is more often poorly-differentiated with high degree of anaplasia (Fig. 25.7).

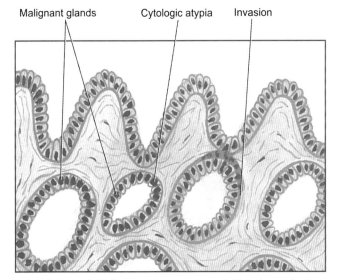

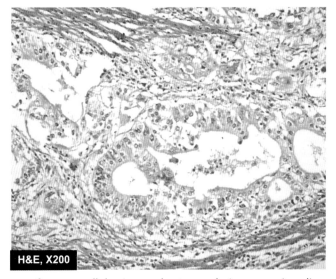

H&E, X200

FIGURE 25.7 ◆ Adenocarcinoma stomach. Tubular and acinar pattern of tumour cells having moderate anaplasia are seen invading the layers of wall of the stomach.

Diseases of Appendix and Large Intestine

Objectives
➢ To learn pathology of common examples of diseases of the appendix (e.g. acute appendicitis) and large intestine (e.g. ulcerative colitis, juvenile polyp rectum and colorectal mucinous carcinoma).
➢ To describe salient gross and microscopic features of these conditions.

An important disease affecting the appendix is acute inflammation called acute appendicitis.

Both small and large bowel may be affected by inflammatory bowel disease (IBD); here we discuss ulcerative colitis as an example. Besides, while small intestine is affected more often by obstruction, large bowel is more common site for development of benign (e.g. colorectal polyps) and malignant tumours (e.g. adenocarcinoma).

Acute Appendicitis

Acute appendicitis is the most common acute abdominal condition confronted by the surgeon.

G/A The appendix is swollen and serosa is hyperaemic and coated with fibrinopurulent exudate. The mucosa is ulcerated and sloughed.

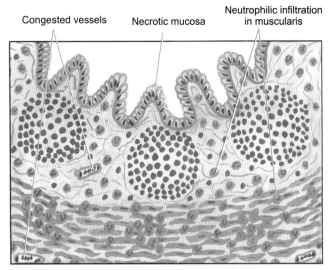

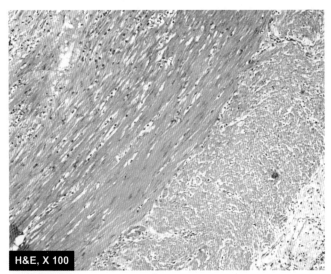

H&E, X 100

FIGURE 26.1 ◆ Acute appendicitis. Microscopic appearance showing diagnostic neutrophilic infiltration into the muscularis layer. The lumen of appendix shows exudates and sloughed mucosa.

M/E

 i. Most important diagnostic feature is neutrophilic infiltration of the muscularis propria.

 ii. Mucosa is sloughed and blood vessels in the wall are thrombosed.

 iii. Periappendiceal inflammation is seen in more severe cases (Fig. 26.1).

Ulcerative Colitis

Ulcerative colitis is an inflammatory bowel disease affecting rectum and extending upwards into the sigmoid colon, descending colon, transverse colon and sometimes may involve the entire colon.

G/A The characteristic feature is the continuous involvement of the rectum and colon without any skip areas. Mucosa shows linear and superficial ulcers while the intervening intact mucosa may form inflammatory pseudopolyps. The muscle layer is thickened due to contraction and produces loss of normal haustral folds giving 'garden-hose appearance' (Fig. 26.2).

M/E The *active disease process* shows following changes (Fig. 26.3):

 i. Focal accumulation of neutrophils in the crypts forming crypt abscess.

 ii. Marked congestion, dilatation and haemorrhages in the lamina propria.

 iii. Superficial mucosal ulcerations with crypt distortion and crypt branching.

 iv. Diminution of goblet cells and mucodepletion.

 v. Regenerating epithelium in some crypts showing flat newly formed layer.

Juvenile Polyp Rectum

Juvenile or retention polyps are hamartomatous and occur more commonly in children under 5 years of age in the region of rectum.

G/A Juvenile polyp is often solitary, spherical, smooth-surfaced, about 2 cm in diameter, and pedunculated.

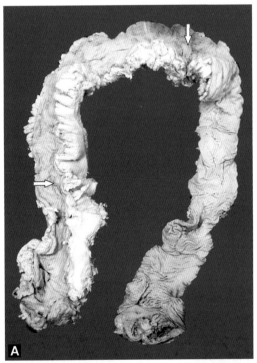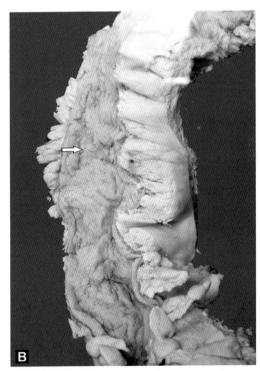

FIGURE 26.2 ◆ Ulcerative colitis. Continuous involvement of the rectum, sigmoid colon and descending colon are seen without any uninvolved skip areas **(A)**. The involved areas show ulcers and formation of mucosal polyps (arrows) with thickened wall and narrowed lumen which is better appreciated in close up **(B)**.

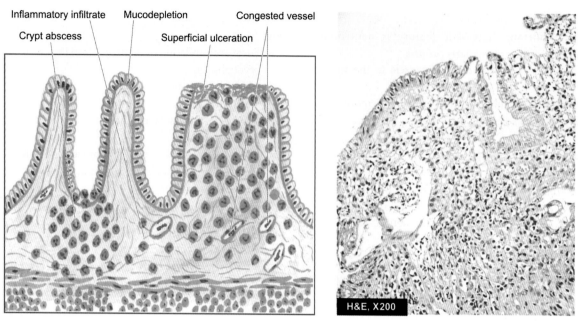

Inflammatory infiltrate   Mucodepletion   Congested vessel

Crypt abscess   Superficial ulceration

H&E, X200

FIGURE 26.3 ◆ Ulcerative colitis in active phase. The microscopic features seen are superficial ulcerations, with mucosal infiltration by inflammatory cells and a 'crypt abscess'.

M/E

i. There are cystically dilated glands containing mucus and lined by normal mucin-secreting epithelium.

ii. The stroma may show chronic inflammatory cell infiltrate.

iii. The surface may show ulceration (Fig. 26.4).

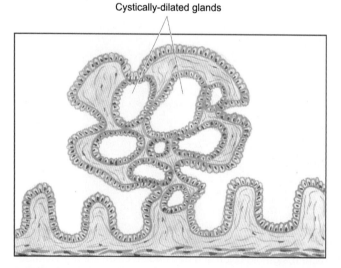

Cystically-dilated glands

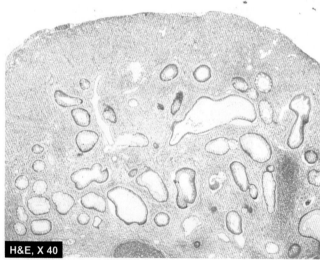

H&E, X 40

FIGURE 26.4 ◆ Juvenile polyp. There are cystically dilated glands while the stroma shows some inflammatory cells. The surface is ulcerated.

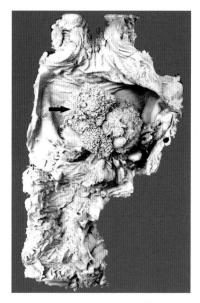

A, RIGHT-SIDED GROWTH

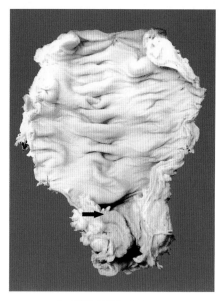

B, LEFT-SIDED GROWTH

FIGURE 26.5 ◆ **A,** Right-sided colonic carcinoma. The colonic wall shows thickening with presence of a luminal growth (arrow). The growth is cauliflower-like, soft and friable projecting into the lumen. **B,** Left-sided colonic carcinoma. Sectioned surface shows napkin ring narrowing of the lumen while the colonic wall shows circumferential firm thickening (arrow).

Colorectal Mucinous Adenocarcinoma

Colorectal carcinoma comprises the most common form of visceral cancer. The most common location is rectum.

G/A The tumour has distinctive features in right and left-sided colonic cancer. *The right-sided growth*, tends to be fungating, large, cauliflower-like, soft and friable mass projecting into the lumen (Fig. 26.5,A). The *left-sided growth*, on the other hand, has napkin-ring configuration, i.e. it

Pleomorphism   Malignant glands   Muscularis propria invaded

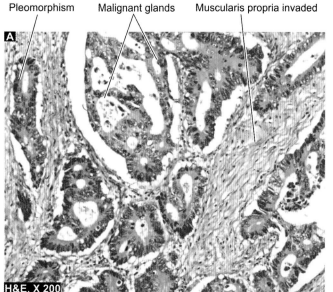

H&E, X 200

Malignant glands   Mucin pools   Muscularis propria invaded

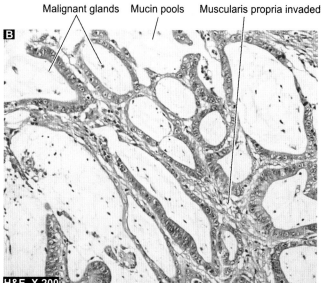

H&E, X 200

FIGURE 26.6 ◆ Colonic adenocarcinoma. **A,** Moderately differentiated. **B,** Mucin-secreting adenocarcinoma.

encircles the bowel wall circumferentially with increased fibrous tissue forming annular ring with central mucosal ulceration (Fig. 26.5,B).

M/E The microscopic appearance on right-sided and left-sided colonic cancer is similar:

i. The tumour has infiltrating glandular pattern in the colonic wall with varying grades of differentiation of tumour cells.

ii. About 10% cases show mucin-secreting colloid carcinoma with pools of mucin (Fig. 26.6).

Hepatitis—Viral, Alcoholic, Fulminant

Objectives
➢ To learn pathology of acute viral, alcoholic and fulminant hepatitis.
➢ To describe salient gross and microscopic features of these conditions.

All forms of liver cell injury (e.g. viruses, alcohol, drugs, etc.) result in necrosis of the liver cells which may be zonal (i.e. centrilobular, midzonal or periportal) or diffuse (i.e. fulminant submassive to massive). A few common and important examples of such forms of liver cell injury discussed in this exercise are acute viral hepatitis, alcoholic hepatitis and fulminant hepatitis.

Acute Viral Hepatitis

The most common consequence of all hepatotropic viruses is acute inflammatory involvement of the entire liver.

G/A The liver is slightly enlarged, soft and greenish.

M/E

i. Earliest hepatocellular injury, most marked in centrilobular zone (zone 3), is ballooning degeneration in which the hepatocytes appear swollen and have granular cytoplasm.

ii. Acidophilic degeneration of hepatocytes produces Councilman body or acidophil body identified by eosinophilic cytoplasm and pyknotic nucleus.

iii. A few areas show dropout necrosis in which isolated or small clusters of hepatocytes undergo lysis (Fig. 27.1).

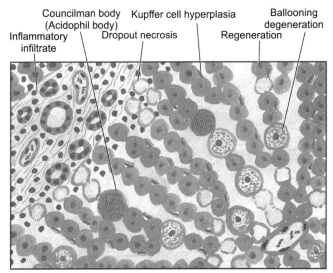

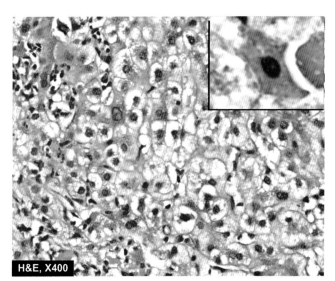

H&E, X400

FIGURE 27.1 ◆ Acute viral hepatitis. Hepatocytes show variable degree of cell injury—ballooning degeneration to necrosis of hepatocytes, more marked in centrilobular zone and lymphocytic infiltrate in the lobule. A few shrunken apoptotic hepatocytes called acidophil body or Councilman body are also seen in the lobule (inbox).

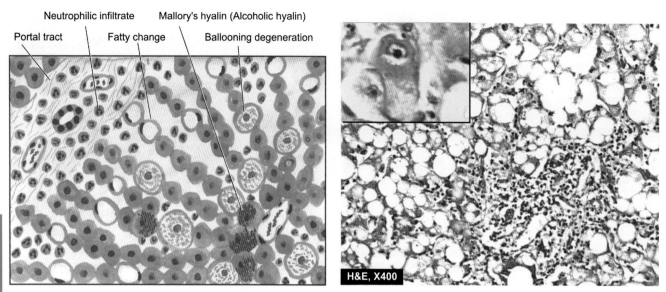

Neutrophilic infiltrate   Mallory's hyalin (Alcoholic hyalin)

Portal tract   Fatty change   Ballooning degeneration

H&E, X400

FIGURE 27.2 ◆ Alcoholic hepatitis. Hepatocytes show ballooning degeneration and necrosis with some containing Mallory's hyalin (inbox). Fatty change and clusters of neutrophils are also seen.

iv. Mononuclear inflammatory cell infiltrate is seen in the portal tracts (zone 1).
v. Kupffer cells show reactive hyperplasia.

Alcoholic Hepatitis

Alcoholic hepatitis develops acutely, usually following a bout of heavy drinking.

G/A The liver is swollen, enlarged, soft and greenish. If repeated attacks of alcoholic hepatitis have superimposed on pre-existing fatty liver, changes of fatty liver in the form of yellow, greasy and smooth appearance may be present.

M/E
i. Hepatocellular necrosis is seen in the form of ballooned out hepatocytes, especially in the centrilobular zone.

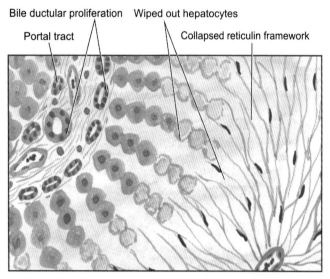

Bile ductular proliferation   Wiped out hepatocytes

Portal tract   Collapsed reticulin framework

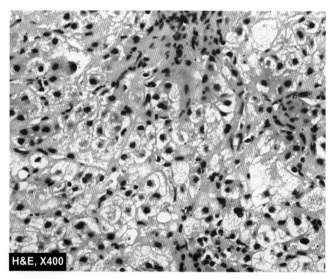

H&E, X400

FIGURE 27.3 ◆ Fulminant hepatitis. There is complete wiping out of liver lobules with only collapsed reticulin framework left out in their place. There is no significant inflammation or fibrosis.

ii. Mallory body or alcoholic hyalin is seen as eosinophilic intracytoplasmic inclusions in the perinuclear location in the swollen and ballooned hepatocytes.

iii. Inflammatory cell infiltrate of polymorphs admixed with some mononuclear cells is seen in the area of necrosis.

iv. There is web-like or chickenwire-like appearance of pericellular and perivenular fibrosis (Fig. 27.2).

Fulminant Hepatitis

Fulminant hepatitis is the most severe form of acute hepatitis of viral or non-viral etiologies and has two patterns—submassive and massive necrosis.

G/A The liver is small and shrunken and weighs 500-700 gm. The capsule is loose and wrinkled. The sectioned surface shows areas of muddy-red and yellow necrosis with patches of green bile staining (older term acute yellow atrophy of liver).

M/E

i. Large groups of hepatocytes are wiped out in centrilobular and mid-zone leading to collapsed reticulin framework (Fig. 27.3).

ii. Areas of attempted regeneration are more orderly in submassive necrosis compared to massive necrosis, best appreciated in reticulin stain (Fig. 27.4).

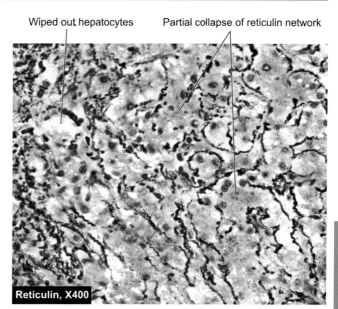

Wiped out hepatocytes　　　Partial collapse of reticulin network

Reticulin, X400

FIGURE 27.4 ◆ Fulminant hepatitis showing regeneration in the lobule while reticulin network is partly collapsed.

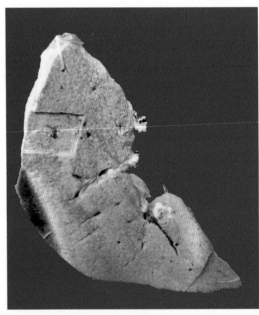

Cirrhosis, Hepatocellular Carcinoma, Gallbladder Diseases

Objectives
➤ To learn pathology of cirrhosis of liver, hepatocellular carcinoma, and common forms of gallbladder diseases.
➤ To describe salient gross and microscopic features of these conditions.

Cirrhosis of the liver is one of the leading causes of death and occurs following hepatocellular necrosis of varying etiology. Hepatocellular carcinoma is the most common primary malignant tumour of the liver, most often following cirrhosis of varying etiology and exposure to chemical carcinogens.

Most common forms of gallbladder diseases are chronic cholecystitis, gallstones, and gallbladder carcinoma.

Cirrhosis Liver

Cirrhosis of the liver is a diffuse disease having disorganised lobular architecture and formation of nodules which are separated from one another by irregular bands of fibrosis.

G/A Cirrhosis is morphologically categorised by the size of nodules—*micronodular,* if the nodules are less than 3 mm (Fig. 28.1), *macronodular* if the nodules are bigger than 3 mm (Fig. 28.2), and *mixed* if both small and large nodules are seen. Etiologically, common forms are postnecrotic, alcoholic, biliary and others. On sectioned surface, the grey-brown nodules are separated from one another by grey-white fibrous septa.

M/E The etiologic diagnosis of cirrhosis in routine microscopy may not be possible. The salient features of cirrhosis are as under:

   i. Lobular architecture of hepatic parenchyma is lost and central veins are hard to find.

FIGURE 28.1 ◆ Alcoholic cirrhosis, showing the typical micronodular pattern. The nodules are smaller than 3 mm diameter on the sectioned surface.

   ii. Fibrous septa divide the hepatic parenchyma into nodules.

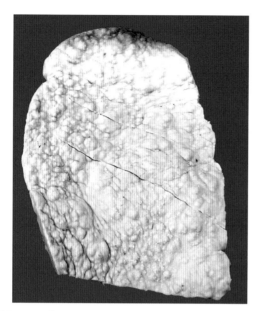

FIGURE 28.2 ◆ Postnecrotic cirrhosis, showing the typical irregular macronodular pattern (nodules larger than 3 mm diameter). The liver is small, distorted and irregularly scarred.

iii. The hepatocytes in the surviving parenchyma form regenerative nodules having disorganised masses of hepatocytes.

iv. Fibrous septa contain some mononuclear inflammatory cell infiltrate and proliferated bile ductules (Fig. 28.3).

Hepatocellular Carcinoma

Hepatocellular carcinoma (HCC) or hepatoma is one of the aggressive primary cancers.

G/A The HCC may form one of the three patterns of growth (in decreasing order of frequency) (Fig. 28.4):

i. *Expanding type* as a single large mass with central necrosis and haemorrhage.

ii. *Multifocal type* as multiple masses scattered throughout the liver.

iii. *Infiltrating type* is a diffusely spreading type and is less common.

M/E The features are as follows (Fig. 28.5):

i. *Histologic patterns.* The tumour cells may be arranged in a variety of patterns. Most common is trabecular or sinusoidal pattern composed of 2-8 cell wide layers of tumour cells separated by endothelium-lined vascular spaces. Other patterns include pseudoglandular or acinar, compact and scirrhous.

ii. *Cytologic features.* The tumour cells show anaplasia but resemble hepatocytes with vesicular nuclei, prominent nucleoli, granular and eosinophilic cytoplasm. These tumour cells have pleomorphism, bizarre giant cell formation, and Mallory's hyalin.

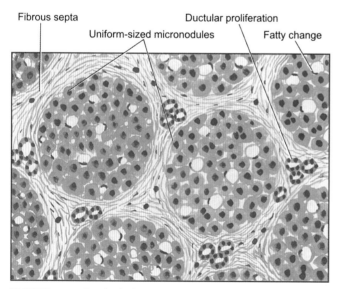

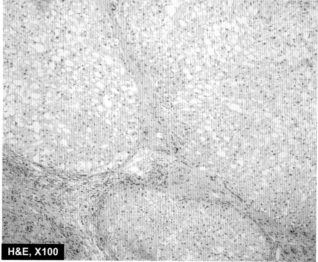

H&E, X100

FIGURE 28.3 ◆ Alcoholic (micronodular) cirrhosis. The field shows dense fibrous septa forming nodules devoid of central veins. Thick fibrous septa divide the nodules. Hepatocytes show fatty change in many cells. There is minimal inflammation and some reactive bile duct proliferation in the septa.

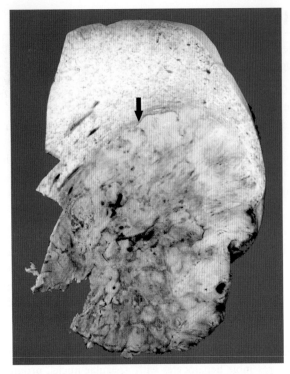

FIGURE 28.4 ◆ Hepatocellular carcinoma. Sectioned surface of the slice of liver shows a single, large mass (arrow) with irregular borders and having central areas of necrosis. The rest of the hepatic parenchyma shows many nodules of variable sizes owing to co-existent macronodular (postnecroitc) cirrhosis.

Chronic Cholecystitis with Cholelithiasis

Chronic cholecystitis is the most common type of gallbladder disease.

G/A The gallbladder is generally contracted and the wall is thickened. Cut section of wall of gallbladder is grey-white due to dense fibrosis. The mucosal folds may be thickened, atrophied or flattened. The lumen commonly contains gallstones, most often multiple multifaceted mixed type; others are pure gallstones (cholesterol, pigment and calcium containing) and combined type gallstones (Figs 28.6 and 28.7).

M/E
  i. Penetration of mucosa deep into the wall of the gallbladder up to the muscularis layer to form Rokitansky-Aschoff sinuses.
  ii. Variable degree of chronic inflammatory cells (lymphocytes, plasma cells and macrophages) in the lamina propria and subserosal layer.
  iii. Variable degree of fibrosis and thickening of perimuscular layer (Fig. 28.8).

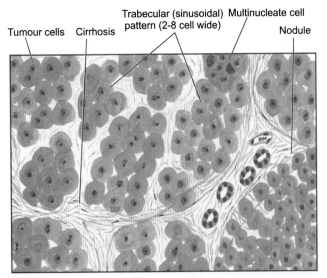

Tumour cells Cirrhosis Trabecular (sinusoidal) pattern (2-8 cell wide) Multinucleate cell Nodule

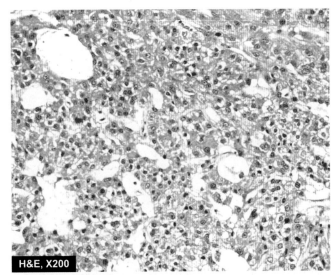

H&E, X200

FIGURE 28.5 ◆ Hepatocellular carcinoma. It shows 2-8 cell wide trabeculae of malignant hepatocytes separated by endothelium-lined sinusoidal spaces.

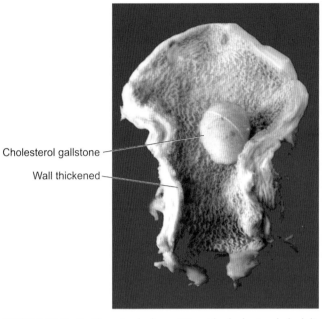

FIGURE 28.6 ◆ Chronic cholecystitis with cholesterol cholelithiasis. The wall of the gallbladder is thickened externally. Cut surface shows that gallbladder wall is thickened, fibrotic and grey-white. The mucosa is velvety. The lumen contains a single large, oval, hard, yellowish-white cholesterol gallstone.

Carcinoma Gallbladder

Primary carcinoma of the gallbladder is more common than cancer of the extra-hepatic biliary sytem.

G/A The most common site for cancer of gallbladder is the fundus, followed next in frequency by the neck of the gallbladder. The tumour may be infiltrating type seen as irregular area of diffuse thickening and induration in the gallbladder wall, or fungating type growing as irregular, friable, papillary or cauliflower-like growth into the lumen. Gallstones may coexist with carcinoma (Fig. 28.9).

M/E

i. Most common is adenocarcinoma, i.e. glandular pattern with features of anaplasia of tumour cells.
ii. The tumour may have papillary or infiltrative growth pattern (Fig. 28.10).
iii. The tumour may be well-differentiated to poorly-differentiated, non-mucin secreting, or less commonly mucin-secreting type.

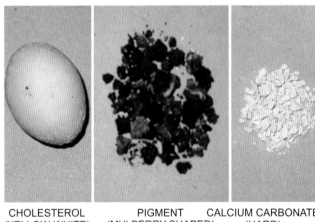
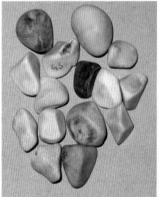
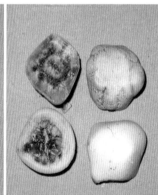

CHOLESTEROL (YELLOW-WHITE) PIGMENT (MULBERRY-SHAPED) CALCIUM CARBONATE (HARD) MIXED GALLSTONES (MULTIFACETED) COMBINED GALLSTONES (SMOOTH-SURFACED)

FIGURE 28.7 ◆ Gallstones of different types.

Rokitansky-Aschoff sinus   Mononuclear inflammatory infiltrate

Hypertrophied muscularis   Perimuscular fibrosis

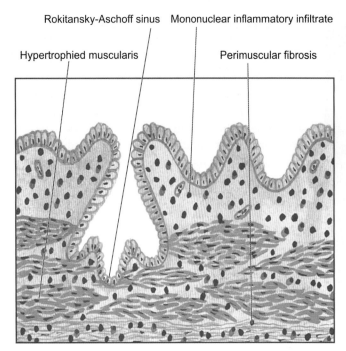
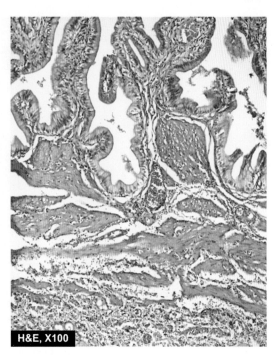

H&E, X100

FIGURE 28.8 ◆ Chronic cholecystitis. There is perimuscular hyperplasia, chronic inflammatory cells in the wall and Rokitansky-Aschoff sinus in the mucosa.

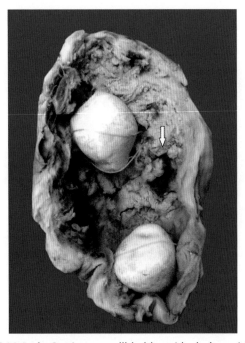

FIGURE 28.9 ◆ Carcinoma gallbladder with cholecystitis and mixed cholelithiasis. The wall of the gallbladder is thickened. The lumen contains irregular, friable papillary growth arising from mucosa (arrow). The lumen also contains multiple, multifaceted, mixed gallstones.

Papillary pattern   Invaded muscle   Anaplastic cells

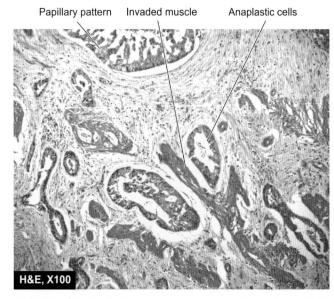

H&E, X100

FIGURE 28.10 ◆ Adenocarcinoma gallbladder. Well-differentiated glands lined by anaplastic cells are seen invading the wall of the gallbladder.

Primary Glomerulonephritis and Tubulointerstitial Disease

Objectives
➢ To learn pathology of common and important forms of primary glomerulonephritis (GN) (e.g. acute GN, rapidly progressive GN, chronic GN) and tubulointerstitial disease (e.g. chronic pyelonephritis).
➢ To describe salient gross and microscopic features of these conditions.

Glomerular diseases involve mainly renal glomeruli and may be further of 2 types:

◆ *Primary glomerulonephritis* (GN) in which glomeruli are the primary site of involvement (e.g. various forms of GN such as acute GN, rapidly progressive GN, chronic GN, etc.).

◆ *Secondary glomerular diseases* in which glomeruli are involved as a part of systemic disease (e.g. in diabetes mellitus, SLE, amyloidosis, etc.).

Renal tubules and interstitial tissues are involved together in inflammatory disease of the kidneys, e.g. pyelonephritis of various types.

Acute Glomerulonephritis

Acute post-streptococcal GN is the most common form of GN in children 6 to 16 years of age in the developing countries.

G/A The kidneys are symmetrically enlarged, weighing one and a half to twice the normal weight. The cortical as well as sectioned surface show petechial haemorrhages giving the characteristic appearance of flea-bitten kidney (Fig. 29.1).

M/E
  i. Glomeruli are affected diffusely. They are enlarged and hypercellular.
  ii. The diffuse hypercellularity of the tuft is due to proliferation of mesangial, endothelial and occasional

epithelial cells *(acute proliferative lesions)* as well as due to infiltration by polymorphs and monocytes *(acute exudative lesions).*

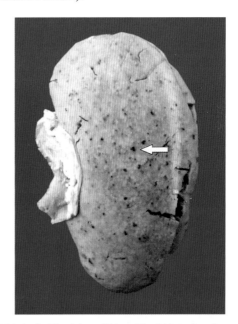

FIGURE 29.1 ◆ Flea-bitten kidney. The kidney is enlarged in size and weight. The cortex shows tiny petechial haemorrhages visible through the capsule (arrow). Sectioned surface (not shown here) would show pale mottled appearance.

Proliferated mesangial cells Endothelial cells
Hypercellular glomerulus Acute inflammatory cells

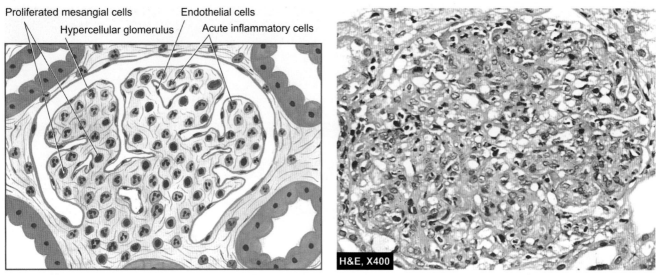

H&E, X400

FIGURE 29.2 ◆ Acute glomerulonephritis. There is increased cellularity by proliferation of mesangial cells, endothelial cells and infiltration of the tuft by polymorphs and monocytes.

iii. Tubules may show swelling of lining cells and their lumina may contain red cell casts.

iv. There may be some degree of interstitial oedema and leucocytic infiltration (Fig. 29.2).

Rapidly Progressive Glomerulonephritis (RPGN)

RPGN presents with acute renal failure in a few weeks to a few months of onset and has a dismal prognosis.

Hypercellular glomerulus Neutrophilic infiltration
Crescent Adhesion between tuft and capsule

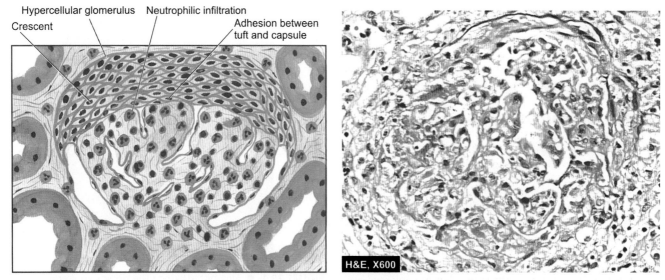

H&E, X600

FIGURE 29.3 ◆ Post-infectious RPGN, light microscopic appearance. There are crescents in Bowman's space due to proliferation of visceral epithelial cells. These form adhesions between the glomerular tuft and Bowman's capsule.

G/A The kidneys are usually enlarged and pale with smooth outer surface (large white kidney). Cut surface shows pale cortex and congested medulla.

M/E

i. Pathognomonic *crescents* are seen on the inside of Bowman's capsule. Crescents are collections of pale-staining polygonal cells formed from the proliferation of parietal epithelial cells.

ii. Glomerular tufts frequently contain fibrin thrombi.

iii. Tubular epithelial cells may show hyaline droplets and tubular lumina may contain casts, red blood cells and fibrin.

iv. The interstitium is oedematous and may show early fibrosis.

v. Arteries and arterioles may show associated changes of hypertension (Fig. 29.3).

Chronic Glomerulonephritis

Chronic GN or chronic kidney disease (CKD) is the final stage of a variety of glomerular diseases.

G/A The kidneys are usually small and contracted weighing as low as 50 gm each. The capsule is adherent to the cortex and the cortical surface is generally diffusely granular (Fig. 29.4). On cut section, the cortex is narrow and atrophic while the medulla is unremarkable.

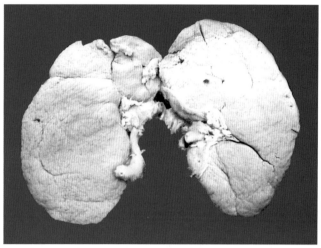

FIGURE 29.4 ◆ Short contracted kidney in chronic glomerulonephritis (chronic kidney disease). The kidney is small and contracted, weighing less than normal. The capsule is adherent to the cortex and has granular surface.

M/E

i. *Glomeruli* are reduced in number and most of them show completely hyalinised tufts appearing as acellular eosinophilic masses.

ii. Many *tubules* completely disappear, there may be atrophy of tubules close to scarred glomeruli and tubular lumina contain eosinophilic homogeneous casts.

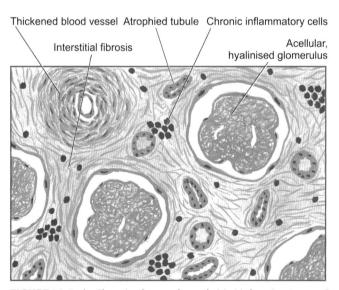

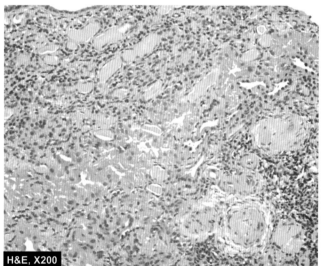

H&E, X200

FIGURE 29.5 ◆ Chronic glomerulonephritis. Light microscopy shows acellular and completely hyalinised glomerular tufts. The blood vessels in the interstitium are hyalinised and thickened and there is fine interstitial fibrosis with a few chronic inflammatory cells. Tubule are atrophied.

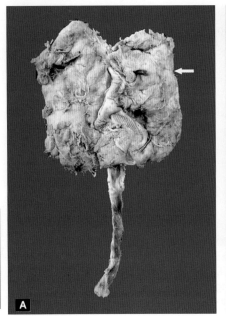 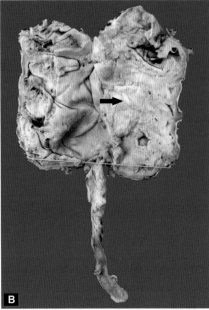 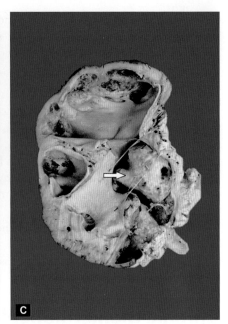

FIGURE 29.6 ◆ Short contracted kidney in chronic pyelonephritis. The kidney is small, contracted weighing less than normal. **A**, (External surface): the capsule is adherent to the cortex and has irregular scars on the surface. **B**, (Sectioned surface): shows dilated pelvicalyceal system with atrophied and thin peripheral cortex and increased hilar fat extending inside (arrow). **C**, Staghorn stone (arrow) lying in dilated pelvicalyceal system.

iii. There is fine delicate fibrosis of the *interstitial tissue* and varying number of chronic inflammatory cells in the interstitium (Fig. 29.5).

iv. Advanced cases associated with hypertension show conspicuous *arterial* and *arteriolar sclerosis*.

Chronic Pyelonephritis

Chronic pyelonephritis is a chronic tubulointerstitial disease resulting from repeated attacks of inflammation and scarring due to infection.

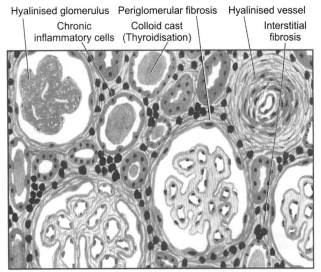 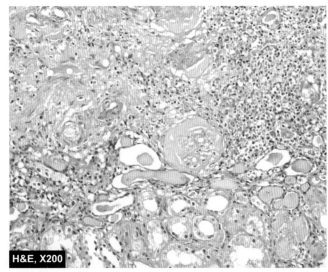

FIGURE 29.7 ◆ Chronic pyelonephritis. The tubules show atrophy of some tubules and dilatation of some others which contain colloid-like casts (thyroidisation). The interstitium shows chronic inflammatory cells and fibrosis. The blood vessels are thick-walled and the glomeruli show periglomerular fibrosis.

G/A The kidneys are usually small and contracted, weighing less than 100 gm each, showing unequal reduction. The outer surface of the kidneys is irregularly scarred. These scars are of variable size and show irregular depressions on the cortical surface. The pelvis of the kidney is dilated and calyces are blunted and may contain renal stone taking the shape of pelvicalyceal system called staghorn stone (Fig. 29.6).

M/E The predominant microscopic changes are seen in the interstitium and tubules:

i. The *interstitium* shows chronic inflammatory infiltrate, chiefly composed of lymphocytes, plasma cells and macrophages with pronounced interstitial fibrosis.

ii. The *tubules* show varying degree of atrophy and dilatation. Dilated tubules may contain colloid casts producing thyroidisation of tubules.

iii. The wall of *dilated pelvicalyceal system* shows marked chronic inflammation and scarring.

iv. There is often *periglomerular fibrosis* and hyalinisation of some glomeruli (Fig. 29.7).

Diabetic Nephropathy and Tumours of Renal System

Objectives

> To learn pathology of glomerular disease in diabetes and some examples of common primary tumours of renal system (e.g. renal cell carcinoma, Wilms' tumour, transitional cell carcinoma).
> To describe salient gross and microscopic features of these conditions.

As stated in previous exercise, glomerular diseases may be *primary glomerulonephritis* (GN) and *secondary glomerular diseases* in which glomeruli are involved as a part of systemic disease (e.g. in diabetes mellitus, SLE, amyloidosis, etc.). Out of these, diabetic nephropathy is discussed here.

Tumours of renal system are classified based on the cell of origin. A few common examples of such tumours are renal cell carcinoma (arising from renal tubular cells), Wilms' tumour (arising from primitive renal tissue) and transitional cell (or urothelial) carcinoma (arising from urothelium that extends from the pelvis of kidney to the urethra).

Diabetic Nephropathy

Renal involvement is an important complication of diabetes mellitus.

G/A The kidneys are often small and contracted. Depending upon the nature of underlying renal lesions, the external surface shows irregular or granular appearance. The cut surface shows narrowed cortex.

M/E Diabetic nephropathy encompasses 4 types of renal lesions—diabetic glomerulosclerosis, vascular lesions, diabetic pyelonephritis, and tubular lesions.

i. **Diabetic glomerulosclerosis**. These lesions may be diffuse or nodular.
   - *Diffuse glomerular lesions* are the most common. These include: diffuse involvement of all parts of glomeruli, thickening of GBM, diffuse increase in mesangial matrix and exudative lesions. *Exudative lesions* include capsular drops and fibrin caps. Capsular drop is an eosinophilic hyaline thickening of the parietal layer of Bowman's capsule and bulges into the glomerular space. Fibrin cap is homogeneous brightly eosinophilic material on the wall of a peripheral capillary of a lobule.
   - *Nodular lesions* of diabetic glomerulosclerosis (or Kimmelstiel-Wilson lesions) are seen in type 1 diabetes and show one or more nodules in some glomeruli. Nodule is spherical, laminated, hyaline acellular mass within a lobule of the glomerulus. The nodule is surrounded peripherally by glomerular capillary loops having thickened GBM (Fig. 30.1).
ii. **Vascular lesions** consist or hyaline arteriolosclerosis affecting afferent and efferent arterioles of the glomeruli.
iii. **Chronic pyelonephritis** is more common in diabetics than in others.
iv. **Tubular lesions** (Armanni-Ebstein lesions) consist of glycogen deposits as cytoplasmic vacuoles.

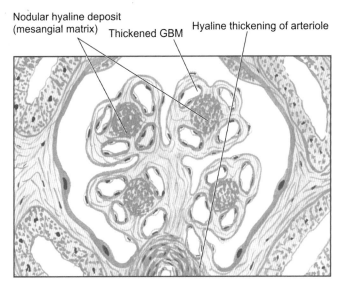

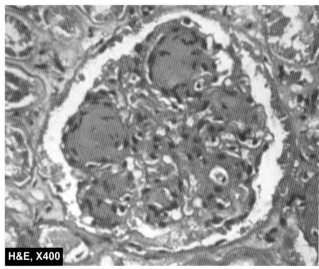

Nodular hyaline deposit (mesangial matrix)   Thickened GBM   Hyaline thickening of arteriole

H&E, X400

FIGURE 30.1 ◆ Diabetic glomerulosclerosis, microscopic appearance of nodular lesion *(Kimmelstiel-Wilson lesion)*. There are hyaline nodules within the lobules of glomeruli, surrounded peripherally by glomerular capillaries with thickened walls.

Renal Cell Carcinoma

Renal cell carcinoma (RCC) or hypernephroma or adeno-carcinoma comprises 70-80% of all renal cancers and occurs most commonly in 50 to 70 years of age.

G/A The tumour commonly arises from a pole, most often upper pole, of the kidney as a solitary and unilateral tumour. The tumour is generally large, golden yellow and circum-scribed. Cut section of the tumour commonly shows large areas of ischaemic necrosis, cystic change and foci of haemorrhages. Another feature is the frequent presence of tumour thrombus in the renal vein (Fig. 30.2).

M/E
  i. A variety of patterns of tumour cells are seen such as solid, acinar, tubular, trabecular, cord and papillary arrangements in a delicate fibrous stroma.
  ii. Tumour cells are generally of 2 types—clear and granular. *Clear cells* comprise 70% of RCC and are large cells with well-defined borders, abundant clear cytoplasm and regular pyknotic nuclei. *Granular cells* have similar features but have moderate amount of pink granular cytoplasm (Fig. 30.3).

Wilms' Tumour

Wilms' tumour or nephroblastoma is an embryonic tumour commonly seen in children between 1 and 6 years of age.

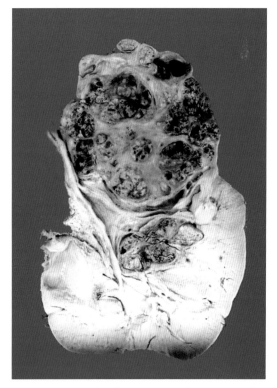

FIGURE 30.2 ◆ Renal cell carcinoma. The upper pole of the kidney shows a large and tan mass while rest of the kidney has reniform contour. Sectioned surface shows irregular, circumscribed, yellowish mass with areas of haemorrhages and necrosis. The residual kidney shows compressed calyces and renal pelvis.

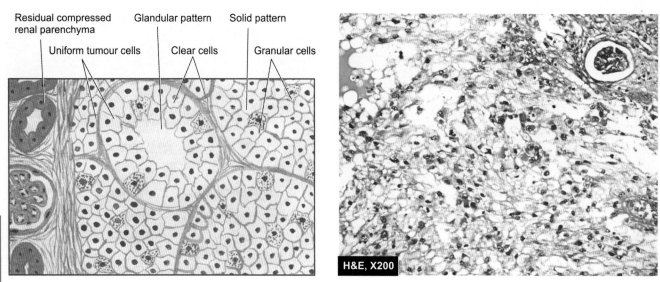

FIGURE 30.3 ◆ Adenocarcinoma kidney. Solid masses and glandular pattern of malignant cells having features of clear cells. The stroma is composed of delicate fibrovascular tissue.

G/A The tumour is generally quite large, spheroidal replacing most of the kidney. It is generally solitary and unilateral. On cut section, the tumour shows soft, fish-flesh like, grey-white appearance with foci of necrosis and haemorrhages. Sometimes, myxomatous and cartilaginous elements are identified (Fig. 30.4).

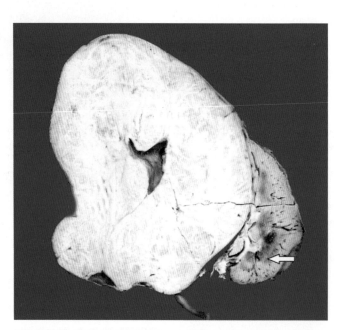

FIGURE 30.4 ◆ Nephroblastoma (Wilms' tumour). The kidney is enlarged and has ovoid and nodular appearance. The sectioned surface shows replacement of almost whole kidney by the tumour leaving a thin strip of compressed renal tissue at lower end (white arrow). Cut section of the tumour is grey-white, fleshy and has small areas of haemorrhages and necrosis.

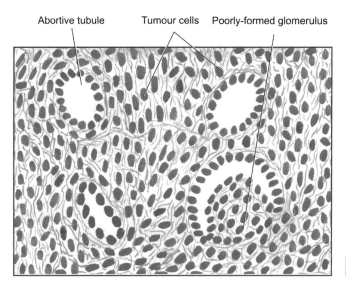

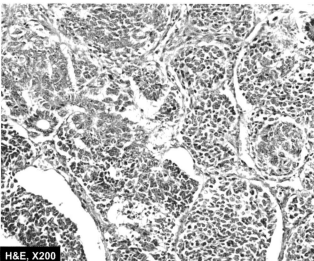

FIGURE 30.5 ◆ Nephroblastoma (Wilms' tumour), showing predominance of small round to spindled sarcomatoid tumour cells. A few abortive tubules and poorly-formed glomerular structures are present in it.

M/E
  i. The tumour shows mixture of primitive epithelial and mesenchymal elements.
  ii. The tumour largely consists of small, round to spindled, anaplastic, sarcomatoid tumour cells.
  iii. Abortive tubules and poorly formed glomerular structures are seen in these areas.
  iv. Sometimes, mesenchymal elements such as smooth muscle, cartilage, bone and fat cells may be seen (Fig. 30.5).

Transitional Cell (Urothelial) Carcinoma

More than 90% of bladder tumours are transitional cell type.

G/A The tumour may be single or multiple. About 90% of the tumours are papillary (non-invasive or invasive) whereas remaining 10% are flat indurated (non-invasive or invasive). The papillary tumour has free floating fern-like arrangement with broad or narrow pedicle (Fig. 30.6). The non-papillary tumours are bulkier with ulcerated surface.

M/E The tumour is divided into 3 histologic grades according the Mostqfi classification (grades I, II and III). Type II transitional cell carcinoma presents classic features (Fig. 30.7):
  i. There is increase in the number of layers of cells (compared to normal 6-7 layers).

  ii. The tumour cells are still recognisable as transitional cells in grade I and II tumours but they have features of

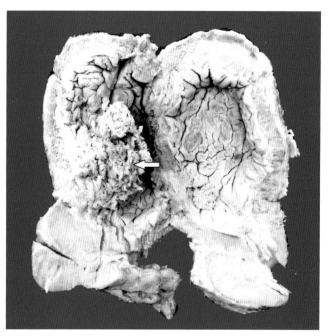

FIGURE 30.6 ◆ Transitional cell (urothelial) carcinoma urinary bladder. The urinary bladder wall is identified by thick muscular wall, narrow lumen and portions of ureters attached above. The mucosal surface shows papillary tumour floating in the lumen (arrow).

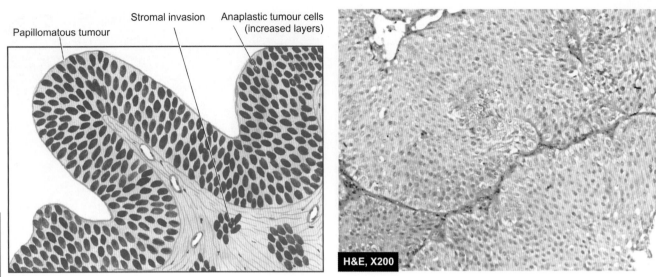

Papillomatous tumour

Stromal invasion

Anaplastic tumour cells (increased layers)

H&E, X200

FIGURE 30.7 ◆ Microscopic features of grade II transitional cell carcinoma. The tumour has papillary pattern and marked increase in the layers of transitional cells depicting features of cytologic atypia.

anaplasia such as nuclear crowding, nuclear hyperchromatism, mitotic activity and loss of polarity.

iii. The tumour may or may not show invasion beyond the basement membrane of urothelium.

Testicular Tumours and Diseases of Prostate

Objectives
➤ To learn pathology of seminoma testis and major forms of prostatic diseases (i.e. nodular hyperplasia and carcinoma).
➤ To describe salient gross and microscopic features of these conditions.

Amongst all the germ cell tumours of the testis, seminoma is the most common. Two of the major diseases of the prostate are nodular hyperplasia (affecting periurethral part of the prostate) and carcinoma of the prostate (arising more commonly in the outer subcapsular part).

Seminoma Testis

Seminoma is the most common malignant tumour of the testis, constituting 45% of all testicular germ cell tumours and corresponds to dysgerminoma in the female gonad.

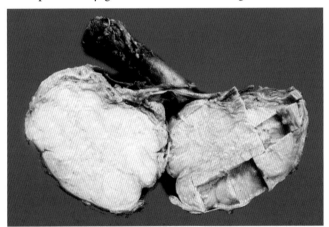

FIGURE 31.1 ◆ Seminoma testis. The testis is enlarged (normal weight 20-27 gm) but the testicular contour is maintained. Sectioned surface shows replacement of the entire testis by lobulated, homogeneous, grey-white mass.

G/A The involved testis is enlarged (up to 10 times) but tends to maintain its normal contour since the tumour rarely invades the tunica. Cut section of the affected testis shows homogeneous, grey-white lobulated appearance (Fig. 31.1).

M/E
i. *Tumour cells.* The seminoma cells generally lie in cords, sheets or columns forming lobules. The tumor cells are typically uniform in size with clear cytoplasm and well-defined cell borders. The nuclei are central, large, hyperchromatic and usually contain 1-2 prominent nucleoli.
ii. *Stroma.* The stroma is delicate fibrous tissue which divides the tumour into lobules. The stroma shows characteristic lymphocytic infiltration (Fig. 31.2).

Nodular Hyperplasia Prostate

Non-neoplastic tumour-like enlargement of the prostate is a very common condition in men, frequently above the age of 50 years.

G/A The enlarged prostate is nodular, smooth and firm and weighs 2-4 times its normal weight (normal average weight 20 gm). The appearance on cut section shows nodularity having varying admixture of yellowish-pink, soft, honey-combed appearance (glandular hyperplasia) and firm homogeneous appearance (fibromuscular hyperplasia) (Fig. 31.3).

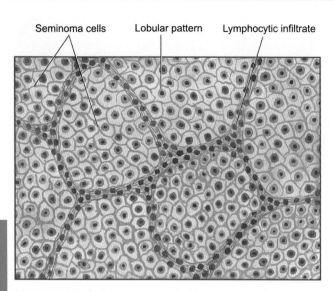
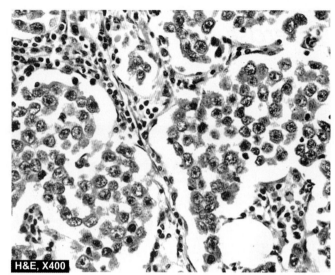

FIGURE 31.2 ◆ Seminoma testis. The tumour cells are monomorphic and uniform and forming lobular pattern with lymphocytic infiltrate.

M/E There is hyperplasia of all three tissue elements in varying proportions—glandular, fibrous and muscular (Fig. 31.4):

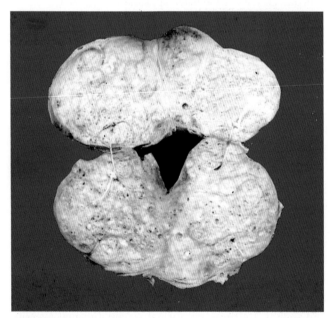

FIGURE 31.3 ◆ Nodular hyperplasia of the prostate. The prostate is enlarged (normal weight 20 gm). Sectioned surface shows soft to firm, grey-white, nodularity with microcystic areas.

i. *Glandular hyperplasia* predominates in most cases and is characterised by exaggerated intra-acinar papillary infolding with delicate fibrovascular cores. Glands are lined by two layers of epithelium.
ii. *Fibromuscular hyperplasia* appears as aggregates of spindle cells giving an appearance similar to fibromyoma of the uterus.

Adenocarcinoma Prostate

Cancer of the prostate is second most common form of cancer in males, next in frequency to lung cancer.

G/A The prostate is often enlarged, firm and fibrous. Cut section is homogeneous and contains irregular yellowish areas.

M/E
i. *Architectural disturbance.* There is loss of intra-acinar papillary infoldings. Instead, the groups of acini are either closely packed in back-to-back arrangement, or are haphazardly distributed.
ii. *Stroma.* Malignant acini have little or no stroma between them.
iii. *Gland pattern.* Often the glands are small or medium-sized, lined by a single layer of cuboidal or low columnar cells.

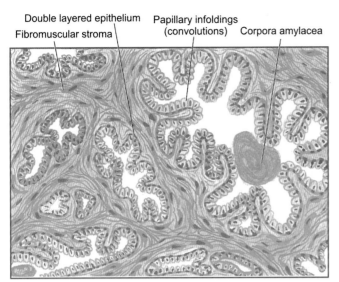

Double layered epithelium
Fibromuscular stroma
Papillary infoldings (convolutions)
Corpora amylacea

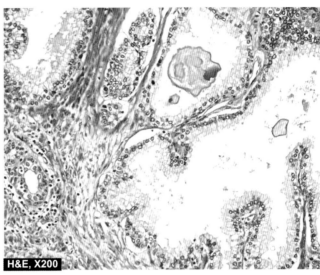

H&E, X200

FIGURE 31.4 ◆ Nodular hyperplasia prostate. There are intra-acinar papillary infoldings (convolutions) lined by two layers of epithelium with basal polarity of nuclei and fibromuscular stromal hyperplasia.

iv. *Tumour cells.* The individual tumour cells may be clear, dark and eosinophilic type and do not show usual morphologic features of malignancy (Fig. 31.5).

v. *Invasion.* There is often early and frequent invasion of intraprostatic perineural spaces (Fig. 31.5, inbox).

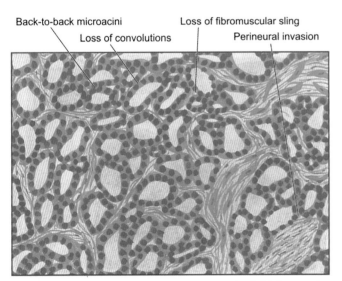

Back-to-back microacini
Loss of convolutions
Loss of fibromuscular sling
Perineural invasion

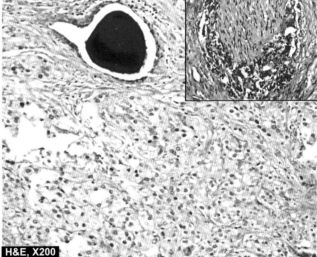

H&E, X200

FIGURE 31.5 ◆ Adenocarcinoma prostate. The field shows microacini of small malignant cells infiltrating the prostatic stroma. Inbox shows perineural invasion by the tumour.

Diseases of Endometrium, Placenta, Cervix

Objectives
➢ To learn pathology of simple hyperplasia endometrium, hydatidiform mole and cervical cancer.
➢ To describe salient gross and microscopic features of these conditions.

Amongst various forms of endometrial hyperplasias, simple (or cystic) hyperplasia is by far the most common. Hydatidiform mole is considered by some as a benign tumour of the palcenta while others describe it as a degenerative condition. Uterine cervical cancer is the most common cancer in females in developing countries of the world.

Simple (Cystic Glandular) Hyperplasia

Endometrial hyperplasia is a condition characterised by proliferative patterns of glandular and stromal tissues.

Compact stroma   Cystic dilatation of gland   Nuclear stratification

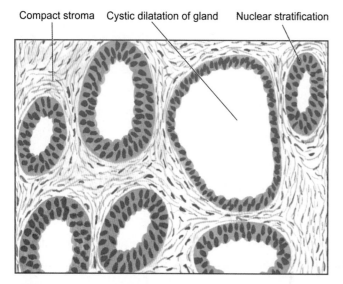
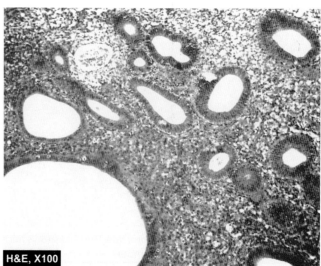

H&E, X100

FIGURE 32.1 ◆ Simple hyperplasia endometrium. Varying-sized glands, some cystically dilated, are lined by atrophied epithelium.

Currently employed classification of endometrial hyperplasia divides it into 3 types—simple (cystic) hyperplasia, complex hyperplasia without atypia (adenomatous hyperplasia), and complex hyperplasia with atypia (atypical hyperplasia).

M/E The features of *simple hyperplasia* are as under:
  i. Presence of varying-sized glands, many of which are large and cystically dilated and are lined by atrophic epithelium.
  ii. The stroma is sparsely cellular and oedematous (Fig. 32.1).

Hydatidiform Mole

The word hydatidiform means drop of water and mole for a shapeless mass. Though benign or degenerative condition of placental tissue, it has potential for developing into choriocarcinoma.

G/A Molar tissue consists of grape-like vesicles up to 3 cm in diameter. The vesicles contain clear watery fluid (Fig. 32.2).

M/E
  i. Large, round oedematous chorionic villi.
  ii. Hydropic degeneration and decreased vascularity of villous stroma.

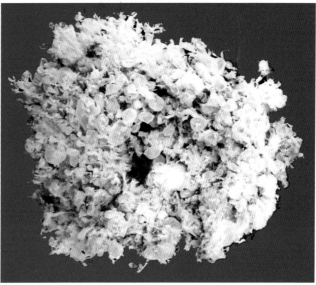

FIGURE 32.2 ◆ Hydatidiform mole. The specimen shows numerous, variable-sized, grape-like translucent vesicles containing clear fluid. Tan areas of haemorrhage are also seen.

  iii. Trophoblastic proliferation as masses and sheets of both cytotrophoblast and syncytiotrophoblast seen circumferentially around the villi (Fig. 32.3).

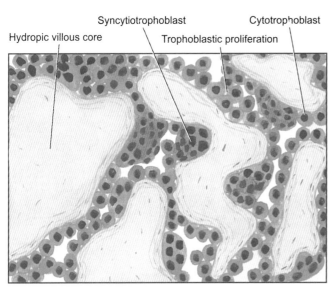

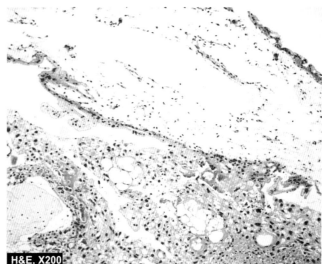

FIGURE 32.3 ◆ Hydatidiform mole characterised by hydropic and avascular enlarged villi with trophoblastic proliferation in the form of masses and sheets.

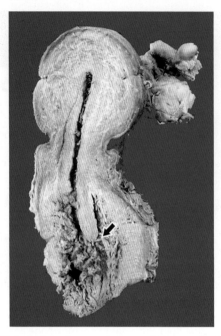

FIGURE 32.4 ◆ Invasive carcinoma of the cervix. Sectioned surface shows normal uterine cavity while the cervix is replaced by irregular grey-white friable growth (arrow) extending into cervical canal as well as distally into attached vaginal cuff.

Invasive Cervical Cancer

Invasive cervical cancer in about 80% of cases is epidermoid (squamous cell) carcinoma, with peak incidence in 4th to 6th decade.

G/A Invasive cervical carcinoma may present 3 types of patterns—fungating, ulcerating and infiltrating. The fungating or exophytic pattern appears as cauliflower-like growth infiltrating the adjacent vaginal wall (Fig. 32.4).

M/E
  i. Most commonly, the tumour is moderately-differentiated, non-keratinising, large cell type.
 ii. The tumour cells are seen as masses of anaplastic cells of varying size and have abundant cytoplasm.
iii. Keratin formation may be seen in some cells.
 iv. Intervening stroma shows prominent inflammatory cell infiltrate (Fig. 32.5).

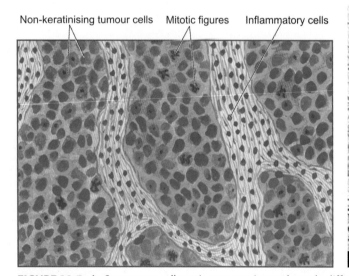

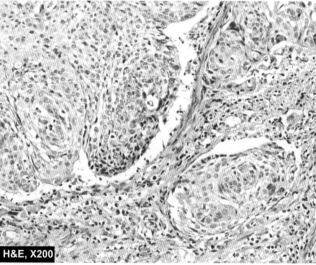

FIGURE 32.5 ◆ Squamous cell carcinoma cervix, moderately differentiated, large cell type, non-keratinising.

Ovarian Tumours

Objectives
➤ To learn pathology of common examples of benign and malignant tumours of ovaries (e.g. serous cystadenoma, papillary serous cystadenocarcinoma, mucinous cystadenoma, and benign cystic teratoma).
➤ To describe salient gross and microscopic features of these conditions.

Ovarian tumours arise from normally-occurring cellular components of the ovaries. Two of the largest groups of primary ovarian tumours are those arising from surface epithelium and those originating from ovarian germ cells. The examples discussed in this exercise in the first group are serous cystadenoma, papillary serous cystadenocarcinoma, and mucinous cystadenoma, while benign cystic teratoma is discussed below as an example of germ cell tumours of ovaries.

Serous Ovarian Tumours

Serous tumours comprise the largest group constituting about 20% of all ovarian tumours. These tumours arise from the ovarian surface (coelomic) epithelium which differentiates along tubal-type of epithelium.

G/A Serous tumours of benign, borderline and malignant type are large and spherical masses. Cut section of benign tumours is unilocular while larger cysts are multilocular with daughter loculi in their walls containing clear watery fluid. Malignant serous tumours have solid areas in the cystic mass and may contain exophytic as well as intracystic papillary projections (Fig. 33.1).

M/E Features of benign and malignant serous tumours are as follows:

SEROUS CYSTADENOMA OVARY
i. The cyst is lined by properly-oriented low columnar epithelium.

ii. The lining cells may be ciliated and resemble tubal epithelium (Fig. 33.2).

PAPILLARY SEROUS CYSTADENOCARCINOMA OVARY
i. Lining of the cyst is by multilayered malignant cells having features such as loss of polarity, presence of solid sheets of anaplastic epithelial cells.

ii. There is definite evidence of stromal invasion by malignant cells.

iii. Papillae formations are more frequent in malignant variety and may be associated with psammoma bodies (Fig. 33.3).

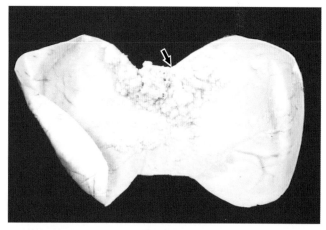

FIGURE 33.1 ◆ Papillary serous cystadenoma of the ovary. Cut surface shows a large unilocular cyst containing numerous papillary structures projecting into it (arrow).

(127)

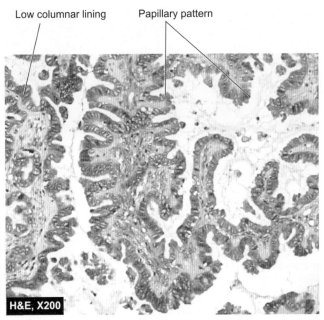

H&E, X200

FIGURE 33.2 ◆ Papillary serous cystadenoma of the ovary. Microscopic features include single layer of low columnar, at places ciliated, epithelium lining with pronounced papillary pattern.

Mucinous Ovarian Tumours

Mucinous tumours are more commonly unilateral than serous tumours. These tumours arise from coelomic epithelium that differentiates along endocervical type or intestinal type of mucosa. Like serous ovarian tumours, mucinous tumours too may be benign, borderline and malignant. However, bilateral mucinous cystadenocarcinoma of the ovary is rare and is frequently due to metastasis.

MUCINOUS CYSTADENOMA OVARY

G/A Mucinous tumours are larger than serous type. They are smooth-surfaced cysts with characteristic multiloculations containing thick and viscid gelatinous fluid (Fig. 33.4). Benign tumours have thin wall and septa which are translucent while malignant variety has thickened areas.

M/E The features of *mucinous cystadenoma* are as follows (Fig. 33.5):
   i. The cyst is lined by a single layer of cells having basal nuclei and apical mucinous vacuoles, resembling intestinal mucosa.
   ii. There is no invasion or papillae formation.

Benign Cystic Teratoma Ovary

Benign cystic teratoma or dermoid cyst of the ovary is more frequent in young women in their active reproductive life. Teratoma is a tumour composed of tissue derived from three germ cell layers—ectoderm, mesoderm and endoderm.

G/A Benign cystic teratoma is characteristically a unilocular cyst, 10-15 cm in diameter. On sectioning, the cyst is filled

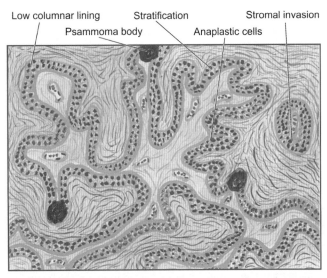

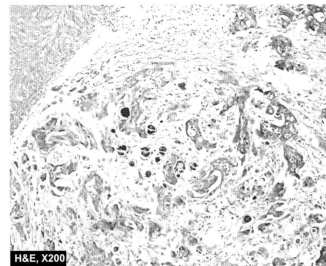

H&E, X200

FIGURE 33.3 ◆ Papillary serous cystadenocarcinoma of the ovary. There is stratification of lining epithelium with features of anaplasia. There is stromal invasion by anaplastic cells. A few psammoma bodies are also seen.

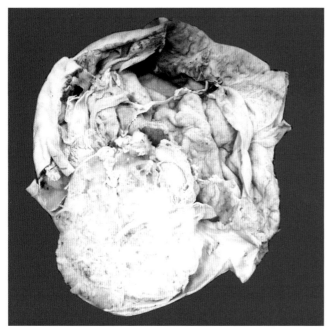

FIGURE 33.4 ◆ Mucinous cystadenoma of the ovary. Cut surface shows a large, multiloculated cyst without papillae. The loculi contain gelatinous material.

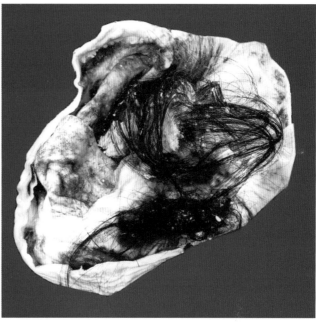

FIGURE 33.6 ◆ Benign cystic teratoma (dermoid cyst) of the ovary. Cut surface shows a large unilocular cyst containing hair, pultaceous material and bony tissue.

with paste-like sebaceous secretions and desquamated keratin admixed with masses of hair. The cyst wall is thin and opaque grey-white. Quite often, the cyst wall shows a solid prominence

where tissue elements such as tooth, bone, cartilage and other odd tissues are present (Fig. 33.6).

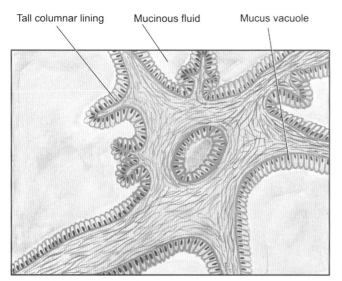

Tall columnar lining   Mucinous fluid   Mucus vacuole

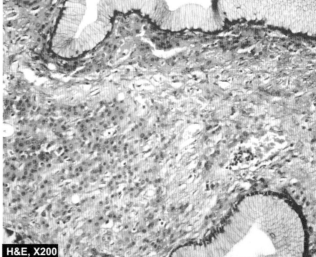

H&E, X200

FIGURE 33.5 ◆ Mucinous cystadenoma of the ovary. The cyst wall and the septa are lined by a single layer of tall columnar mucin-secreting epithelium with basally-placed nuclei and large apical mucinous vacuoles.

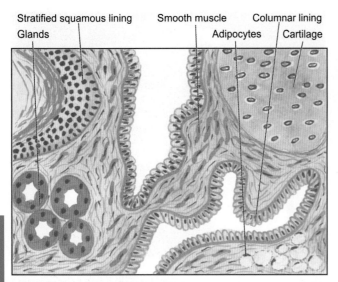
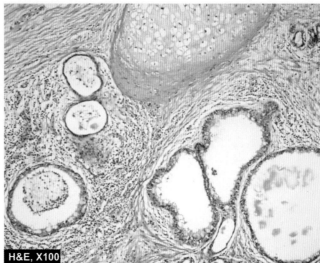

Stratified squamous lining   Smooth muscle   Columnar lining
Glands   Adipocytes   Cartilage

H&E, X100

FIGURE 33.7 ◆ Benign cystic teratoma ovary. The field shows epidermis-lined cyst, islands of cartilage and some adipose tissue.

M/E

i. Viewing a benign cystic teratoma in different microscopic fields reveals a variety of mature differentiated tissues, producing kaleidoscopic appearance.

ii. Ectodermal derivatives are most prominent. The lining of the cyst wall is by stratified squamous epithelium and its adnexal structures such as sebaceous glands, sweat glands and hair follicles.

iii. Tissues of mesodermal and endodermal origin are commonly present and include bronchus, intestinal epithelium, cartilage, bone, smooth muscle, neural tissue, salivary gland, retina, pancreas and thyroid tissue (Fig. 33.7).

Diseases of Breast

Objectives
> To learn pathology of fibrocystic change and an example each of common benign (e.g. fibroadenoma) and malignant (e.g. infiltrating duct carcinoma) tumour.
> To describe salient gross and microscopic features of these conditions.

Fibrocystic change is the most common form of change (and not disease) in the breast producing vague lumpiness in 3rd to 5th decade of life. Fibroadenoma is an example of the most common benign breast tumour in young girls. Invasive breast cancer has many histologic subtypes but infiltrating duct carcinoma is by far the most common type of breast cancer.

Fibrocystic Change

Fibrocystic change is a histologic entity characterised by 3 changes: cystic dilatation of terminal ducts, relative increase in intra- and interlobular fibrous tissue, and variable degree of epithelial proliferation in the terminal ducts. Based on last

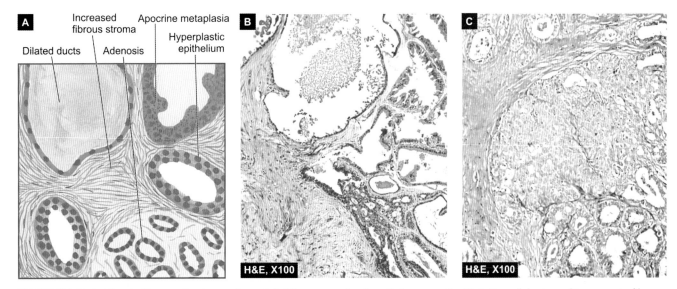

FIGURE 34.1 ◆ Simple fibrocystic change breast. **A,** Diagrammatic view. It shows cystic dilatation of ducts and increase in fibrous stroma. There is mild epithelial hyperplasia in terminal ducts. **B,** Non-proliferative fibrocystic changes—fibrosis, cyst formation, adenosis and apocrine metaplasia. **C,** Proliferative fibrocystic changes showing moderate epithelial hyperplasia.

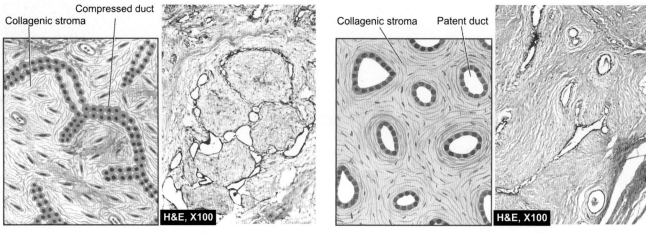

A, INTRACANALICULAR PATTERN   B, PERICANALICULAR PATTERN

FIGURE 34.2 ◆ Fibroadenoma breast. The tumour is encapsulated and composed of intracanalicular growth pattern of stroma and compressed ducts (**A**) and pericanalicular pattern (**B**) showing fibrous tissue encircling the ducts.

feature, fibrocystic change is further of 2 types: non-proliferative (or simple) and proliferative fibrocystic change.

G/A The cysts are usually multifocal and bilateral, varying in size from microcysts to 5-6 cm in diameter. On sectioning, the cysts contain thin serous to haemorrhagic fluid.

M/E

i. The cysts are often lined by flattened or atrophic epithelium.

ii. Apocrine change in the lining of the cyst is frequently present.

iii. In proliferative fibrocystic change, there is epithelial hyperplasia forming tiny intracystic papillary projections.

iv. There is increased fibrous stroma surrounding the cyst and varying degree of lymphocytic infiltrate (Fig. 34.1).

Fibroadenoma

Fibroadenoma is a benign tumour of fibrous and epithelial elements of the breast. It is the most common benign tumour of the breast in reproductive life.

G/A Typically fibroadenoma is a small (2-4 cm diameter), solitary, well-encapsulated, spherical or discoid mass. The cut surface is firm, grey-white, slightly myxoid and may show slit-like spaces.

M/E The arrangement between fibrous overgrowth and ducts may produce 2 types of patterns: intracanalicular and pericanalicular (Fig. 34.2):

i. *Intracanalicular pattern* is one in which the stroma compresses the ducts so that they are reduced to slit-like clefts lined by ductal epithelium and may appear as cords of epithelial elements surrounding masses of fibrous tissue.

ii. *Pericanalicular pattern* is characterised by encircling masses of fibrous tissue around the patent or dilated ducts.

Infiltrating Duct Carcinoma-*NOS*

Infiltrating duct carcinoma–*NOS* (not otherwise specified) is the classic breast cancer and is the most common histologic pattern accounting for 70% cases of breast cancer.

G/A The tumour is irregular, 1-5 cm in diameter, hard, cartilage-like mass that cuts with a grating sound. Sectioned surface of the tumour is grey-white to yellowish with chalky streaks and often extends irregularly into the surrounding fat (Fig. 34.3).

M/E

i. Anaplastic tumour cells form various patterns—solid nests, cords, poorly-formed glandular structures and some intraductal foci.

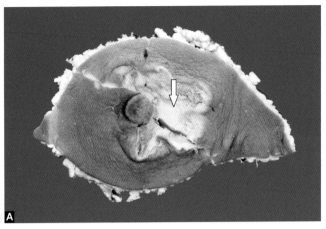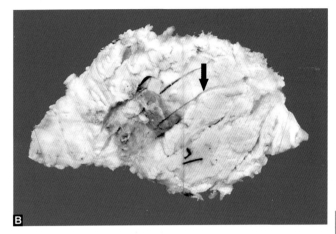

FIGURE 34.3 ◆ Infiltrating duct carcinoma—*NOS*. **A,** Specimen of the breast shows a tumour extending upto nipple and areola (white arrow). **B,** Cut surface shows a grey-white firm tumour (black arrow) extending irregularly into adjacent breast parenchyma.

ii. Infiltration by these patterns of tumour cells into diffuse fibrous stroma and fat.

iii. Invasion by the tumour cells into perivascular and perineural space, besides lymphatic and vascular emboli (Fig. 34.4).

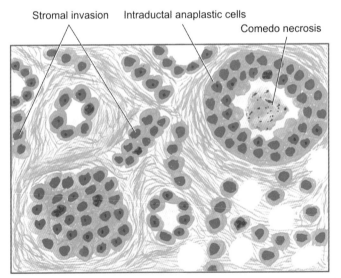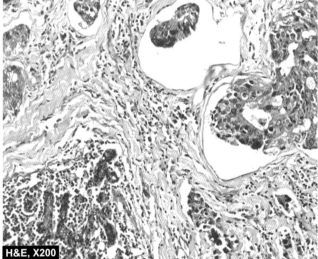

FIGURE 34.4 ◆ Infiltrating duct carcinoma breast—*NOS*. Anaplastic tumour cells proliferating in the ducts with central areas of necrosis termed comedo pattern and areas showing ductal carcinoma *in situ.*

Diseases of Thyroid

Objectives
➢ To learn pathology of a few common non-neoplastic (e.g. Hashimoto's thyroiditis, nodular goitre) and neoplastic (e.g. follicular adenoma, papillary carcinoma) conditions of thyroid.
➢ To describe salient gross and microscopic features of these conditions.

Hashimoto's thyroiditis is characterised by a triad of features: thyroid enlargement, lymphocytic infiltration of thyroid and presence of serum autoantibodies. Goitre is a quite common non-neoplastic condition occurring due to iodine deficiency and presents with enlargement of thyroid. Follicular adenoma is singular important example of benign thyroid tumour that requires distinction from nodular goitre. Among various histologic types of thyroid cancers, papillary carcinoma is most common and is discussed here.

Hashimoto's Thyroiditis

Hashimoto's thyroiditis, also called diffuse lymphocytic thyroiditis, occurs more frequently between the age of 30 and 50 years and shows about 10 times higher preponderance in females. Pathologically, two types of Hashimoto's thyroiditis are seen: classic and fibrosing.

G/A The classic form is characterised by diffuse, symmetric, firm and rubbery enlargement of the thyroid. Sectioned surface

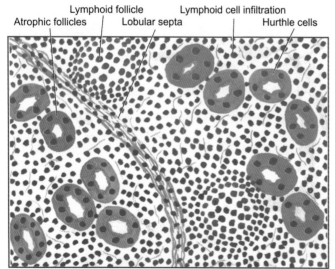

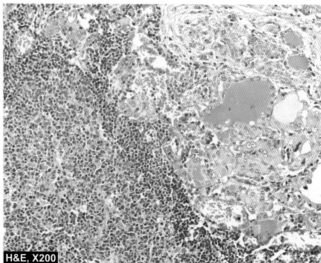

FIGURE 35.1 ◆ Hashimoto's thyroiditis. The features include infiltration by lymphocytes and formation of lymphoid follicles with germinal centres, atrophic and colloid-deficient thyroid follicles and presence of a few Hurthle cells.

(134)

of the gland is fleshy with accentuation of normal lobulations. The fibrosing variant has a firm enlarged gland with compression of the surrounding tissues.

M/E

i. Extensive infiltration of the gland by lymphocytes, plasma cells, immunoblasts and macrophages with formation of lymphoid follicles having germinal centres.

ii. Decreased number of thyroid follicles, atrophic follicles which are often devoid of colloid.

iii. Follicular epithelial cells are transformed into their degenerated state termed Hurthle's cells (oxyphil cells or oncocytes). These cells have abundant eosinophilic and granular cytoplasm due to numerous mitochondria.

iv. Variable amount of fibrous replacement of thyroid parenchyma (Fig. 35.1).

Nodular Goitre

Nodular goitre is regarded as end-stage of long-standing simple (or diffuse or colloid) goitre. It presents with tumour-like enlargement of the thyroid gland that has characteristic nodularity.

G/A The thyroid shows asymmetric and extreme enlargement weighing 100-500 gm (normal weight 15-40 gm). The *5 cardinal gross features* are: nodularity with poor encapsulation, fibrous scarring, haemorrhages, focal calcification, and cystic degeneration. Cut surface of the gland shows multinodularity (Fig. 35.2).

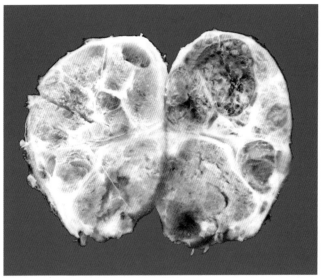

FIGURE 35.2 ◆ Nodular goitre. The thyroid gland is enlarged and nodular (normal weight 15-40 gm). Cut surface shows multiple nodules separated from each other by incomplete fibrous septa. Areas of haemorrhage and cystic change are also seen.

M/E

i. Partial or incomplete encapsulation.

ii. The follicles of varying size from small to large and lined by flat to high epithelium.

iii. Areas of haemorrhages, haemosiderin-laden macrophages and cholesterol crystals.

iv. Fibrous scarring and calcification in the nodules.

v. Cystic degeneration (Fig. 35.3).

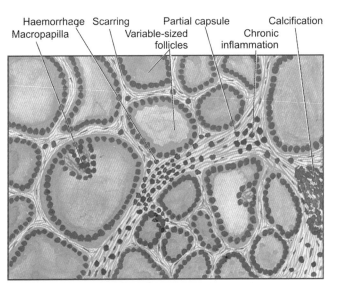

Haemorrhage Scarring Partial capsule Calcification
Macropapilla Variable-sized Chronic
follicles inflammation

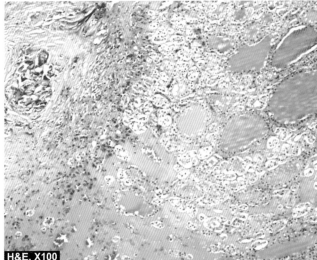

H&E, X100

FIGURE 35.3 ◆ Nodular goitre. The predominant histologic features are: nodularity, extensive scarring with foci of calcification, areas of haemorrhages and variable-sized follicles lined by flat to high epithelium and containing abundant colloid.

Follicular Adenoma

Follicular adenoma is the most common benign thyroid tumour seen more frequently in adult women.

G/A Follicular adenoma is characterised by *4 cardinal features:* solitary nodule, complete encapsulation, clearly distinct architecture inside and outside the capsule, and compressed thyroid parenchyma outside the capsule. Usually, the adenoma is small (up to 3 cm in diameter) and spherical. On cut section, the tumour is grey-white to red-brown, and less colloidal than the surrounding thyroid parenchyma (Fig. 35.4). Less commonly, secondary changes such as fibrous scarring, focal calcification, haemorrhages and cyst formation are seen.

M/E

  i. The tumour shows complete fibrous encapsulation.
 ii. The tumour cells are benign follicular epithelial cells lining the follicles of varying size.
iii. Variety of patterns of growth may be seen, most commonly being microfollicular (foetal) pattern characterised by small follicles containing little or no colloid (Fig. 35.5). Other patterns include macrofollicular, Hurthle cell type, trabecular and atypical.

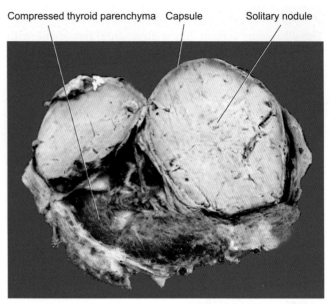

Compressed thyroid parenchyma   Capsule   Solitary nodule

FIGURE 35.4 ◆ Follicular adenoma. Sectioned surface shows a solitary nodule having complete encapsulation. The nodule is grey-white and is distinct from the adjoining thyroid parenchyma. Lower part of the specimen shows thyroid tissue identified by light brown colloid.

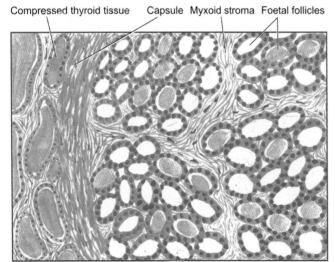

Compressed thyroid tissue   Capsule Myxoid stroma Foetal follicles

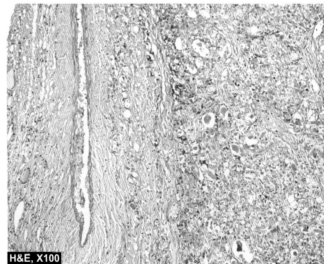

H&E, X100

FIGURE 35.5 ◆ Follicular adenoma thyroid, foetal (microfollicular) type. The tumour is well-encapsulated with compression of surrounding thyroid parenchyma. The tumour consists of small follicles lined by cuboidal epithelium and contain little or no colloid and separated by abundant loose stroma.

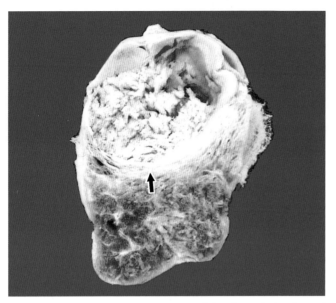

FIGURE 35.6 ◆ Papillary carcinoma of the thyroid. The thyroid gland is enlarged and nodular (normal weight 15-40 gm). Cut surface shows a single nodule separated from the rest of thyroid parenchyma by incomplete fibrous septa. The nodule on cut section shows grey-white soft papillary tumour (arrow).

Papillary Carcinoma

Papillary carcinoma is the most common type of thyroid cancer comprising about 60% of cases, seen more frequently in females.

G/A Papillary carcinoma may range from microscopic foci to nodules up to 10 cm in diameter and is generally poorly delineated. Cut surface of the tumour is greyish-white, hard to scar-like (Fig. 35.6).

M/E

  i. *Papillary pattern:* Papillae composed of fibrovascular stalk and covered by single layer of tumour cells.
  ii. *Tumour cells:* The tumour cells have overlapping pale nuclei imparting it a ground-glass appearance or optically clear appearnace and clear or oxyphil cytoplasm.
  iii. *Invasion:* The tumour cells invade the capsule, and intrathyroid lymphatics.
  iv. *Psammoma bodies:* Almost half of papillary carcinomas show typical, small concentric calcified spherules in the stroma (Fig. 35.7).

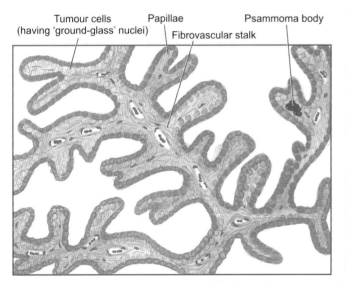
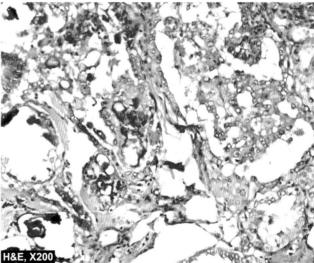

Tumour cells (having 'ground-glass' nuclei)   Papillae   Psammoma body
Fibrovascular stalk

H&E, X200

FIGURE 35.7 ◆ Papillary carcinoma of the thyroid. Microscopy shows branching papillae having fibrovascular stalk covered by a single layer of cuboidal cells having ground-glass nuclei. Colloid-filled follicles and solid sheets of tumour cells are also present.

Osteomyelitis and Benign Bone Tumours

Objectives
➢ To learn pathology of common examples of inflammatory (e.g. chronic osteomyelitis, tuberculous osteomyelitis) and common benign neoplastic (e.g. osteoclastoma, osteochondroma) lesions of bones.
➢ To describe salient gross and microscopic features of these conditions.

Infection of the bones is termed osteomyelitis. It may occur following systemic or local infection (e.g. bacterial, fungal, tuberculous).

Bone tumours may be benign or malignant; each of these may arise from epiphysis, metaphysis or diaphysis. These tumours may be bone-forming, cartilage-forming and from other tissues. Two common examples of benign bone tumours discussed here are osteochondroma and osteoclastoma.

Pyogenic Osteomyelitis

Chronic osteomyelitis is pyogenic or suppurative infection of the bone. Infection may occur by haematogenous route or by direct penetration or extension of bacteria.

G/A Residual and fragmented necrotic bone is seen as sequestrum while the surrounding reactive new bone is involucrum.

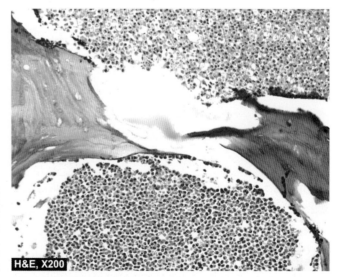

FIGURE 36.1 ◆ Chronic suppurative osteomyelitis. Histologic appearance shows necrotic bone and mixed inflammatory cells infiltrate of extensive purulent inflammatory exudates and inflammatory granulation tissue.

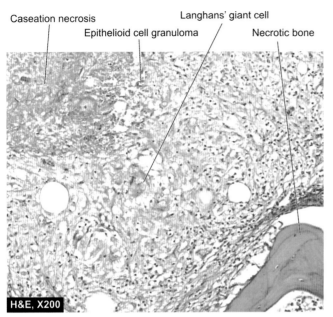

Caseation necrosis   Langhans' giant cell
Epithelioid cell granuloma   Necrotic bone

H&E, X200

FIGURE 36.2 ◆ Tuberculous osteomyelitis consisting of epithelioid cell granulomas with minute areas of caseation necrosis and necrotic bone.

M/E
  i. There is marked mixed infiltrate of polymorphs and chronic inflammatory cells (lymphocytes, plasma cells and macrophages).
  ii. Chips of necrotic bone are seen in the pus.

iii. Repair reaction consisting of osteoclasts, fibroblastic proliferation and new bone formation (Fig. 36.1).

Tuberculous Osteomyelitis

Infection of the bone marrow by tubercle bacilli is a common condition in the underdeveloped and developing countries of the world. It occurs secondary to pulmonary tuberculosis by haematogenous spread. Tuberculosis of the vertebral bodies or Pott's disease is one of the important forms of tuberculous osteomyelitis.

G/A The appearance of necrotic bone (sequestrum) and surrounding new bone (involucrum) is similar to chronic osteomyelitis but foci of caseation necrosis may at times be evident.

M/E
  i. Presence of epithelioid cell granulomas with Langhans' and foreign body giant cells and foci of caseation necrosis.
  ii. Admixture of acute and chronic inflammatory cells.
  iii. Chips of necrotic bone.
  iv. Formation of granulation tissue (Fig. 36.2).

Osteochondroma

Osteochondromas or osteocartilaginous exostoses are common benign cartilage-forming lesions. They arise from metaphysis of long bones as exophytic lesions, most commonly lower femur or upper tibia (i.e. around knee joint) and upper humerus.

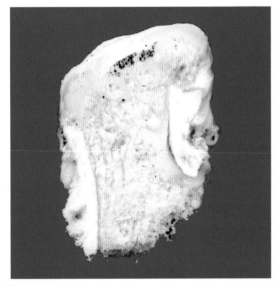

FIGURE 36.3 ◆ Osteochondromas. The amputated head of the long bone shows multiple mushroom-shaped elevated nodular areas. These nodules have cartilaginous caps and inner osseous tissue.

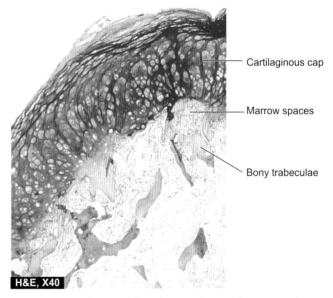

Cartilaginous cap

Marrow spaces

Bony trabeculae

H&E, X40

FIGURE 36.4 ◆ Osteochondroma. The overlying cap shows mature cartilage covering underlying lamellar bone containing marrow spaces.

G/A Osteochondromas have a broad or narrow base (i.e. either sessile or pedunculated) which is continuous with the cortex. They protrude exophytically as mushroom-shaped, cartilage-capped lesions enclosing well-formed cortical bone and marrow (Fig. 36.3).

M/E

i. The outer part consists of mature cartilage resembling epiphyseal cartilage.

ii. The inner part is composed of mature lamellar bone enclosing marrow spaces (Fig. 36.4).

Osteoclastoma

Osteoclastoma or giant cell tumour is a tumour arising in the epiphysis of the long bones, more common in the age range of 20 to 40 years. Common sites of involvement are: lower end of femur and upper end of tibia (i.e. about the knee), lower end of radius, and upper end of fibula.

G/A Giant cell tumour is eccentrically located in the epiphyseal end of a long bone which is expanded. The tumour is well-circumscribed, dark-tan and covered by thin shell of subperiosteal bone. Cut surface of the tumour is characteristically haemorrhagic, necrotic and honey-combed (Fig. 36.5).

M/E

i. Large number of osteoclast-like giant cells which are regularly scattered throughout the stroma.

ii. Giant cells may contain as many as 100 benign nuclei and are similar to normal osteoclasts.

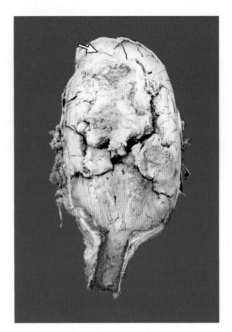

FIGURE 36.5 ◆ Giant cell tumour (osteoclastoma). The end of the long bone is expanded in the region of epiphysis (white arrow). Sectioned surface shows circumscribed, dark-tan and necrotic tumour.

iii. Stromal cells are mononuclear cells and are the real tumour cells and determine the behaviour of the tumour. They are uniform, plump, spindle-shaped or round to oval but may have varying degree of atypia and mitosis (Fig. 36.6).

Osteoclastic giant cells   Stromal cells

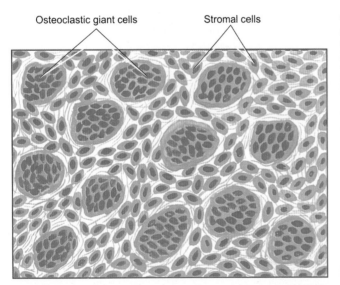

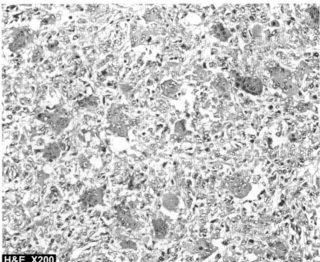

H&E, X200

FIGURE 36.6 ◆ Osteoclastoma. The tumour shows spindle-shaped tumour cells, with uniformly distributed osteoclastic giant cells.

Malignant Bone Tumours

Objectives

➢ To learn pathology of common examples of malignant primary bone tumours (e.g. Ewing's sarcoma, osteosarcoma, chondrosarcoma).

➢ To describe salient gross and microscopic features of these conditions.

Like benign bone tumours, malignant primary bone tumours may be located in epiphysis, metaphysis or diaphysis. These may be bone-forming, cartilage-forming and from other tissues. A few common examples discussed here are Ewing's sarcoma (commonly diaphyseal), osteosarcoma (bone forming tumour, commonly metaphyseal) and chondrosarcoma (cartilage-forming tumour, commonly metaphyseal).

Ewing's Sarcoma

Ewing's sarcoma is a highly malignant round cell tumour arising in the medullary canal of diaphysis or metaphysis. The common sites are shafts of long bones, particularly femur, tibia, humerus and fibula. Common age for occurrence is between 5 to 20 years with predilection in females.

G/A Ewing's sarcoma is typically located in the medullary cavity and produces expansion of the affected diaphysis (shaft) or metaphysis. The tumour often extends into adjacent soft tissues. Cut surface of the tumour is characteristically grey-white, soft and friable (Fig. 37.1).

M/E

i. The tumour is divided by fibrous septa into irregular lobules of closely-packed cells.

ii. The tumour cells comprising the lobules are small and uniform resembling lymphocytes and have round nuclei with frequent mitosis.

iii. The tumour cells may be arranged around blood vessels forming pseudorosettes.

iv. Areas of acute inflammatory cell reaction and necrosis are often seen (Fig. 37.2).

v. The cytoplasm is scanty and contains glycogen positive for PAS stain (Fig. 37.3).

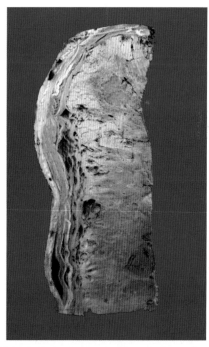

FIGURE 37.1 ◆ Ewing's sarcoma. The specimen shows a tumour extending into soft tissues including the skeletal muscle. Cut surface of the tumour is grey-white, cystic, soft and friable.

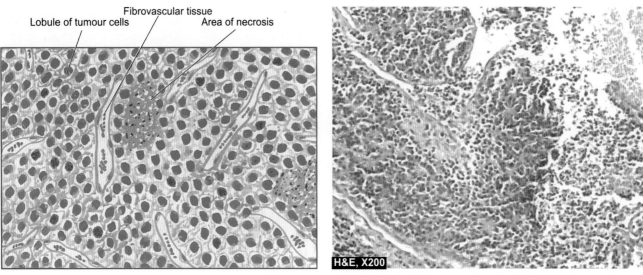

FIGURE 37.2 ◆ Ewing's sarcoma. Characteristic microscopic features are irregular lobules of uniform small tumour cells with indistinct cytoplasmic outlines which are separated by fibrous tissue septa having rich vascularity. Areas of necrosis and inflammatory infiltrate are also included.

Osteosarcoma

Osteogenic sarcoma or osteosarcoma is the most common primary malignant bone tumour. Classically, the tumour occurs in young patients between the age of 10 to 20 years. The tumour arises in the metaphysis of long bones, most commonly in the lower end of femur and upper end of tibia (i.e. around knee joint).

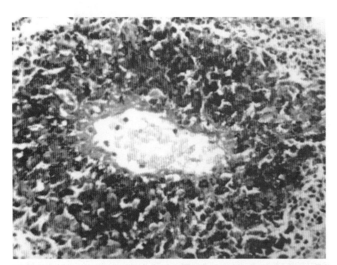

FIGURE 37.3 ◆ Ewing's sarcoma. The figure shows tumour cells containing scanty ill-defined cytoplasm having glycogen stained positive with PAS.

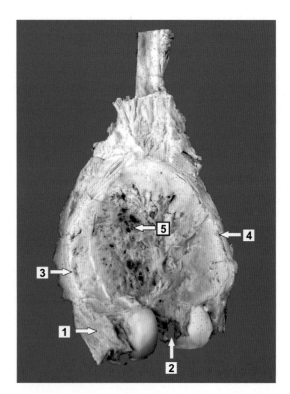

FIGURE 37.4 ◆ Osteosarcoma. The lower end of the femur shows a bulky expanded tumour in the region of metaphysis (1) sparing the epiphyseal cartilage (2). Sectioned surface of the tumour shows lifting of the periosteum by the tumour (3) and eroded cortical bone (4). Cut surface of the tumour is grey-white with areas of haemorrhage and necrosis (5).

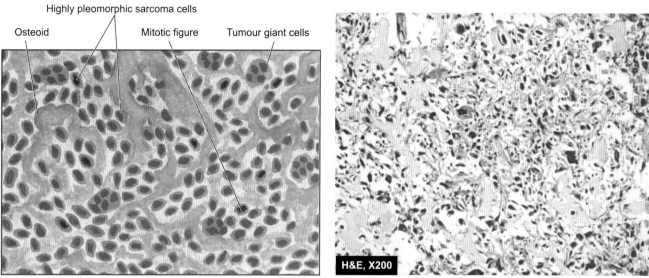

FIGURE 37.5 ◆ Osteosarcoma. The tumour cells show pleomorphic and polymorphic features with direct formation of osteoid by tumour cells.

G/A The tumour appears as a grey-white, bulky mass at the metaphyseal end of a long bone of the extremity, generally sparing the articular end of the bone. Codman's triangle formed by the angle between lifting of periosteum and underlying surface of the cortex may be grossly identified. Cut surface of the tumour is grey-white with areas of haemorrhages and necrotic bone (Fig. 37.4).

M/E

i. *Sarcoma cells.* The tumour cells are anaplastic mesenchymal stromal cells which show marked pleomorphism and polymorphism, i.e. variation in size as well as shape. The tumour cells may be spindled, round, oval, polygonal or bizarre tumour giant cells. They show hyperchromatism and atypical mitoses.

ii. *Osteogenesis.* The anaplastic sarcoma cells form osteoid matrix and bone directly, which lies interspersed in the areas of tumour cells (Fig. 37.5).

Chondrosarcoma

Chondrosarcoma is a malignant tumour of chondroblasts. However, it is much slow growing than osteosarcoma. The tumour usually occurs between 3rd and 6th decades of life. The tumour has 2 varieties—*central form* occurring in medullary cavity of the diaphysis or metaphysis (most commonly femur), and *peripheral form* that may be cortical or parosteal (most often in the vicinity of hip joint and shoulder).

G/A The tumour may vary in size from a few centimetres to extremely large and lobulated masses of firm consistency. Cut section of the tumour shows translucent, bluish-white, gelatinous or myxoid appearance with foci of spotty calcification (Fig. 37.6).

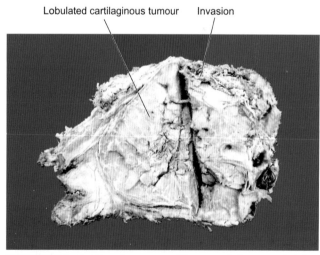

FIGURE 37.6 ◆ Chondrosarcoma. The scapula is expanded due to a gelatinous tumour. Sectioned surface shows lobulated mass with bluish cartilaginous hue infiltrating the soft tissues.

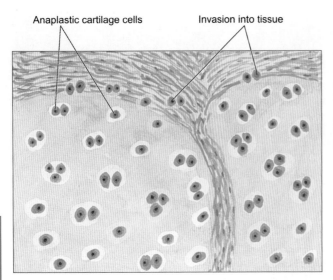

Anaplastic cartilage cells   Invasion into tissue

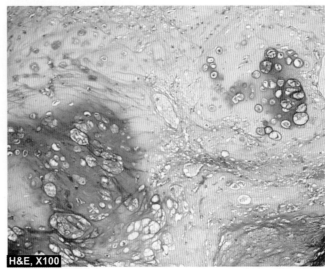

H&E, X100

FIGURE 37.7 ◆ Chondrosarcoma. Histologic features include invasion of the tumour into adjacent soft tissues and cytologic anaplasia in the tumour cells.

M/E

i. Lobular pattern of anaplastic cartilage cells.

ii. Cartilage cells have cytologic features of malignancy such as hyperchromatism, pleomorphism, two or more cells in the lacunae and tumour giant cells.

iii. Invasive character of the tumour into the adjoining soft tissues (Fig. 37.7).

Meningitis and CNS Tumours

Objectives
➢ To learn pathology of pyogenic meningitis and common examples of CNS tumours (e.g. meningioma, schwannoma, astrocytoma).
➢ To describe salient gross and microscopic features of these conditions.

Meningitis is inflammatory involvement of the meninges, most commonly due to infection. Infectious meningitis may be acute pyogenic (discussed here), acute lymphocytic (mostly viral) and chronic (tuberculous or fungal).

The tumours of nervous system are classified based on the cells of origin, for example meningiomas arise from pia-arachnoid layer, schwannomas arise from nerve sheath, and gliomas arise from neuroglia.

Acute Pyogenic Meningitis

Acute pyogenic or purulent meningitis is acute infection of the pia-arachnoid and of the CSF.

G/A Pus accumulates in the subarachnoid space and the CSF becomes turbid or frankly purulent. The meninges are coated with exudate.

M/E
  i. The meninges, particularly around blood vessels, show numerous polymorphs and fibrinous material.
  ii. There may be formation of granulation tissue of nonspecific type (Fig. 38.1).
  iii. Bacteria may be identified in routine or Gram staining.

Meningioma

The most common tumour arising from the pia-arachnoid is meningioma. The most frequent sites are in the front half of

the head—lateral cerebral convexities, midline along the falx cerebri adjacent to the major venous sinuses parasagittally.

G/A Meningioma is well circumscribed, solid, spherical or hemispherical mass of variable size (1 to 10 cm in diameter). The tumour is generally firmly attached to the dura while the overlying bone may show hyperostosis. Cut surface of the

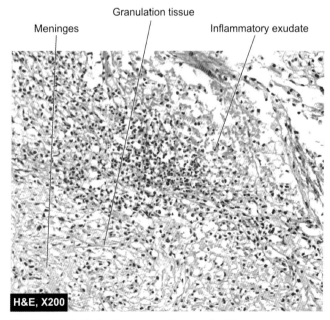

Granulation tissue

Meninges

Inflammatory exudate

H&E, X200

FIGURE 38.1 ◆ Acute suppurative meningitis.

(145)

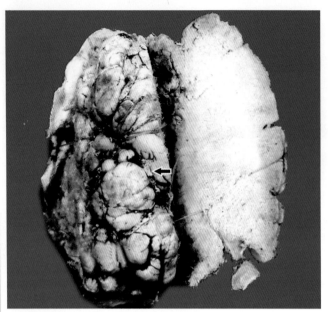

FIGURE 38.2 ◆ Meningioma. The tumour mass is circumscribed with irregular surface convolutions and prominent blood vessels. It is firm in consistency with peripherally adherent thick firm dural tissue. Cut surface of the mass is firm and fibrous (black arrow).

i. There is conspicuous whorled pattern of tumour cells, often around central capillary-sized blood vessels.
ii. There is combination of cells with syncytial and fibroblastic features. Syncytial cells resemble normal arachnoid cap cells and are polygonal cells with poorly-defined cell membranes (i.e. syncytial appearance).
iii. Many of the whorls may show psammoma bodies.
iv. Other secondary changes like xanthomatous and myxomatous degeneration may be seen.

Schwannoma

Schwannoma or neurilemmoma arises from the cranial or spinal nerve roots. It may occur as an intraspinal tumour or a peripheral nerve sheath tumour. Multiple schwannomas are uncommon and occur in von Recklinghausen's disease.

G/A A schwannoma is an encapsulated, solid, sometimes cystic tumour, that produces eccentric enlargement of the nerve root from where it arises.

M/E
i. The tumour is composed of fibrocellular bundles forming whorled pattern.
ii. There are areas of dense and compact cellularity (Antoni A pattern) alternating with loose acellular areas (Antoni B pattern).
iii. Areas of Antoni A show palisaded nuclei called Verocay bodies.

tumour is firm and fibrous, sometimes with foci of calcification (Fig. 38.2).

M/E The most common microscopic type is mixed or transitional type. The features are as follows (Fig. 38.3):

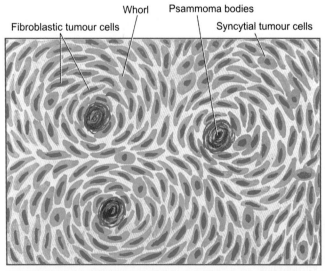

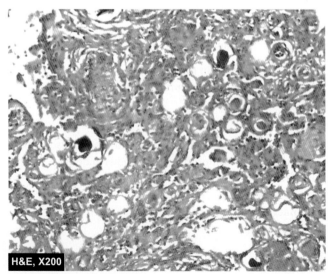

FIGURE 38.3 ◆ Meningioma. The tumour cells have features of both syncytial and fibroblastic type forming whorls which contain central laminated areas of calcification called psammoma bodies.

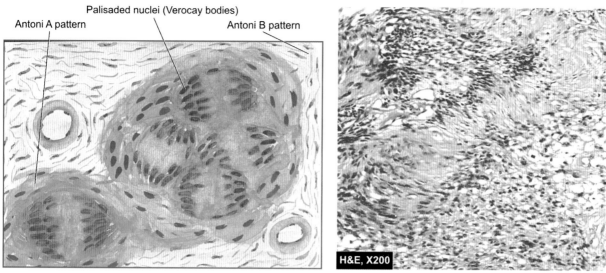

FIGURE 38.4 ◆ Schwannoma (neurilemmoma), showing whorls of densely cellular (Antoni A) and loosely cellular (Antoni B) areas with characteristic nuclear palisading (Verocay bodies).

iv. Areas of degeneration containing haemosiderin and lipid-laden macrophages are often present (Fig. 38.4).

Astrocytoma

Astrocytomas are the most common type of glioma. They are most frequent in late middle life and occur predominantly in the cerebral hemispheres. Depending upon the degree of anaplasia, they vary from low grade to high grade, the higher grades being labelled as anaplastic astrocytoma (grade III) and glioblastoma multiforme (grade IV).

G/A The tumour is poorly-defined, grey-white tumour of variable size. The tumour merges with the adjoining brain tissue. Cut section of higher grades of the tumour may show variegated appearance with areas of necrosis and haemorrhages.

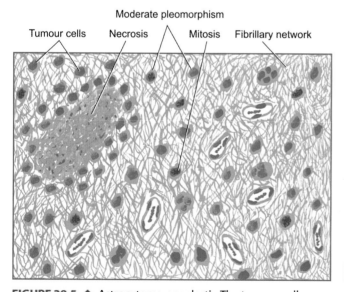

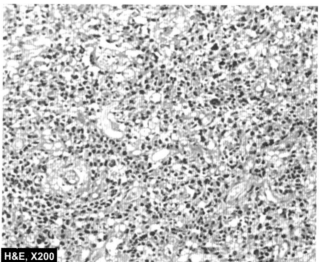

FIGURE 38.5 ◆ Astrocytoma, anaplastic. The tumour cells are anaplastic and there is proliferation of vascular endothelium.

M/E Microscopic features of higher grade of astrocytoma are as under:

i.   Highly cellular.

ii. The tumour cells have features of anaplasia such as pleomorphism, nuclear hyperchromatism and mitoses.

iii. Proliferation of blood vessels and endothelial cells (Fig. 38.5).

iv. Glioblastoma multiforme (grade IV glioma), in addition, shows pseudopalisading of tumour cells around area of necrosis and multinucleate tumour giant cells and bizarre cells (Fig. 38.6).

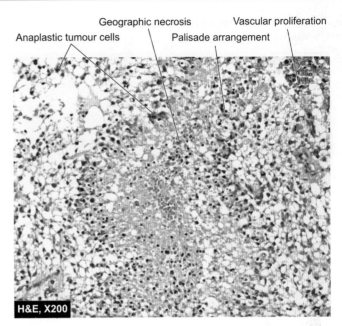

FIGURE 38.6 ◆ Glioblastoma multiforme (grade IV astrocytoma). The tumour is densely cellular having marked pleomorphism. Characteristically, the tumour has areas of necrosis which are surrounded by palisade layer of tumour cells.

Section Four

CYTOPATHOLOGY

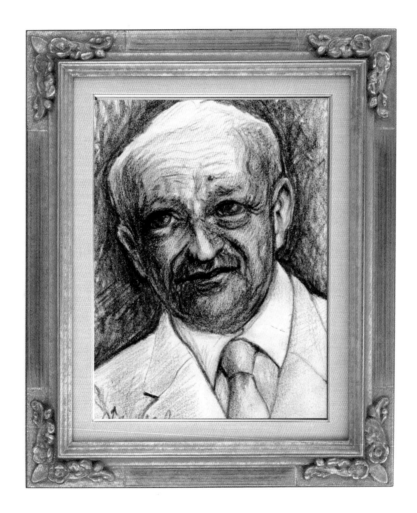

GEORGE N PAPANICOLAOU (1883–1962)
'Father of Exfoliative Cytology'

American pathologist, who developed Pap test
for detection and early diagnosis of uterine cervical cancer.

Section Contents

Basic Cytopathologic Techniques and their Applications

Objectives
- To learn the types of cytopathologic techniques and their applications.
- To get familiar with procedure and staining of exfoliative cytology, aspiration cytology and imprint cytology.

Cytology is the study of body cells that are either exfoliated spontaneously from epithelial surfaces or are obtained from various body tissues and organs by different techniques. Accordingly, cytology has following branches:

A. Exfoliative cytology
B. Aspiration cytology
C. Imprint cytology

Exfoliative Cytology

This is the study of cells which are spontaneously shed off from epithelial surfaces into body cavities or into fluid. The cells can also be obtained by scraping, brushing or wash of body surfaces. The principle of this technique is that there is increased rate of exfoliation of cells in diseased states.

APPLICATIONS OF EXFOLIATIVE CYTOLOGY

Exfoliative cytology is applied in diagnosing diseases of the following:

1. Female genital tract
2. Respiratory tract
3. Gastrointestinal tract
4. Urinary tract
5. Body fluids (pleural, peritoneal, pericardial, CSF and semen)
6. Buccal smears for sex chromatin

Female Genital Tract

Smears from female genital tract are known as 'Pap smears'. These smears are prepared by different methods depending upon the purpose for which they are intended:

i. *Cervical smear* is obtained by Ayre's spatula (Fig. 39.1) from portio of the cervix by rotating the spatula through 360° to sample the entire cervix. The scraped material is placed on a clean glass slide and smear prepared. It is ideal for detection of cervical carcinoma.

ii. *Lateral vaginal smear (LVS)* is obtained by scraping upper third of lateral walls of the vagina and is ideal for cytohormonal assessment.

iii. *Vaginal pool smear* is obtained by aspirating material from posterior fornix of vagina and is done for detecting endometrial and ovarian carcinoma.

Combined (fast) smears are a combination of vaginal pool and cervical scrapings and are used for routine population screening.

Respiratory Tract

Material from respiratory tract may be obtained during bronchoscopic procedures as expectorant (sputum), or by brushing (BB), by washing (BW) and bronchioalveolar lavage (BAL). Sputum examination is advantageous as samples are easily obtained and cellular content is representative of entire

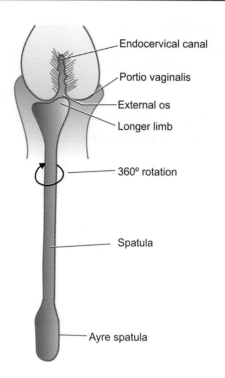

FIGURE 39.1 ◆ Method of obtaining cervical material by Ayre's spatula (Fast smear).

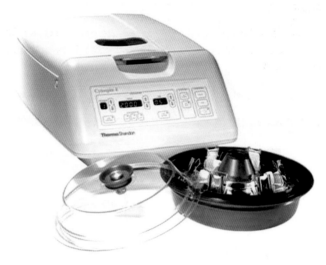

FIGURE 39.2 ◆ Cytospin used for making smears in cases with small volume of fluid (Photograph courtesy of Thermo Shandon, UK through Towa Optics India Pvt. Ltd., Delhi).

respiratory tract. At least three samples of sputum, preferably early morning samples, should be examined.

Gastrointestinal Tract

Lesions in the oral cavity can be sampled by scraping the surface with a metallic or wooden spatula. Samples can be obtained from the oesophagus, stomach, small and large intestine either by brushing or lavage during fibreoptic endoscopy.

Urinary Tract

Samples from lesions in the urinary tract are either urinary sediment examined from voided urine/catheterised urine or washings of the urinary bladder obtained at cystoscopy.

Body Fluids

Fluid from pleural, peritoneal or pericardial cavity is obtained by paracentesis. At least 50-100 ml of fluid is aspirated. The sample is examined fresh but if delay is anticipated then fluid should be anticoagulated either in EDTA 1 mg/ml or 3.8% sodium citrate 1 ml/10 ml. Fluid should be centrifuged and smears are prepared from the sediment. If amount of fluid is less (less than 1 ml), then it can be subjected to cytospin centrifuged smear preparation (Fig. 39.2).

Buccal Smears for Sex Chromatin

Smears are prepared from the oral cavity after cleaning the area. Vaginal smears can also be used. In normal females, Barr bodies are present in 4-20% nuclei. In males their count is in less than 2% nuclei.

FIXATION OF SMEARS IN EXFOLIATIVE CYTOLOGY

Methods of fixation depend upon type of staining employed. Pap smears are wet-fixed (i.e. smears are immersed in fixative without allowing them to dry). Smears to be stained by Romanowsky stains are air-dried as fixation is affected during the staining procedure. Fixative used is either equal parts of ether and 95% ethanol, or 95% ethanol alone, 100% methanol, or 85% isopropyl alcohol. Fixation time of 10-15 minutes at room temperature is adequate. Smears may be left in fixative for 24 hours or more. Smears should be transported to the laboratory in fixative solution in coplin jars.

STAINING OF SMEARS IN EXFOLIATIVE CYTOLOGY

Three staining procedures are commonly employed: Papanicolaou and H & E stains are used for *wet-fixed smears* while Romanowsky stains are used for *air-dried smears*.

Papanicolaou Stain

This is the best stain for routine cytodiagnostic studies. In this, haematoxylin gives nuclear stain while OG-6 and EA-50 are two cytoplasmic counterstains.

H & E Stain

This stain is the same as that used for histological sections. In this, haematoxylin is nuclear stain and eosin is cytoplasmic counterstain.

Romanowsky Stain

Leishman's stain, Giemsa and May-Grunwald-Giemsa (MGG) are usually used; the last one is most commonly used.

Aspiration Cytology

In this study, samples are obtained from diseased tissue by fine needle aspiration (FNA).

APPLICATIONS OF FNA

FNA is applied for diagnosis of palpable as well as non-palpable lesions.

I.   Palpable Mass Lesions in

1. Lymph nodes
2. Breast
3. Thyroid
4. Salivary glands
5. Soft tissue masses
6. Bones

II.   Non-Palpable Mass Lesions in

1. Abdominal cavity
2. Thoracic cavity
3. Retroperitoneum

Procedure for FNA

Materials. For performing FNA, a Franzen's handle, syringe with needles, clean glass slides and suitable fixative are required (Fig. 39.3).

Method

♦ No anaesthesia is required.
♦ Ask the patient to lie down in comfortable position exposing the target area.
♦ Palpate the target area.
♦ Clean the overlying skin with spirit.
♦ Fix 10/20 ml disposable syringe in Franzen's handle. Insert 20-25 gauge disposable needle into syringe (Fig. 39.4,A, B).
♦ Fix the mass by palpating hand and insert needle into target area (Fig. 39.4, C). Apply suction while moving needle back and forth within the lesion and change the direction of the needle.
♦ Terminate the aspiration when aspirated material or blood is visible at the base/hub of the needle.
♦ Release the suction before withdrawing the needle to equalise pressure within the syringe (Fig. 39.4,D).
♦ After withdrawal of needle, apply pressure for 2-3 minutes at the site of puncture to arrest bleeding and prevent haematoma formation.
♦ Aspirated material from the needle is expressed on to clean glass slides by first detaching the needle and filling the syringe with air and expressing it with pressure.
♦ Smears are prepared as for blood smears. If the material is semi-solid, it is first crushed by gentle pressure with a glass slide and smears prepared (Fig. 39.5).

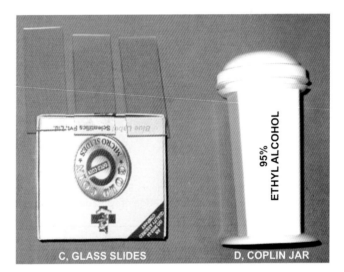

FIGURE 39.3 ♦ Equipment required for transcutaneous FNAC.

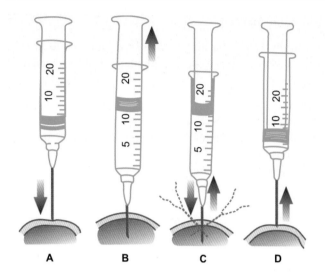

FIGURE 39.4 ◆ Procedure of FNAC of palpable masses. Needle is introduced into the mass (A). Plunger is retracted after needle enters the mass (B). Suction is maintained while needle is moved back and forth within the mass (C). Suction is released and plunger returned to original position before needle is withdrawn (D).

◆ Fixation and staining are the same as for exfoliative cytology.

RADIOLOGICAL IMAGING AIDS FOR FNA

Non-palpable lesions require some form of localisation by radiological aids for FNA to be carried out. While plain X-ray is usually adequate for lesions in bones and chest, ultrasonography (USG) allows direct visualisation of needle in intra-abdominal and soft tissue masses and hence US-guided FNA can be carried out. CT-guided FNA can also be used for lesions in chest and abdomen.

ADVANTAGES OF FNA OVER SURGICAL BIOPSY

  i. Outdoor procedure
 ii. No anaesthesia required
iii. Results obtained within hours
 iv. Procedure can be repeated
  v. Low cost procedure

Imprint Cytology

In imprint cytology touch preparations from cut surfaces of fresh unfixed surgically excised tissue are prepared on clean glass slides. These are fixed, stained and examined immediately. It is considered complementary to frozen section.

APPLICATIONS OF IMPRINT CYTOLOGY

Imprint cytology is useful in following situations:
  i. Lymph node biopsy
 ii. Surgically resected tumours

ADVANTAGES OF IMPRINT CYTOLOGY

  i. Tissue and cell architecture is retained
 ii. Useful as an intraoperative pathologic consult

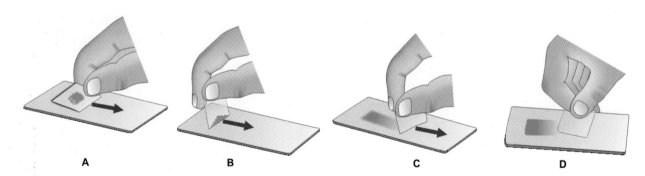

FIGURE 39.5 ◆ Preparation of smears. Semisolid aspirates are crush-smeared by flat pressure with cover slip or glass slide (A). Fluid or blood droplet is collected along edge of spreader (B), and pulled as for peripheral blood films (C). Particles at the end of the smear are crush-smeared (D).

Interpretation of Pap Smears and Fluid Cytology

Objectives
➢ To learn the types of exfoliative cytology methods (Pap and body fluids) and identification of normal cells.
➢ To get familiar with abnormal cells in Pap smears (e.g. inflammatory smear, trichomoniasis, cervical cancer) and in body fluids (e.g. in visceral cancer) in major diseases.

A normal Pap smear shows the following cells:
  i. Superficial cells
 ii. Intermediate cells
iii. Parabasal cells

    The features of these cells are summarised in Table 40.1.

Inflammatory Pap Smear

    In inflammatory smear, the superficial and intermediate cells show features as under (Fig. 40.1):
  i. Cytoplasmic eosinophilia.
 ii. Cytoplasmic vacuolisation.

Table 40.1: Squamous epithelial cells found in normal combined *(Fast)* smears				
Cell type	Size	Nuclei	Cytoplasm	Morphology
Superficial	30-60 µm	< 6 µm dark, pyknotic	Polyhedral, thin, broad, acidophilic or cyanophilic with keratohyaline granules.	
Intermediate	20-40 µm	6-9 µm vesicular	Polyhedral or elongated, thin, cyanophilic with folded edges.	
Parabasal	15-25 µm	6-11 µm vesicular	Round to oval, thick, well-defined, basophilic with occasional small vacuoles.	
Basal	13-20 µm	Large, (> one-half of cell volume), hyperchromatic, may have small nucleoli	Round to oval, deeply basophilic.	

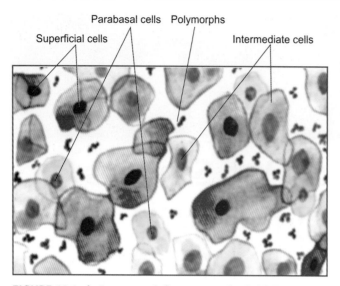

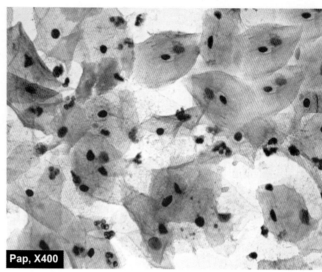

Pap, X400

FIGURE 40.1 ◆ Pap smear, inflammatory. The field shows mainly superficial and some intermediate cells, and a few polymorphs.

iii. Large number of leucocytes in the background.

iv. Leucocytes into cytoplasm of epithelial cells.

v. Perinuclear halos.

vi. Clumping of chromatin.

vii. Nuclear enlargement and pyknosis.

viii. Increase in the number of parabasal cells.

The specific inflammation could be caused by the following microbial infections:

i. *Trichomonas vaginalis*

ii. *Candida albicans*

Pap, X1000 Oil

FIGURE 40.2 ◆ Pap smear showing *Trichomonas* vaginitis. Trophozoite of Trichomonas is shown by arrows.

iii. Herpes simplex virus

iv. Human papilloma virus

The following morphological features are used to diagnose *Trichomonas vaginalis* vaginal infection (Fig. 40.2):

1. Presence of trophozoites of the protozoa in the smear are seen as fuzzy grey-green, round or elliptical structure 8 to 20 μm in size and contain an eccentric, small round vesicular nucleus. Flagella are, however, rarely seen.

2. Other non-specific inflammatory changes as described above are seen.

Pap Smear in Carcinoma Cervix

Pap smear has become one of the key screening procedures for diagnosing precursor lesions as well as for carcinoma of the cervix. Compared to earlier system of categorizing Pap smears into mild, moderate and severe dysplasias, currently the cytological diagnosis of cervical lesions is based commonly on the *Bethesda system* which divides the precursor lesions into two tiers:

1. LSIL (low grade squamous intraepithelial lesions)

2. HSIL (high grade squamous intraepithelial lesions).

The characteristic cytological features of invasive squamous cell carcinoma are as follows (Fig. 40.3):

i. Cells present singly, in sheets and syncytium-like aggregates.

ii. Marked variation in cell size and shape.

iii. Altered nuclear-cytoplasmic ratio.

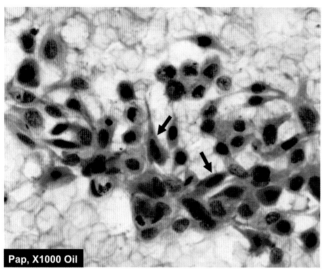

Pap, X1000 Oil

FIGURE 40.3 ◆ Pap smear in invasive carcinoma cervix. The field shows pleomorphic squamous cells in a sheet having coarse nuclear chromatin. A few fibre cells and caudate cells also seen (arrows). The background shows abundant haemorrhage and some necrotic debris.

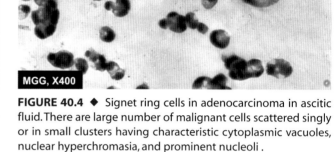

MGG, X400

FIGURE 40.4 ◆ Signet ring cells in adenocarcinoma in ascitic fluid. There are large number of malignant cells scattered singly or in small clusters having characteristic cytoplasmic vacuoles, nuclear hyperchromasia, and prominent nucleoli .

iv. Nuclei having irregular membranes, prominent macro-nucleoli, irregularly distributed coarse chromatin and parachromatin clearing.

v. Tadpole/caudate cells and spindled squamous cells are seen.

vi. Associated tumour diathesis in the background (necrosis and old, degenerated blood).

Fluid Cytology for Malignant Cells

Accumulation of fluid in the body cavities may be due to:

A. Benign conditions

B. Malignant conditions

In benign conditions the fluid shows presence of mesothelial cells which can be confused with malignant cells. The characteristics of *mesothelial cells* are as under:

i. Seen in small clusters, papillae, pseudoacini or singly.

ii. Round to oval 30 to 90 μm in size.

iii. Cytoplasm is basophilic and is usually abundant.

iv. Central nuclei with perinuclear halo.

v. Clumped chromatin with 1-4 distinct nucleoli.

Malignant cells (adenocarcinoma) in effusion show following characteristics in smears (Fig. 40.4):

i. Seen in acini, papillae or singly.

ii. Cells are variable-sized.

iii. Cytoplasm is abundant deep purple.

iv. Cytoplasmic vacuoles in some forming signet ring cells.

v. Nuclei irregular shaped, well-defined nuclear border, hyperchromatic and nuclear overlapping.

vi. Chromatin clumping with prominent nucleoli.

vii. Frequent mitosis.

Interpretation of FNA Smears

Objectives
➢ To learn the interpretation of FNA smears in common infective (e.g. tuberculous lymphadenitis) and benign (e.g. fibroadenoma breast) and malignant tumours (e.g. infiltrating duct carcinoma breast).

While fine needle aspiration cytology (FNAC) is increasingly being applied to a wide variety of conditions, both non-neoplastic and neoplastic, by direct aspiration as well as by guidance (ultrasound or CT), a few common examples of interpretation of FNA findings on smears prepared by direct aspiration are illustrated below where a diagnosis can be made readily.

FNA in Tuberculous Lymphadenitis

Fine needle aspiration of lymph nodes has become the primary tool in diagnosing tuberculosis. The characteristic findings (one or more) are as under (Fig. 41.1):
　i. Multiple epithelioid cell granulomas are seen. Epithelioid cells have an elongated slipper-shaped vesicular nuclei and pale cytoplasm with indistinct cell borders.

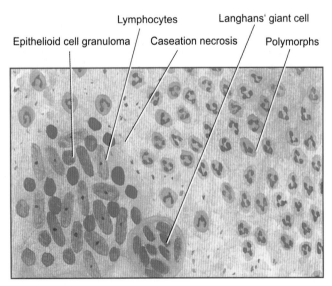
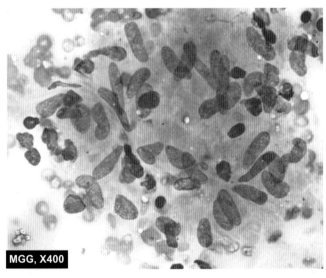

FIGURE 41.1 ◆ FNA smear from tuberculous lymphadenitis. There are epithelioid cell clusters and necrotic debris in the background.

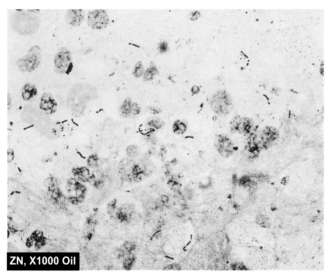

ZN, X1000 Oil

FIGURE 41.2 ◆ FNA smear from tuberculous lymphadenitis stained with Ziehl-Neelsen stain. The field shows acid-fast bacilli.

ii. Variable number of Langhans' and foreign body type of giant cells.

iii. Background shows eosinophilic granular material (caseous necrosis).

iv. Ziehl-Neelsen stain for acid-fast bacilli may be positive (Fig. 41.2).

v. Not infrequently, the smears may show only polymorphs and necrotic debris, especially in immunocompromised patients.

FNA in Fibroadenoma Breast

Fibroadenoma is a common benign biphasic tumour of the breast in young females presenting as a movable firm lump. The cytological smears show the following features (Fig. 41.3):

i. Cellular smears.

ii. Monolayered sheets of uniform epithelial cells having antler horn configuration.

iii. Sheets show both epithelial and myoepithelial cells.

iv. Numerous single, bipolar benign nuclei.

v. Fragments of fibromyxoid stroma.

FNA in Duct Carcinoma Breast

The characteristic features of infiltrating duct carcinoma breast in smear are as under (Fig. 41.4):

i. Highly cellular smears.

ii. Cells are less cohesive.

iii. Cells disorderly arranged with over-lapping.

iv. Altered nuclear-cytoplasmic ratio.

v. Cytoplasm is mild to moderate and well-defined.

vi. Nuclei are large, irregular, hyperchromatic, some show prominent nucleoli.

vii. Background shows necrotic debris.

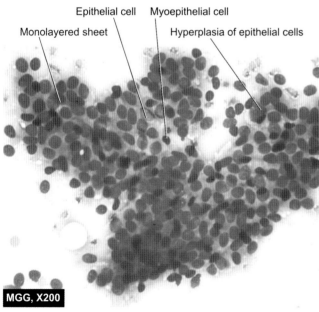

Epithelial cell   Myoepithelial cell
Monolayered sheet   Hyperplasia of epithelial cells

MGG, X200

FIGURE 41.3 ◆ FNA breast from fibroadenoma breast. The field shows monolayered sheet of monomorphic cells and some fibromyxoid stromal fragment.

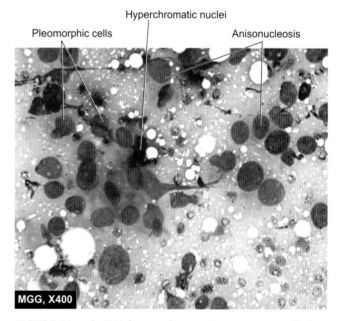

Hyperchromatic nuclei
Pleomorphic cells   Anisonucleosis

MGG, X400

FIGURE 41.4 ◆ FNA breast, duct carcinoma. Scattered pleomorphic malignant cells with hyperchromatic nuclei.

Section Five

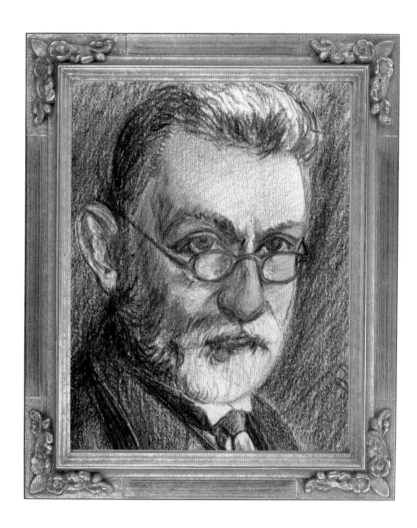

PAUL EHRLICH (1854–1915)
'Immunologist and Clinical Pathologist'

German Physician, winner of Nobel Prize for his work in immunology;
described Ehrlich's test for urobilinogen; staining
techniques of cells and bacteria, and laid the foundations of haematology.

Section Contents

Urine Examination I: Physical and Chemical

Objectives
➤ To learn the physical characteristics of normal and abnormal urine.
➤ To learn the principle, perform the procedure and interpret the results of various routine tests for chemical constituents of a urinary sample.

Examination of urine is important for diagnosis and assistance in the diagnosis of various diseases. Routine (complete) examination of urine is divided into four parts:

A. Adequacy of specimen
B. Physical/gross examination
C. Chemical examination
D. Microscopic examination

The last named, microscopic examination, is discussed separately in the next exercise.

A. Adequacy of Specimen

The specimen should be properly collected in a clean container which should be properly labelled with name of the patient, age, sex, identity number with date and time of collection. It should not show signs of contamination.

SPECIMEN COLLECTION

For routine examination a clean glass tube or capped jar is used; for bacteriologic examination a sterilised container is required. For routine urinanalysis, first morning sample is best since it is most concentrated. For bacteriologic examination, mid-stream sample is preferable, i.e. first part of urine is discarded and mid-stream sample is collected. For 24-hour sample, collection of urine is started in the morning

at 8 AM (first voided sample is discarded) and all subsequent samples are collected till next day 8 AM.

METHODS OF PRESERVATION OF URINE

Urine should be examined fresh or within one hour of voiding. But if it has to be delayed then following preservatives can be used which prevent its decomposition:

i. *Refrigeration* at 4°C.
ii. *Toluene.* Toluene is used 1 ml per 50 ml of urine. It acts by forming a surface layer and it preserves the chemical constituents of urine.
iii. *Formalin.* 6-8 drops of 40% formalin per 100 ml of urine is used. It preserves RBCs and pus cells. However, its use has the disadvantage that it gives false-positive test for sugar.
iv. *Thymol.* It is a good preservative; 1% solution of thymol is used. Its use has the disadvantage that it gives false-positive test for proteins.
v. *Acids.* Hydrochloric acid, sulphuric acid and boric acid can also be used as a preservative.

B. Physical Examination

Physical examination of urine consists of volume, colour, odour, reaction/pH and specific gravity.

VOLUME

Normally 700-2500 ml (average 1200 ml) of urine is passed in 24 hours and most of it is passed during day time.

i) Nocturia. Nocturia means when urine is passed in excess of 500 ml during night with specific gravity of less than 1.018. This is a sign of early renal failure.

ii) Polyuria. Polyuria is when excess of urine is passed in 24 hours (> 2000 ml) with low specific gravity. Polyuria can be physiological due to excess water intake, may be seasonal (e.g. in winter), or can be pathological (e.g. in diabetes insipidus, diabetes mellitus).

iii) Oliguria. When less than 500 ml of urine is passed in 24 hours, it is termed as oliguria. It can be due to less intake of water, dehydration, renal ischaemia.

iv) Anuria. When there is almost complete suppression of urine (< 150 ml in 24 hours), it is termed as anuria. It can be due to renal stones, tumours, renal ischaemia.

COLOUR

Normally, urine is clear, pale or straw-coloured due to pigment urochrome.

i) Colourless in diabetes mellitus, diabetes insipidus, excess intake of water.

ii) Deep amber colour due to good muscular exercise, high grade fever.

iii) Orange colour due to increased urobilinogen, concentrated urine.

iv) Smoky urine due to small amount of blood, administration of vitamin B12, aniline dye.

v) Red due to haematuria, haemoglobinuria.

vi) Yellow-brown due to bile and its derivatives.

vii) Milky due to pus, fat.

viii) Green due to putreficd sample, phenol poisoning.

ODOUR

Normally urine has faint aromatic odour.

i) Pungent due to ammonia produced by bacterial contamination.

ii) Putrid due to UTI.

iii) Fruity due to ketoacidosis.

iv) Mousy due to phenylketonuria.

REACTION/pH

It reflects ability of the kidney to maintain H^+ ion concentration in extracellular fluid and plasma. It can be measured by pH indicator paper or by electronic pH meter.

Freshly voided normal urine is slightly acidic and its pH ranges from 4.6-7.0 (average 6.0).

◆ *Acidic urine* is due to the following:
   i. High protein intake, e.g. meats.
   ii. Ingestion of acidic fruits.
   iii. Respiratory and metabolic acidosis.
   iv. UTI by *E. coli.*

◆ *Alkaline urine* is due to following:
   i. Citrus fruits.
   ii. Vegetables.
   iii. Respiratory and metabolic alkalosis.
   iv. UTI by *Proteus, Pseudomonas.*

SPECIFIC GRAVITY

This is the ratio of weight of 1 ml volume of urine to that of weight of 1 ml of distilled water. It depends upon the concentration of various particles/solutes in the urine. Specific gravity is used to measure the concentrating and diluting power of the kidneys. It can be measured by urinometer, refractometer or reagent strips.

1. Urinometer

Procedure
◆ Fill urinometer container 3/4th with urine.
◆ Insert urinometer into it so that it floats in urine without touching the wall and bottom of container (Fig. 42.1).
◆ Read the graduation on the arm of urinometer at lower urinary meniscus.
◆ Add or substract 0.001 from the final reading for each 3°C above or below the calibration temperature respectively marked on the urinometer.

2. Refractometer

It measures the refractive index of urine. This procedure requires only a few drops of urine in contrast to urinometer where approximately 100 ml of urine is required.

3. Reagent Strip Method

This method employs the use of chemical reagent strip (see Fig. 42.3).

Significance of Specific Gravity

The normal specific gravity of urine is 1.003 to 1.030.

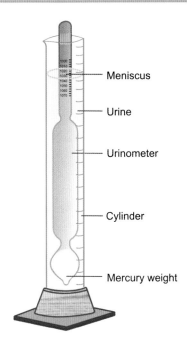

FIGURE 42.1 ◆ Urinometer and the container for floating it for measuring specific gravity.

Low specific gravity urine occurs in:
  i. Excess water intake
  ii. Diabetes insipidus

High specific gravity urine is seen in:
  i. Dehydration
  ii. Albuminuria
  iii. Glycosuria

Fixed specific gravity (1.010) of urine is seen in:
  i. ADH deficiency
  ii. Chronic nephritis

C. Chemical Examination

Chemical constituents frequently tested in urine are: proteins, glucose, ketones, bile derivatives and blood.

TESTS FOR PROTEINURIA

If urine is not clear, it should be filtered or centrifuged before testing. Urine may be tested for proteinuria by qualitative tests and quantitative methods.

Qualitative Tests for Proteinuria

1. Heat and acetic acid test
2. Sulphosalicylic acid test
3. Heller's test
4. Reagent strip method.

1. Heat and Acetic Acid Test

Heat causes coagulation of proteins. The procedure is as under:
◆ Take a 5 ml test tube.
◆ Fill 2/3rd with urine.
◆ Acidify by adding a few drops of 3% acetic acid if urine is alkaline.
◆ Boil upper portion for 2 minutes (lower part acts as control).
◆ If precipitation or turbidity appears, add a few drops of 3% acetic acid.

Interpretation. If turbidity or precipitation disappears on addition of acetic acid, it is due to phosphates; if it persists after addition of acetic acid, then it is due to proteins. The test is semiquantitative and can be graded from traces to 4+ depending upon amount of protein as under (Fig. 42.2):

No cloudiness	=	Negative
Faint cloudiness	=	Traces (less than 0.1 g/dl).
Cloudiness without granularity	=	+(0.1 g/dl).
Granular cloudiness	=	++(0.1-0.2 g/dl)
Precipitation and flocculation	=	+++(0.2-0.4 g/dl).
Thick solid precipitation	=	++++ (≥ 0.5 g/dl).

2. Sulphosalicylic Acid Test

This is a very reliable test. The procedure is as under:
◆ Make urine acidic by adding 3% acetic acid.
◆ To 2 ml of urine add a few drops (4-5) of 20% sulphosalicylic acid.

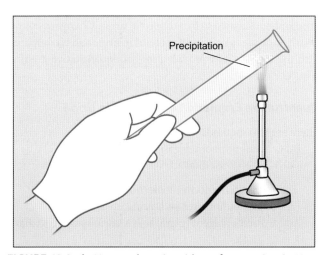

FIGURE 42.2 ◆ Heat and acetic acid test for proteinuria. Note the method of holding the tube from the bottom while heating the upper part.

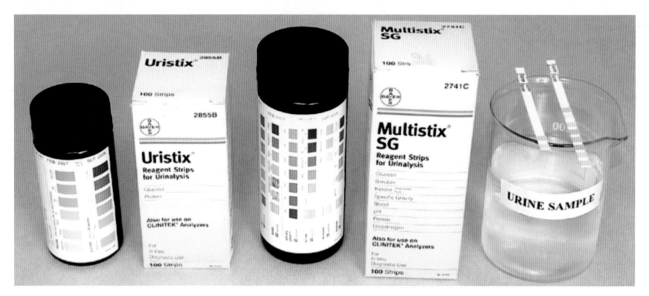

FIGURE 42.3 ◆ Strip method for testing various constituents in urine. Multistix 10 SG, and Uristix (Photograph courtesy of Bayer Diagnostics, Baroda, India).

Interpretation. Appearance of turbidity which persists after heating indicates presence of proteins.

3. Heller's Test

◆ Take 2 ml of concentrated nitric acid in a test tube.
◆ Add urine drop by drop by the side of test tube.

Interpretation. Appearance of white ring at the junction indicates presence of protein.

4. Reagent Strip Method

Bromophenol coated strip is dipped in urine. Change in colour of strip indicates presence of proteins in urine and is compared with the colour chart provided for semiquantitative grading (Fig. 42.3).

Quantitative Estimation of Proteins in Urine

There are two methods:
1. Esbach's albuminometer method
2. Turbidimetric method

1. Esbach's albuminometer method
◆ Fill the albuminometer with urine up to mark U.
◆ Add Esbach's reagent (picric acid + citric acid) up to mark R (Fig. 42.4).
◆ Stopper the tube, mix it and let it stand for 24 hours.
◆ Take the reading from the level of precipitation in the albuminometer tube and divide it by 10 to get the percentage of proteins.

2. Turbidimetric method
◆ Take 1 ml of urine and 1 ml standard in two separate tubes.
◆ Add 4 ml of trichloroacetic acid to each tube.
◆ After 5 minutes take the reading with red filter (680 nm).

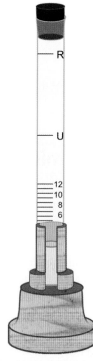

FIGURE 42.4 ◆ Esbach's albuminometer for quantitative estimation of proteins (U = urine; R = Esbach's reagent).

Causes of Proteinuria

Normally, there is a very scanty amount of protein in urine (< 150 mg/day).

- *Heavy proteinuria* (> 3 gm/day) occurs due to:
  i. Nephrotic syndrome
  ii. Renal vein thrombosis
  iii. Diabetes mellitus
  iv. SLE
- *Moderate proteinuria* (1-3 gm/day) is seen in:
  i. Chronic glomerulonephritis
  ii. Nephrosclerosis
  iii. Multiple myeloma
  iv. Pyelonephritis
- *Mild proteinuria* (< 1.0 gm/day) occurs in:
  i. Hypertension
  ii. Polycystic kidney
  iii. Chronic pyelonephritis
  iv. UTI
  v. Fever.
- *Microalbuminuria* is excretion of albumin 30-300 mg/day or random urine albumin/creatinine ratio of 30-300 mg/ gm creatinine and is indicative of early and possibly reversible glomerular damage from hypertension and risk factor for cardiovascular disease. *Microalbuminuria* is estimated by radioimmunoassay.

Test for Bence Jones Proteinuria

Bence Jones proteins are light chains of γ-globulin. These are excreted in multiple myeloma and other paraproteinaemias.

In heat and acetic acid test performed under temperature control, these proteins are precipitated at lower temperature (56°C) and disappear on further heating above 90°C but reappear on cooling to lower temperature again. In case both albumin and Bence Jones proteins are present in urine, the sample of urine is heated to boiling. Precipitates so formed due to albumin are filtered out and the test for Bence Jones proteins is repeated under temperature control as above.

TEST FOR GLUCOSURIA

Glucose is by far the most important of the sugars which may appear in urine. Normally, approximately 130 mg of glucose in urine is passed per 24 hours which is undetectable by qualitative tests.

Tests for glucosuria may be qualitative or quantitative.

Qualitative Tests

These are as under:
1. Benedict's test
2. Reagent strip test

1. *Benedict's test*

In this test cupric ion is reduced by glucose to cuprous oxide and a coloured precipitate is formed.

Procedure
- Take 5 ml of Benedict's qualitative reagent in a test tube.
- Add 8 drops (or 0.5 ml) of urine.
- Heat to boiling for 2 minutes (Fig. 42.5).
- Cool in water bath or in running tap water and look for colour change and precipitation.

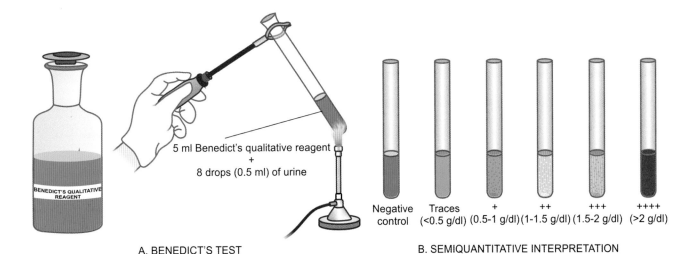

5 ml Benedict's qualitative reagent
+
8 drops (0.5 ml) of urine

BENEDICT'S QUALITATIVE REAGENT

A. BENEDICT'S TEST

Negative control | Traces (<0.5 g/dl) | + (0.5-1 g/dl) | ++ (1-1.5 g/dl) | +++ (1.5-2 g/dl) | ++++ (>2 g/dl)

B. SEMIQUANTITATIVE INTERPRETATION

FIGURE 42.5 ◆ **A,** Method for Benedict's test (qualitative) for glucosuria. The test sample shows brick red precipitation (++++). **B,** Semiquantitative interpretation of glucosuria by Benedict's test.

Interpretation

No change of blue colour	=	Negative
Greenish colour	=	Traces (< 0.5 g/dl)
Green/cloudy green ppt	=	+ (0.5-1 g/dl)
Yellow ppt	=	++ (1-1.5 g/dl)
Orange ppt	=	+++ (1.5-2 g/dl)
Brick red ppt	=	++++ (> 2 g/dl)

Since Benedict's test is for reducing substances excreted in the urine, the test is positive for all reducing sugars (glucose, fructose, maltose, lactose *but not for sucrose which is a non-reducing sugar*) and other reducing substances (e.g. ascorbic acid, salicylates, antibiotics, L-dopa).

2. Reagent strip test

These strips are coated with glucose oxidase and the test is based on enzymatic reaction. This test is specific for glucose. The strip is dipped in urine for 10 seconds. If there is change in colour of strip it indicates presence of glucose. The colour change is matched with standard colour chart provided on the label of the reagent strip bottle (see Fig. 42.3).

Quantitative Test for Glucose

Procedure. Take 25 ml of quantitative Benedict's reagent in a conical flask. Add to it 15 gm of sodium carbonate (crystalline) and some pieces of porcelain and heat it to boil. Add urine to it from a burette slowly till there is disappearance of blue colour of Benedict's reagent. Note the volume of urine used. Calculate the amount of glucose present in urine as under:

$$\frac{0.05 \times 100}{\text{Amount of urine}}$$

(0.05 gm of glucose reduces 25 ml of Benedict's reagent).

Causes of Glucosuria

   i. Diabetes mellitus
  ii. Renal glucosuria
 iii. Severe burns
 iv. Administration of corticosteroids
  v. Severe sepsis
 vi. Pregnancy

TESTS FOR KETONURIA

These are products of incomplete fat metabolism. The three ketone bodies excreted in urine are: acetoacetic acid (20%), acetone (2%), and β-hydroxybutyric acid (78%).

Tests for Ketonuria

1. Rothera's test
2. Gerhardt's test
3. Reagent strip test

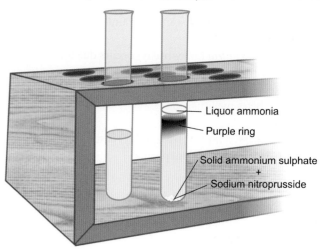

FIGURE 42.6 ◆ Rothera's test for ketone bodies in urine showing purple coloured ring in positive test.

1. Rothera's Test

Principle. Ketone bodies (acetone and acetoacetic acid) combine with alkaline solution of sodium nitroprusside forming purple complex.

Procedure
- Take 5 ml of urine in a test tube.
- Saturate it with solid ammonium sulphate salt; it will start settling to the bottom of the tube when saturated.
- Add a few crystals of sodium nitroprusside and shake.
- Add liquor ammonia from the side of test tube.

Interpretation. Appearance of purple or permanganate coloured ring at the junction indicates presence of ketone bodies (Fig. 42.6).

2. Gerhardt's Test

It is not a very sensitive test.

Procedure
- Take 5 ml of urine in a test tube.
- Add 10% ferric chloride solution drop by drop.
- Filter it and add more ferric chloride.

Interpretation. Brownish-red colour indicates presence of ketone bodies.

3. Reagent Strip Test

These strips are coated with alkaline sodium nitroprusside. When strip is dipped in urine it turns purple if ketone bodies are present (See Fig. 42.3).

Causes of Ketonuria

i. Diabetic ketoacidosis
ii. Dehydration
iii. Hyperemesis gravidarum
iv. Fever
v. Cachexia
vi. After general anaesthesia

TEST FOR BILE DERIVATIVES IN URINE

Three bile derivatives excreted in urine are: urobilinogen, bile salts and bile pigments. While urobilinogen is normally excreted in urine in small amounts, bile salts and bile pigments appear in urine in liver diseases only.

Tests for Bile Salts

Bile salts excreted in urine are cholic acid and chenodeoxycholic acid. Tests for bile salts are Hay's test and strip method.

1. Hay's Test

Principle. Bile salts if present in urine lower the surface tension of the urine.

Procedure
◆ Fill a 50 or 100 ml beaker 2/3rd to 3/4th with urine.
◆ Sprinkle finely powdered sulphur powder over it (Fig. 42.7).

Interpretation. If bile salts are present in the urine then sulphur powder sinks, otherwise it floats.

2. Reagent Strip Method

Coated strips can be used for detecting bile salts as for other constituents in urine (see Fig. 41.3).

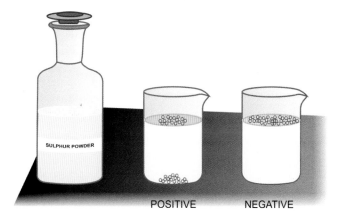

SULPHUR POWDER

POSITIVE   NEGATIVE

FIGURE 42.7 ◆ Hay's test for bile salts in urine. The test is positive in beaker in the centre contrasted with negative control in beaker on right side.

Cause for Bile Salts in Urine

Obstructive jaundice

Tests for Urobilinogen

Normally a small amount of urobilinogen is excreted in urine (4 mg/24 hr). The sample should always be collected in a dark coloured bottle as urobilinogen gets oxidised on exposure to light.

Tests for urobilinogen in urine are Ehrlich's test and reagent strip test.

1. Ehrlich's Test

Principle. Urobilinogen in urine combines with Ehrlich's aldehyde reagent to give a red purple coloured compound.

Procedure
◆ Take 10 ml of urine in a test tube.
◆ Add 1 ml of Ehrlich's aldehyde reagent.
◆ Wait for 3-5 minutes.
◆ If the test is positive, the test is repeated by preparing multiple dilutions, e.g. 1:10, 1:20, 1:40 and so on.

Interpretation. Development of red purple colour indicates presence of urobilinogen. A positive test is subsequently done in dilutions; normally it is positive in up to 1:20 dilution.

2. Reagent Strip Test

These strips are coated with p-dimethyl-amino-benzaldehyde. When strip is dipped in urine, it turns reddish-brown if urobilinogen is present (see Fig. 42.3).

Significance
Causes of increased urobilinogen in urine
    Haemolytic jaundice and haemolytic anaemia

Causes for absent urobilinogen in urine
    Obstructive jaundice

Tests for Bilirubin (Bile Pigment) in Urine

Bilirubin is breakdown product of haemoglobin. Normally, no bilirubin is passed in urine.

Following tests are done for detection of bilirubin in urine:
1. Fouchet's test
2. Foam test
3. Reagent strip test

1. Fouchet's Test

Principle. Ferric chloride oxidises bilirubin to green biliverdin.

Procedure
- Take 10 ml of urine in a test tube.
- Add 3-5 ml of 10% barium chloride.
- Filter through filter paper.
- To the precipitate on filter paper, add a few drops of Fouchet's reagent (ferric chloride + trichloroacetic acid).

Interpretation. Development of green colour indicates bilirubin.

2. Foam Test

It is a non-specific test.

Procedure
- Take 5/10 ml of urine in a test tube.
- Shake it vigorously.

Interpretation. Presence of yellow foam at the top indicates presence of bilirubin.

3. Reagent Strip Test

Principle. It is based on coupling reaction of bilirubin with diazonium salt with which strip is coated. Dip the strip in urine; if it changes to blue colour then bilirubin is present (see Fig. 42.3).

Causes of bilirubinuria
  i. Obstructive jaundice
  ii. Hepatocellular jaundice

TESTS FOR BLOOD IN URINE

Tests for detection of blood in urine are as under:
1. Benzidine test
2. Orthotoluidine test
3. Reagent strip test

1. Benzidine Test

Procedure
- Take 2 ml of urine in a test tube.

- Add 2 ml of saturated solution of benzidine with glacial acetic acid.
- Add 1 ml of H_2O_2 to it.

Interpretation. Appearance of blue colour indicates presence of blood. Benzidine is, however, carcinogenic and this test is not commonly used.

2. Orthotoluidine Test

Procedure
- Take 2 ml of urine in a test tube.
- Add a solution of 1 ml of orthotoluidine in glacial acetic acid.
- Add a few drops of H_2O_2.

Interpretation. Blue or green colour indicates presence of blood in urine.

3. Reagent Strip Test

The reagent strip is coated with orthotoluidine. Dip the strip in urine. If it changes to blue colour then blood is present (see Fig. 42.3).

Causes of blood in urine
  i. Renal stones
  ii. Renal tumours
  iii. Polycystic kidney
  iv. Bleeding disorders
  v. Trauma.

Automated Urinalysis

Currently, fully automated urine chemistry reagent strip analysers are available which are equipped to perform automatic pipetting or test strip dipping, as well as carry out photometric measurement of reagent strip fields. The end result readings can be taken as a printout.

Urine Examination II: Microscopy

Objectives

➤ To learn the method of making wet preparation of urine and its microscopic examination and interpretation.
➤ To be familiar with various formed elements seen in the sediment of urine in routine microscopic examination.

Microscopic examination of urine is discussed under four headings:

A. Collection of sample
B. Preparation of sediment
C. Examination of sediment
D. Automation in urine analysis

A. Collection of Sample

First voided urine sample in the morning is the best specimen. It provides an acidic and concentrated sample which preserves the formed elements (RBCs, WBCs and casts) which otherwise tend to lyse in a hypotonic or alkaline urine. The specimen should be examined fresh or within 1-2 hours of collection. But if some delay is anticipated, the sample should be preserved as described in the preceding exercise.

B. Preparation of Sediment

♦ Take 5-10 ml of urine in a centrifuge tube.
♦ Centrifuge for 5 minutes at 3000 rpm.
♦ Discard the supernatant.
♦ Resuspend the deposit in about one ml of urine left and shake it well.
♦ Place a drop of this on a clean glass slide.
♦ Place a coverslip over it and examine it under the microscope.

C. Examination of Sediment

Urine is an unstained preparation and its microscopic examination is routinely done under reduced light using the light microscope. This is done by keeping the condenser low with partial closure of iris diaphragm. First examine it under low power objective, then under high power and keep on changing the fine adjustment in order to visualise the sediments in different planes and report as number of cells per high power field (cells/HPF). Phase contrast microscopy may be used for more translucent formed elements. Rarely, polarising microscopy is used to distinguish crystals and fibres from cellular or protein casts.

Following categories of constituents are frequently reported in the urine on microscopic examination:

1. Cells (RBCs, WBCs, epithelial cells)
2. Casts
3. Crystals
4. Miscellaneous structures

These are discussed below.

1. CELLS IN URINE

These include RBCs, WBCs, and epithelial cells.

RBCs

These appear as pale or yellowish, biconcave, double-contoured, disc-like structures, and when viewed from side

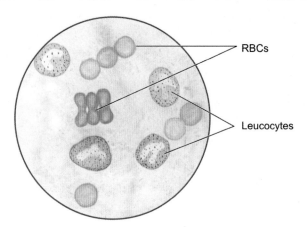

FIGURE 43.1 ◆ RBCs and WBCs in the urine sediment.

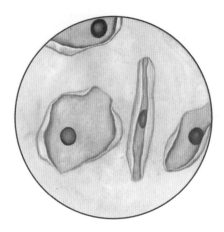

FIGURE 43.2 ◆ Squamous epithelial cells in urine, frequently seen in females.

they have an hourglass appearance. In hypotonic urine, RBCs swell up while in hypertonic urine they are crenated. They can be confused with WBCs, yeast and air bubbles/oil droplets but can be distinguished as under (Fig. 43.1):

i. The WBCs are larger in size than RBCs and are granular.
ii. Yeast cells appear round but show budding.
iii. Air bubbles and oil droplets vary in size. When edge of the coverslip is touched with a pencil, oil droplets tumble while RBCs do not.

Significance. Normally, 0-2 RBCs/HPF may be passed in urine. RBCs in excess of this number are seen in urine in the following conditions:

Physiological
i. Following severe exercise
ii. Smoking
iii. Lumbar lordosis

Pathological
i. Renal stones
ii. Kidney tumours
iii. Glomerulonephritis
iv. Polycystic kidney
v. Urinary tract infection (UTI)
vi. Trauma

WBCs

These appear as round granular 12-14 μm in diameter. In fresh urine nuclear details are well visualised (Fig. 43.1). WBCs can be confused with RBCs. For differentiating, add a drop of dilute acetic acid under coverslip. RBCs are lysed while nuclear details of WBCs become more clear. WBCs can also be stained by adding a drop of supravital stain, crystal violet or safranin stain.

Significance. Normally 0-4 WBCs/HPF may be present in females. WBCs are seen in urine in following conditions:

Pathological
i. UTI
ii. Cystitis
iii. Prostatitis
iv. Chronic pyelonephritis
v. Renal stones
vi. Renal tumours

Epithelial Cells

These are round to polygonal cells with a round to oval, small to large nucleus. Epithelial cells in urine can be squamous epithelial cells, tubular cells and transitional cells, i.e. they can be from lower or upper urinary tract, and sometime it is difficult to distinguish between different types of these cells. At times, these cells can be confused with cancer cells.

Significance. Normally a few epithelial cells are seen in normal urine, more common in females and reflect normal sloughing of these cells (Fig. 43.2).

When these cells are present in large number along with WBCs, they are indicative of inflammation.

2. CASTS IN URINE

These are formed due to moulding in renal tubules of solidified proteins. Their shape depends upon the level of tubules where formed. In general, casts are cylindrical in shape with rounded ends. The basic composition of casts is Tamm-Horsfall protein which is secreted by tubular cells. Casts appear in urine only in renal diseases.

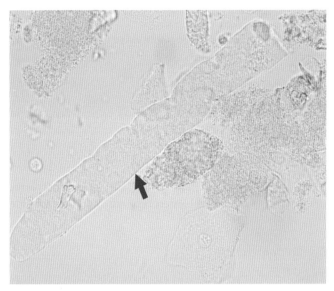

| A, HYALINE CAST | B, RED CELL CAST |

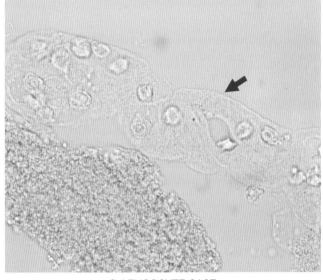

| C, LEUCOCYTE CAST | D, GRANULAR CAST |

FIGURE 43.3 ◆ Various types of casts in urine.

Depending upon the content, casts are of following types: hyaline cast, red cell cast, leucocyte cast, granular cast, waxy cast, fatty cast, epithelial cast and pigment cast (Fig. 43.3):

i.   Hyaline Cast

Hyaline cast is basic protein cast. These are cylindrical, colourless homogeneous and transparent (Fig. 43.3,A). They are passed in urine in the following conditions:

a.   Fever

b.   Exercise

c.   Acute glomerulonephritis

d.   Malignant hypertension

e.   Chronic renal disease

ii.   Red Cell Cast

These casts contain RBCs and have a yellowish-orange colour (Fig. 43.3,B). Glomerular damage results in appearance of RBCs into tubules. They are passed in urine in the following conditions:

a. Acute glomerulonephritis
b. Renal infarct
c. Goodpasture syndrome
d. Lupus nephritis

iii. Leucocyte Cast

These contain granular cells (WBCs) in a clear matrix. WBCs enter the tubular lumina from the interstitium (Fig. 43.3,C). They are passed in urine in the following conditions:
a. Acute pyelonephritis
b. Acute glomerulonephritis
c. Nephrotic syndrome
d. Lupus nephritis
e. Interstitial nephritis

iv. Granular Casts

Granular casts have coarse granules in basic matrix. Granules form from degenerating cells or solidification of plasma proteins (Fig. 43.3,D). They are passed in urine in the following conditions:
a. Pyelonephritis
b. Chronic lead poisoning
c. Viral diseases
d. Renal papillary necrosis

v. Waxy Casts

Waxy casts are yellowish homogeneous with irregular blunt or cracked ends and have high refractive index. These are also known as renal failure casts. They are passed in urine in the following conditions:
a. Chronic renal failure
b. End-stage kidney
c. Renal transplant rejection

vi. Fatty Cast

They contain fat globules of varying size which are highly refractile. Fat in the cast is cholesterol or triglycerides. These are passed in urine in the following conditions:
a. Nephrotic syndrome
b. Fat necrosis

vii. Epithelial Cast

Epithelial casts contain shed off tubular epithelial cells and appear as two parallel rows of cells. Sometimes these are difficult to differentiate from WBC casts. They are passed in urine in following conditions:
a. Acute tubular necrosis
b. Heavy metal poisoning
c. Renal transplant rejection

viii. Pigment Cast

Pigment casts include haemoglobin casts, haemosiderin casts, myoglobin casts, bilirubin cast, etc.

3. CRYSTALS IN URINE

Formation and appearance of crystals in urine depends upon pH of the urine, i.e. acidic or alkaline.

Crystals in Acidic Urine

These are as under: calcium oxalate, uric acid, amorphous urate, tyrosine, cystine, cholesterol crystals and sulphonamide (Fig. 43.4):

i) Calcium oxalate

These are colourless refractile and have octahedral envelope-like structure. They can also be dumb-bell shaped (Fig. 43.4,A).

ii) Uric acid

They are yellow or brown rhomboid-shaped seen singly or in rosettes. They can also be in the form of prism, plates and sheaves (Fig. 43.4,B).

iii) Amorphous urate

They appear as yellowish-brown granules in the form of clumps (Fig. 43.4,C). They dissolve on heating. When they are made of sodium urate, they are needle-like in the form of thorn-apple. They are passed more often in patients having gout.

iv) Tyrosine

They are yellowish in the form of silky needles or sheaves (Fig. 43.4,D). They are passed in urine in jaundice.

v) Cystine

They are colourless, hexagonal plates which are highly refractile (Fig. 43.4,E). They are passed in urine in an inborn error of metabolism, cystinuria.

vi) Cholesterol crystals

These are rare and are seen in urinary tract infection, rupture of lymphatic into renal pelvis or due to blockage of lymphatics (Fig. 43.4,F).

vii) Sulphonamide

They appear as yellowish sheaves, rosettes, or rounded with radial striations (Fig. 43.4,G). They appear in urine after administration of sulphonamide drugs.

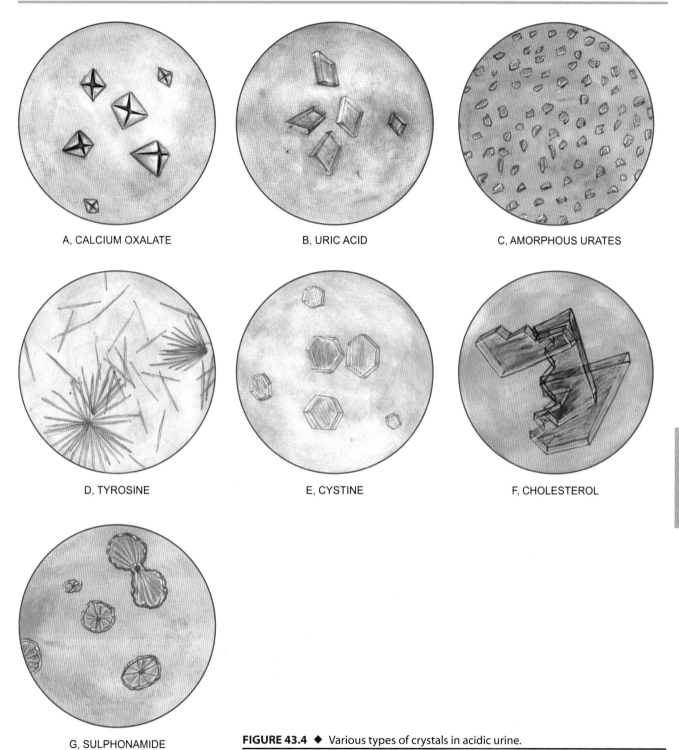

A, CALCIUM OXALATE

B, URIC ACID

C, AMORPHOUS URATES

D, TYROSINE

E, CYSTINE

F, CHOLESTEROL

G, SULPHONAMIDE

FIGURE 43.4 ◆ Various types of crystals in acidic urine.

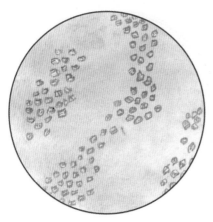

A, AMORPHOUS PHOSPHATES

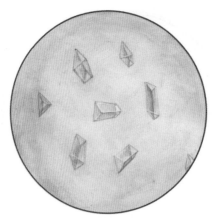

B, TRIPLE PHOSPHATES

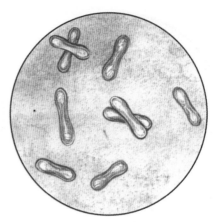

C, CALCIUM CARBONATE

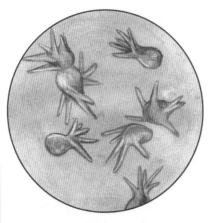

D, AMMONIUM BIURATES

FIGURE 43.5 ◆ Various types of crystals in alkaline urine.

Crystals in Alkaline Urine

These are as under: amorphous phosphate, triple phosphate, calcium carbonate and ammonium biurate (Fig. 43.5):

i) Amorphous phosphate

They are seen as colourless granules in the form of clumps or irregular aggregates (Fig. 43.5,A). They dissolve when urine is made acidic.

ii) Triple phosphate

They are in the form of prisms and sometimes in fern leaf pattern (Fig. 43.5,B). They dissolve when urine is made acidic.

iii) Calcium carbonate

They are in the form of granules, spheres or rarely dumbbell-shaped (Fig. 43.5,C). They again dissolve in acidic urine.

iv) Ammonium biurate

They are round or oval yellowish-brown spheres with thorns on their surface giving 'thorn apple' appearance (Fig. 43.5,D). They dissolve on heating the urine or by making it acidic.

4. MISCELLANEOUS STRUCTURES IN URINE

These include the following: spermatozoa, parasite, fungus and tumour cells (Fig. 43.6):

i) Spermatozoa

They can be seen in normal urine in males. They have a head and tail and can be motile (Fig. 43.6,A).

ii) Parasites

Urine may contain *Trichomonas vaginalis* which is more common in females (Fig. 43.6,B). Eggs of *Schistosoma hematobium* or *Entamoeba histolytica* can also be seen in urine.

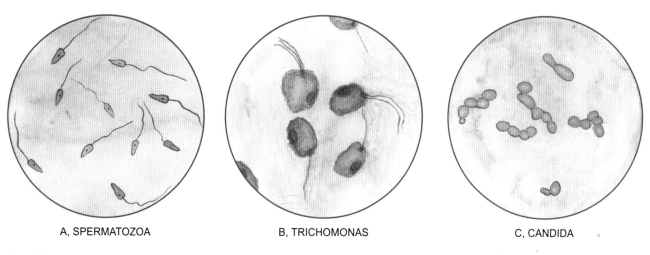

A, SPERMATOZOA   B, TRICHOMONAS   C, CANDIDA

FIGURE 43.6 ◆ Miscellaneous structures in urine.

iii) Fungus

Candida which are budding yeast cells can be seen in urine in patients with UTI or as contaminant (Fig. 43.6,C).

iv) Tumour cells

Tumour cells having all the characteristics of malignancy may be seen singly or in groups in urine. These tumour cells could be from kidney, ureter, bladder or urethra. These cells are examined after staining of urine sediment.

D. Automation in Urine Analysis

In the recent times, automated urine analysis has been made possible by one of the following techniques:

URINE STRIP ANALYSERS

These are commercially available electronic urine strip readers. These strips may include various parameters of physical, chemical and microscopic constituents. After analysis, the results are obtained as printout.

FLOW CYTOMETRY

Just as flow cytometry is used for blood and other body fluids, urine can be analysed by flow cytometry. In this method, DNA and membranes of formed elements are stained and pass as a laminar flow through a laser beam and the light scatter is measured by fluorescence impedance.

Exercise 44

Semen Analysis

Objectives
➢ To learn the method of sample collection, gross inspection and routine microscopic analysis of semen sample.
➢ To be briefly familiar with various chemical, immunological, microbiological and function tests of semen.

Semen examination is an inexpensive test done for the following indications:
1. Infertility (in couples who fail to conceive after 6 months of unprotected coitus)
2. Success of vasectomy
3. Success of varicocele surgery (after 3-4 months of surgery)
4. Medicolegal cases, e.g. rape

Analysis of semen consists of the following:
A. Sample collection
B. Gross examination
C. Microscopic examination
D. Chemical examination
E. Immunological assays
F. Microbiological assays
G. Sperm function tests
H. Semen cryopreservation

Sample Collection

Patient is instructed to collect the specimen by masturbation after 3-5 days of sexual abstinence. The sample is collected in a clean glass tube, wide-mouthed container or in a properly washed dry condom. The sample is submitted in the laboratory immediately but preferably within one hour of collection for examination. Two specimens collected at 2-3 weeks interval are used for evaluation.

Gross Examination

Semen is examined grossly for the following features: colour, volume, viscosity, reaction and liquefaction.

1. Colour. Normally it is whitish, grey-white or slightly yellowish.

2. Volume. Normally, volume of semen is between 2.5 and 5 ml. The volume is slightly more in patients of infertility. The volume does not vary with the period of abstinence.

3. Viscosity. When ejaculated, semen is fairly viscid and it falls drop by drop.

4. Reaction. Normally, it is slightly alkaline with pH between 7 and 8.

5. Liquefaction. Liquefaction occurs because of presence of fibrinolysin. Normally liquefaction occurs at room temperature within 10-30 minutes (average 20 minutes).

Microscopic Examination

Semen is examined microscopically for the following: motility, count and morphology.

MOTILITY

Place a drop of liquefied semen on a clean glass slide. Put a coverslip over it and examine it under the microscope, first under low power and then under high power. Normally within 2 hours of ejaculation, more than 60% of spermatozoa are vigorously motile, and in 6-8 hours 25-40% are still motile. If motility is less than 50%, a stain for viability such as eosin Y with nigrosin as counterstain can be done. Heads of non-motile sperms show red dye.

COUNT

This is done in Neubauer's (haemacytometer) chamber using a WBC pipette. Draw liquefied semen in WBC pipette up to mark 0.5 and then draw the diluting fluid up to mark 11. The composition of diluting fluid is as under:

Sodium bicarbonate	5 gm
Formalin (neutral)	1 ml
Distilled water	100 ml

After mixing it properly, charge the Neubauer's chamber. Allow the spermatozoa to settle down in 2 minutes. Examine under microscope and count the number of spermatozoa in two large peripheral squares (used for TLC counting) and multiply the number by 1 lakh (100,000) which gives number of spermatozoa per millilitre:

In $1 \times 1 \times 0.1$ µl volume,

number of spermatozoa $= n \times 10$

But dilution factor is 10

$\therefore$ Number of spermatozoa per µl $= n \times 10 \times 10$

or Number of spermatozoa per ml $= n \times 10 \times 10 \times 1000$

$= n \times 100,000$

i.e. $n \times 1$ lakh

(where n is the average number of spermatozoa counted in two squares).

Normal value	=	> 60 million/ml
Abnormal value	=	< 20 million/ml.

MORPHOLOGY

Prepare a thin smear from liquefied semen on a glass slide. Stain it with any of the Romanowsky stains, Pap or H & E stain. Observe at least 200 spermatozoa for any abnormality in their morphology. Normally 80% of spermatozoa are normal (Fig. 44.1). The abnormal forms of spermatozoa are with double head, swollen and pointed head, double tail and rudimentery forms. Also look for the presence of RBCs or WBCs, if any. Computer-assisted morphologic screening is particularly useful in samples with very low numbers of normal sperm count which may otherwise remain undetected.

Chemical Examination

Chemical analysis of semen consists of 2 main tests: fructose test and acid phosphatase test.

FRUCTOSE TEST

This test determines androgen deficiency or ejaculatory obstruction to semen; the level of seminal fructose is low in both these conditions. Normal seminal fructose level is 150-600 mg/dl.

Fructose is measured qualitatively by resorcinol test.

Procedure
- Take 5 ml of dilute HCl in a test tube.
- Add 1 ml of semen.
- Add 5 mg of resorcinol.
- Boil.

Interpretation. Appearance of red colour indicates presence of fructose which can be measured by spectrophotometer.

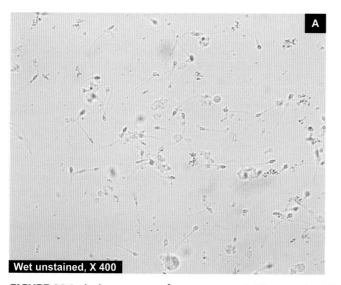
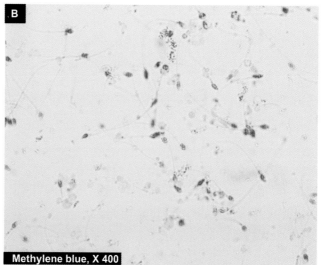

Wet unstained, X 400

Methylene blue, X 400

FIGURE 44.1 ◆ Appearance of spermatozoa. **A,** Wet unstained **B,** Wet preparation stained with methylene blue.

ACID PHOSPHATASE TEST

This test is used for seminal stain and on vaginal aspirate in medicolegal cases. Normally semen has 2500 KA units/ml of acid phosphatase.

Immunological Assays

The presence of sperm antibody binding to head or tail antigens is considered specific for immunologic infertility. The antibodies are usually of immunoglobulin A (IgA) or IgG, and rarely of IgM class. These are detected by direct or indirect mixed agglutination reaction tests.

Microbiological Assays

Genital tract infections by bacteria, yeast and sexually-transmitted diseases may have significant adverse effect on male infertility. If the concentration of bacteria exceeds 1000 CFUs per ml, the colonies should be identified and tested for antibiotic sensitivity.

Sperm Function Tests

Defective sperm function may affect various fertilising functions. Most importantly, it includes transport of sperm in the male and female reproductive tracts, which is responsible for fertilisation activities such as specific zona binding, penetration and formation of male pronucleus. A list of common sperm function tests is as under:

1. *Sperm penetration assay*: to test the success of penetration of egg by the spermatozoa
2. *Hypoosmotic swelling test*: to test the membrane integrity of the sperm
3. *Cervical mucus penetration test*: to test the relative ability of motile sperms to pass through cervical mucus of the partner collected at midcycle.

Semen Cryopreservation

Cryopreservation or semen banking is indicated in the following conditions:

1. For assisted reproduction
2. For donor insemination
3. For men undergoing vasectomy
4. In men before starting cancer therapy
5. In life threatening jobs (e.g. military service)

Examination of CSF

Objectives
➤ To learn the method of specimen collection of CSF and to know the various parameters of normal physical and chemical composition and microscopic findings.
➤ To be familiar with CSF abnormalities of various parameters in different types of meningitis.

Most of the CSF (70%) is produced by choroid plexus in the lateral, third and fourth ventricle while the remainder is produced by the surface of brain and spinal cord. CSF examination is an important part of neurologic evaluation in non-neoplastic and neoplastic diseases of CNS. It includes its physical characters, chemical composition, and microscopic findings, and in some instances microbiologic and immunologic tests.

Normal Composition of CSF

Appearance	:	Clear and colourless
Rate of production	:	500 ml/day
Total volume	:	120-150 ml in adults, 10-60 ml in neonates
Specific gravity	:	1.006-1.008
Normal pressure	:	60-150 mm of water in adults, 10-100 mm water in infants
Sugar	:	50-80 mg/dl (i.e. 60% of plasma value)
Proteins	:	15-45 mg/dl
Chloride	:	720-760 mg% (i.e. same as in plasma)
Cells	:	0-4 leucocytes/ml (0-30 leucocytes/ml in neonates)
Bacteria	:	Nil

Examination of CSF is discussed under the following headings:
A. Specimen collection
B. Microscopic examination
C. Chemical examination
D. Microbiological examination
E. Immunological examination

Specimen Collection

CSF is obtained by the following techniques:
    i. Lumbar puncture
    ii. Cisternal puncture
    iii. Ventricular cannulas or shunts
    iv. Lateral cervical puncture

Normally, up to 2 ml of CSF is withdrawn. Most often, CSF tap is done by lumbar puncture for which indications can be divided into following 4 categories:
a. Meningeal infection
b. Subarachnoid haemorrhage
c. CNS malignant tumours
d. Demyelinating diseases.

The specimen should be transported to the laboratory immediately and processed within one hour, otherwise cellular degradation occurs giving incorrect results. In case delay in examination of CSF is anticipated, the sample may be refrigerated, except for microbial culture. Various parameters of normal CSF in comparison with various types of meningitis are given in Table 45.1.

	Feature	Normal	Acute pyogenic (bacterial meningitis)	Acute lymphocytic (viral meningitis)	Chronic (tuberculosis meningitis)
TABLE 45.1: CSF findings in health and various types of meningitis.					
1.	**Naked eye appearance**	Clear and colourless	Cloudy or frankly purulent	Clear or slightly turbid	Clear of slightly turbid, forms fibrin coagulum on standing
2.	**CSF pressure**	60-150 mm water	Elevated (above 180 mm water)	Elevated (above 250 mm water)	Elevated (above 300 mm water)
3.	**Cells**	0-4 lympho-cytes/ml	1,000-100,000 neutrophils/ml	10-100 mononuclears/ml	100-1,000 mononuclears/ml
4.	**Proteins**	15-45 mg/dl	Raised	Raised	Raised
5.	**Glucose**	50-80 mg/dl	Reduced (usually less than 40 mg/dl)	Normal	Reduced (usually less than 45 mg/dl)
6.	**Bacteriology**	Sterile	Causative organisms present	Sterile	Tubercle bacilli present

Microscopic Examination

It involves TLC and DLC in the CSF.

TOTAL LEUCOCYTE COUNT

TLC in CSF can be done by manual method or automated method.

Manual Method

The number of WBCs in CSF is quite low and hence counting of these cells is done in undiluted sample of CSF. Either of the counting chambers—Fuchs-Rosenthal or improved Neubauer's chamber, may be used; the former being better since its depth is 0.2 mm and hence cells are counted in greater volume of CSF. WBC counting is done in all the peripheral squares (1 mm² area in each).

Calculations for Fuchs-Rosenthal chamber (counting in 18 squares):

Number of WBCs in 18 mm² × 0.2 mm depth (i.e. 3.6 μl)

$$= n$$

$$\text{Number of WBC in 1 } \mu l = \frac{n}{3.6}$$

Calculations for improved Neubauer's chamber (counting in 4 squares):

Number of WBCs in 4 mm² × 0.1 mm depth (i.e. 0.4 μl)

$$= n$$

$$\text{Number of WBC in 1 } \mu l = \frac{n}{0.4}$$

Automated Method

Automated method employs use of electronic particle counter as for TLC in blood. In these methods, results are not good if counts are too low.

DIFFERENTIAL LEUCOCYTE COUNT

Centrifuge or cytocentrifuge a small amount of CSF; prepare smears from the sediment. Stain one of the smears with any of the Romanowsky stain and examine under high power and oil immersion of microscope for the presence of various cells. The various cells which may be seen in CSF are as under:

   i. neutrophils,
   ii. lymphocytes,
   iii. plasma cells,
   iv. monocytes, and
   v. malignant cells.

Conditions causing increased neutrophils in CSF
   i. Bacterial meningitis
   ii. Brain abscess
   iii. Brain infarct
   iv. Repeated lumbar puncture

Conditions causing increased lymphocytes in CSF
   i. Viral meningitis
   ii. Tuberculous meningitis
   iii. Parasitic meningitis
   iv. Fungal infections

Conditions causing plasma cells in CSF
   i. Tuberculous meningitis
   ii. Syphilitic meningoencephalitis

iii. Multiple myeloma
iv. Malignant brain tumours

Conditions causing lymphocytes and monocytes in CSF
i. Viral meningitis
ii. Degenerative brain disorders
iii. Tuberculous meningitis
iv. Fungal meningitis
v. Sarcoidosis of meninges

Conditions causing malignant cells in CSF
i. Metastatic cancers
ii. Leukaemias
iii. Lymphomas
iv. Medulloblastoma
v. Ependymoma

Chemical Examination

Sugar, proteins, chloride and enzymes, ammonia and amines, electrolytes and acid-base balance and tumour markers can be estimated in CSF.

CSF findings in various types of meningitis are summarised in Table 45.1.

Microbiological Examination

Smears from CSF can also be stained with Gram's stain for bacteria and Ziehl-Neelsen's stain for AFB and India ink for the capsule of *Cryptococcus*.

CSF can be subjected to culture of the following:
i. Bacteria
ii. Tubercle bacilli
iii. Fungus

Immunological Examination

CSF can be required for demonstration of the following:
i. Viral inclusions by immunostains
ii. PCR for viral DNA and tuberculosis
iii. ELISA for tuberculosis
iv. VDRL for syphilis.

Section Six

HAEMATOLOGY

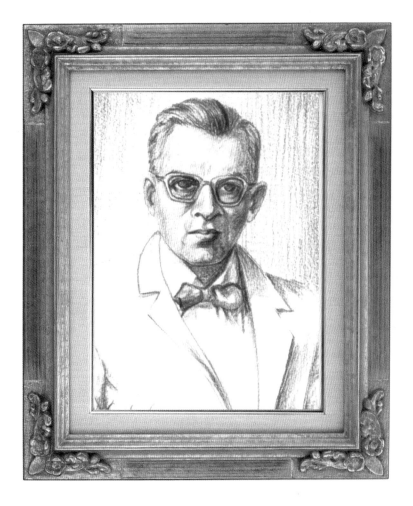

MM WINTROBE (1901–1986)

American physician, who devised Wintrobe haematocrit tube for estimation of
PCV and ESR and thus enabled measuring red cell indices.
Wintrobe was a pupil of William Loyd, a pioneering teacher
and eminent author of last century.

Section Contents

Types of Blood Samples, Anticoagulants and Blood Collection

Objectives
➢ To learn the types of blood samples for investigations and various anticoagulants used in a haematology laboratory.
➢ To learn method of collection of blood samples for various haematologic tests.

Before discussing anticoagulants and methods of blood sample collection, it is desirable to know the various types of blood samples submitted for investigations. Knowledge of anticoagulants used in haematology laboratory and the skill of blood collection for different tests are the basic requirements for the laboratory staff performing these tests. However, these are equally essential for all those who are sending samples and requests for such investigations.

Types of Blood Samples

There are 3 main types of blood samples submitted for tests: whole blood, serum and plasma (Fig. 46.1).

WHOLE BLOOD

Whole blood sample is the anticoagulated blood sample containing all formed elements as well as plasma.

Uses

  i. For complete haemogram or complete blood counts (CBC)
 ii. Foetal haemoglobin determination
iii. Osmotic fragility
 iv. Hb electrophoresis
  v. Coombs' test
 vi. Biochemical estimation of glucose, urea

SERUM

When freshly collected blood (without any anticoagulant) is allowed to stand in a tube for at least one hour, serum separates on the top while clotted blood retracts at the bottom of the tube. The yield of serum can be increased by centrifugation at 3000 rpm for 15 minutes. Serum does not contain most of the coagulation factors.

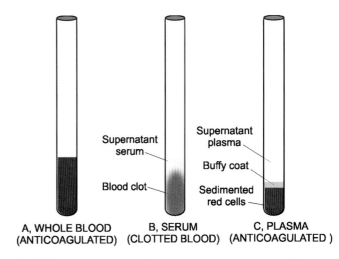

FIGURE 46.1 ◆ Tubes showing three main types of blood samples used for patient's investigations.

(187)

Uses

i. For quantitative biochemical determinations of most components of metabolism, enzymes, hormones, markers
ii. For electrophoresis of proteins and immunoglobulins
iii. Serum antibody tests.

PLASMA

Plasma is obtained by centrifugation of anticoagulated blood (compared from serum which is centrifugation of clotted blood). After centrifugation, the plasma lies as a supernatant in the tube, the bottom of the tube contains RBCs while other formed elements of blood (leucocytes, platelets) lie at the junction of plasma with sedimented RBCs.

Uses

i. Used for coagulation studies
ii. For factor assays
iii. For tests of products of coagulation, e.g. FDP, D-dimer test.

Anticoagulants

Anticoagulants are used to prevent clotting of the blood specimen in such a way that the anticoagulant does not cause any alteration in the blood plasma or formed elements. Although the choice of anticoagulant to be used depends upon the determination to be made, some of the commonly used anticoagulants in haematology laboratory are: ethylene-diaminetetraacetate (EDTA), sodium citrate, double oxalate, heparin and sodium fluoride.

1. EDTA

EDTA is by far the most commonly used anticoagulant in haematology laboratory. Generally, a dipotassium salt of EDTA is preferred over disodium salt due to higher solubility of the former. The mechanism of action of K_2EDTA as anticoagulant is by removal of free calcium from blood by chelation.

EDTA can be either used as a solid salt (2 mg/ml of blood), or as a 1% solution in distilled water (0.5 ml per 5 ml of blood) for anticoagulation.

Uses

i. Smears can be prepared from EDTA blood up to 4 hours after collection.
ii. Complete blood counts (CBC) (i.e. Hb, TLC, DLC, platelet count, RBC count, eosinophil count) can be done from EDTA sample within one hour.

iii. Can be used for ESR and PCV by Wintrobe's method.
iv. Ideal for use in cell counters.

However, EDTA blood sample is not used for coagulation studies.

2. SODIUM CITRATE

Sodium citrate is another commonly used anticoagulant. The salt used is trisodium citrate pentahydrate; 3.8% solution of this salt is prepared in distilled water. It prevents coagulation by loosely binding free calcium ions of the blood in a soluble complex, calcium citrate complex.

Uses

i. Citrate is anticoagulant of choice for coagulation studies; it is used as 3.8% in the ratio 1:9 between anticoagulant and the whole blood.
ii. Citrated blood is used for Westergren method of ESR determination; a ratio of 1:4 between citrate and blood is used (0.4 ml citrate+1.6 ml blood).

However, citrated blood is not suitable for other routine haematologic tests such as CBC, blood smear, etc. due to dilution of blood.

3. DOUBLE OXALATE

In haematology laboratory, a double oxalate is used as anticoagulant; sodium or potassium and ammonium oxalate in the ratio of 2:3 is used (4 mg sodium or potassium oxalate +6 mg ammonium oxalate per 10 ml of blood). Oxalate combines with calcium in the blood to form insoluble calcium oxalate, thereby preventing coagulation. Although both oxalates are independent anticoagulants, double oxalate is used in haematology since sodium oxalate causes cell shrinkage and ammonium oxalate causes swelling; hence net effect on the cell is counteracted by each other.

Uses

i. Widely used in coagulation studies
ii. Can be used for CBC and ESR and PCV by Wintrobe method as well.

4. HEPARIN

Heparin is more expensive and dissolves less readily in blood than double oxalate. However, it does not cause any cell distortion. Approximately, 0.5 to 1.0 mg is required per 5 ml of blood for anticoagulation.

Uses

i. Used for coagulation studies
ii. For red cell enzyme studies, e.g. G6PD and PK deficiency

iii. For osmotic fragility test

iv. Ideal for comparison of cellular distortion by any anticoagulant.

5. SODIUM FLUORIDE

Sodium fluoride is used for estimation of blood glucose and is not used for haematologic tests. It acts by inhibiting red cell glycolytic enzyme pathway.

Blood Collection

In most hospitals, there is common blood collection centre so that a patient does not have to visit different laboratories and does not have to suffer needle pricks again and again. The blood sample is collected by a trained phlebotomist or a trainee doctor. Blood may be collected by venipuncture or by prick for capillary blood. In general, following prerequisites need to be followed before venepuncture is done:

i. Patient's identity is available.

ii. A proper request form (or more than one request form) tallying with patient's identity is available.

iii. Appropriate test tubes for sample collection is labeled.

iv. For biochemical tests, the patient should be made aware to come fasting (after overnight fast) to avoid errors in reading due to ingested food.

v. Correct volume of blood sample should be collected in appropriate vacutainer meant for particular tests. These are generally colour-coded (Fig. 46.2).

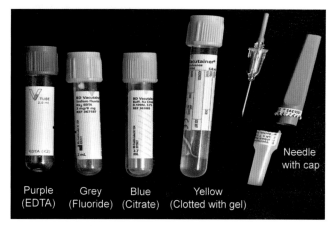

Purple (EDTA)   Grey (Fluoride)   Blue (Citrate)   Yellow (Clotted with gel)   Needle with cap

FIGURE 46.2 ◆ Colour-coded caps of vacutainers used in laboratory. In addition to coloured caps shown, vacutainer with red cap is also available which is used for collection of clotted blood but without gel in it.

vi. Capillary blood is collected by puncture of heal in infants or children, and by pricking ring fingertip in older patients. Capillary blood can be used for routine blood tests (e.g. Hb, preparing blood smear, for blood counts, etc).

vii. Arterial blood is collected for blood gas analysis, most often from femoral artery.

Haemoglobin Estimation

Objectives
➢ To learn the various methods of haemoglobin estimation.
➢ To have an overview of quality control in haemoglobin estimation.

Haemoglobin (Hb) is the main component of red blood cells and is a conjugated protein. A molecule of Hb contains two pairs of polypeptide chains $\alpha_2 \beta_2$ and four haem groups each having an atom of ferrous iron. Approximately 34% of the RBCs by weight is Hb. Iron content of Hb is 0.347 gm/100 g. The main function of Hb is to transport oxygen from lungs to the tissues. There are various forms of Hb as under:

  i. Oxyhaemoglobin (Hb O_2)
  ii. Carboxy haemoglobin (Hb CO)
  iii. Sulfhaemoglobin (SHb)
  iv. Methaemoglobin (Hi)

The mass of red blood cells can be measured by Hb estimation; the measurement of Hb concentration in the blood is known as haemoglobinometry.

Two types of blood samples can be used for Hb estimation:
  i. *Capillary blood* from finger prick.
  ii. *Intravenous sample.* It should be well anticoagulated, preferably in EDTA. Liquid anticoagulants should not be used at all as these dilute and decrease Hb concentration.

Methods for Estimation of Haemoglobin

Various methods used for estimation of Hb are divided into 4 groups as under:

I. Colorimetric method. Colorimetric method is based on colorimetric measurement of the intensity of colour developed on addition of some substance to the blood. Colorimetric methods include the following:
1. Cyanmethaemoglobin method
2. Oxyhaemoglobin method
3. Electronic counter method
4. Direct reading electronic haemoglobinometer
5. Sahli's method

II. Measurement of O_2 carrying capacity of Hb. Measurement of O_2 carrying capacity of Hb cannot be used for mass screening but is used in referral or research laboratories only.

III. Measurement of iron content of Hb. Measurement of iron content of Hb is used only for research purpose.

IV. Specific gravity method. It is a very rapid method and is useful for screening blood donors for anaemia in blood donation programme. Normal specific gravity of blood ranges from 1.048-1.066.

Some of the commonly used methods are discussed below.

CYANMETHAEMOGLOBIN METHOD

This is the best method for Hb estimation and it has been recommended by International Committee for Standardisation in Haematology (ICSH).

Principle. Blood is diluted in a solution called Drabkin's fluid containing potassium ferricyanide and potassium cyanide (KCN). The oxy, carboxy and metHb are all converted into cyanmethaemoglobin (HiCN) and there is development of pink colour. The intensity of pink colour can be measured in a spectrophotometer or photoelectric colorimeter at 540 nm and this is compared with that of a standard cyanmethaemoglobin solution.

Reagents. Drabkin's fluid can be prepared as under:

Potassium ferricyanide	:	0.2 g
Potassium cyanide	:	0.05 g
Dihydrogen potassium phosphate	:	0.14 g
Distilled water	:	1000 ml

Drabkin's fluid should be clear and pale yellow having a pH of 7.0-7.4.

Procedure

- Add 20 μl (0.02 ml) of blood to 5 ml of Drabkin's solution in a test tube (1:251 dilution).
- Mix well and allow it to stand for 3-5 minutes.
- Take reading of test and standard in a spectrophotometer or photoelectric colorimeter at 540 nm (Fig. 47.1).

Calculations

Hb concentration in test (g%) =

$$\frac{\text{Absorbance of test}}{\text{Absorbance of standard}} \times \frac{\text{Hb concentration of standard (mg / dl)} \times 251}{100 \text{ mg / g}}$$

Where 251 is the dilution factor.

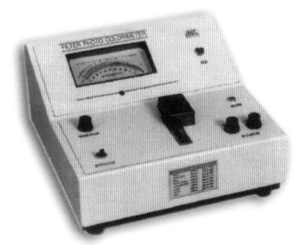

FIGURE 47.1 ◆ Photoelectric colorimeter used for taking reading of haemoglobin in cyanmethaemoglobin method and oxyhaemoglobin method. (Photograph courtesy of Max Electronics India, Chandigarh).

Advantages

i. There is no chance of visual error.
ii. All forms of Hb except sulfhaemoglobin can be measured.
iii. The standard is very stable.

Disadvantages

i. We cannot take the reading immediately.
ii. If blood is turbid due to plasma proteins, hyperlipidaemia, leukaemias, the absorbance is more and hence incorrect results may be obtained.
iii. Results are affected due to hyperbilirubinaemia.

OXYHAEMOGLOBIN METHOD

This is a simple and quick method and results are not affected by hyperbilirubinaemia.

Principle. Blood is diluted in a solution of ammonia. There is development of reddish pink-colour which is measured in a spectrophotometer or photoelectric colorimeter at 625 nm and compared with that of a standard oxyHb solution.

Procedure

- Add 20 μl (0.02 ml) of blood to 4 ml of 0.4 ml/l ammonia solution in a test tube.
- Use a tight fitting stopper and mix by inverting the tube several times.
- Take reading of test and standard in a spectrophotometer or photoelectric colorimeter with a yellow or green filter (625 nm).

Calculations. As for cyanmet method.

Advantages

i. The method is simple and quick.
ii. Result is not affected by rise of plasma bilirubin.
iii. Most forms of haemoglobins (i.e. HbO, Hi, and HbCO) are measured in this method.

Disadvantages

i. It does not measure sulfhaemoglobin.
ii. The standard is not stable.
iii. Increased absorbance may be caused by turbidity due to hyperlipidaemia, leucocytosis ($> 30 \times 10^9$/l) and abnormal plasma proteins.

ELECTRONIC COUNTER METHOD

This is a multiparameter determining electronic equipment.

Principle. The method is based on electrical impedance principle. The blood is diluted with isoton and lysate which lyses the RBCs converting Hb into cyanmethaemoglobin and its concentration is measured in the spectrophotometer at

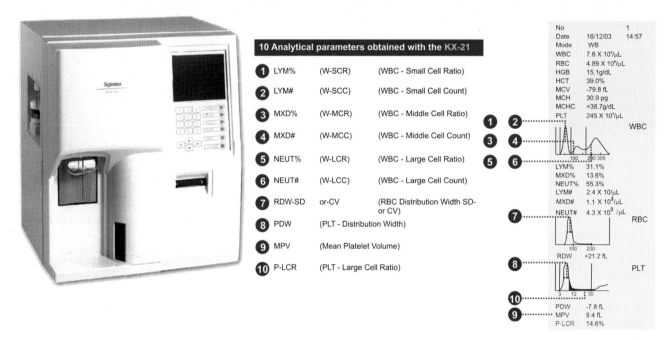

FIGURE 47.2 ◆ Electronic particle counter (Haematology Analyser) Model K X–21 (Photograph courtesy of Sysmex Corporation, Japan through Transasia Biomedicals Ltd., Mumbai).

540 nm. In some instruments, cyanmethaemoglobin method is replaced with another method employing a non-toxic chemical, sodium lauryl sulphate.

Disadvantage

High white cell count (> 30,000/μl) produces false elevation of Hb.

DIRECT READING ELECTRONIC HAEMOGLOBINOMETERS

These instruments have inbuilt filters. Reading of Hb in g/dl is visualised on the screen which may have light emitting diode (LED) display or analog meter. These equipments work on the principle of cyanmethaemoglobin, oxyhaemoglobin method or colour comparators in which colour of blood is compared without conversion to a derivative, against a range of colours which represent haemoglobin concentration (Fig. 47.2).

Disadvantage

Calibration of the instrument can be faulty.

SAHLI'S METHOD

Principle. Hb is converted into acid haematin with the action of dilute hydrochloric acid (N/10 HCl). The acid haematin is brown in colour and its intensity is matched with a standard brown glass comparator in a visual colorimeter called Sahli's colorimeter.

Procedure

◆ Fill Sahli's Hb tube up to mark 2 with N/10 HCl.
◆ Deliver 20 μl (0.02 ml) of blood from a Hb pipette into it.
◆ Stir with a stirrer and wait for 10 minutes.

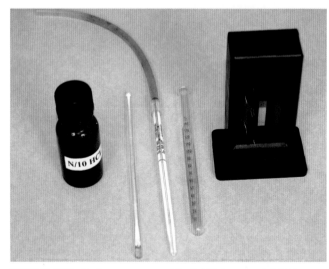

FIGURE 47.3 ◆ Apparatus used for Sahli's haemoglobinometry.

◆ Add distilled water drop by drop and stir till colour matches with the comparator.

◆ Take the reading at upper meniscus (Fig. 47.3).

Advantages

i. Simple bedside test.

ii. Reagents and apparatus are cheap.

Disadvantages

i. There can be visual error.

ii. Carboxy, met and sulfhaemoglobins cannot be converted to acid haematin.

iii. Comparator can fade over the years.

iv. Colour of acid haematin also fades quickly.

OTHER METHODS

Following methods are not in common use these days:

1. *Alkali haematin method* in which diluting fluid is a strong alkali such as N/10 NaOH and the colour so produced is compared with the standard.

2. *Haldane method* (or carboxy Hb method) in which the RBCs are lysed by carbon monoxide to form carboxy Hb. The colour so produced is compared with the standard.

NORMAL VALUES OF HAEMOGLOBIN

Men	15 ± 2 g/dl
Women	13.5 ± 1.5 g/dl
Infants	16.5 ± 3 g/dl

ERRORS IN HAEMOGLOBINOMETRY

1. *Sampling error.* Improper venipuncture technique, e.g. more squeezing can alter the results, or the reading may be affected by type of anticoagulant used.

2. *Error in method.* Results are better with cyanmet and oxyHb method. In Sahli's method chances of error are more.

3. *Error in equipment.* These could be due to quality of material of the equipment or calibration of the equipment.

4. *Operator's error.* This could be because of improper training, lack of familiarity with the equipment or over-worked operator.

Quality Control in Haemoglobin Estimation

For reliability of the results, quality assurance or quality control is a must. It includes proficiency in collection, labelling, storage and results of the test. Quality control has three components: *internal quality control, standardisation* and *external quality control.* Precision refers to reproducibility of a result but a test may be precise without being accurate. Inaccuracy occurs as a result of improper standard, reagents, calibration of equipment and poor technique. Accuracy is attained by use of reference material which has been assayed by different methods and in different laboratories. The reference materials with known values of results are commercially available, or can also be prepared in the laboratory.

Counting of Blood Cells

Objectives
➢ To learn the principle, techniques and interpretation of counting of WBCs, RBCs, platelets and eosinophils.
➢ To know their normal values and conditions producing abnormal counts of these blood cells.

Counting of circulating blood cells is a basic screening blood test and includes counting of leucocytes (total and differential, i.e. TLC, DLC), red cells and platelets, and sometimes, eosinophils. However, the term *complete blood counts (CBC)* is commonly used these days for the following panel of tests determined by electronic particle counter:

1. *Evaluation of WBCs*: TLC, DLC
2. *Evaluation of RBCs*: RBC count, haemoglobin, haematocrit, red cell indices (MCV, MCH, MCHC, red cell distribution width or RDW)
3. *Evaluation of platelets*: Platelet count, mean platelet volume (MPV) and platelet distribution width (PDV).

WBC Count

This is determination of number of white blood cells per μl of blood.

METHODS

There are two methods:
1. Visual haemacytometer method
2. Electronic method

Visual Haemacytometer Method

Principle. This is counting of WBCs in a calibrated chamber by diluting of blood to 1:20 dilution with diluent which causes lysis of RBCs and stains WBCs.

Diluting fluid. Turk's fluid is used which has the following composition:

Glacial acetic acid	:	3.0 ml
1% Aqueous gentian violet	:	2.0 ml
Distilled water	:	195 ml

Procedure
◆ Suck anticoagulated blood or blood from finger prick up to mark 0.5 in WBC pipette (Fig. 48.1,A).
◆ Wipe tip and outside of the pipette.
◆ Draw diluting fluid up to mark 11 in the WBC pipette to get dilution of 1:20.
◆ Mix well by rotating the pipette for 2-3 minutes.
◆ Charge the Neubauer's chamber (haemacytometer) after discarding 1-2 drops of the mixture from the WBC pipette.

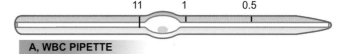

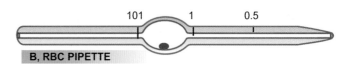

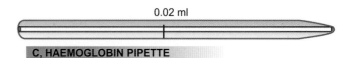

FIGURE 48.1 ◆ Pipettes for WBC **(A)** and RBC counting **(B)** contrasted with haemoglobin pipette **(C)**.

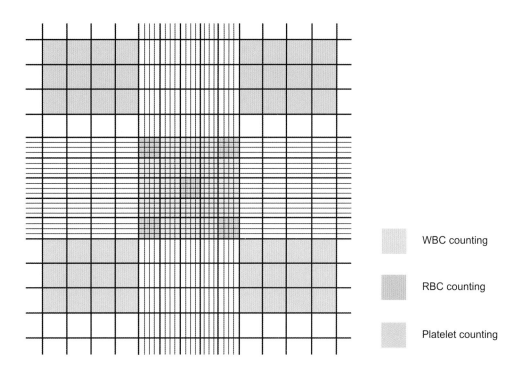

FIGURE 48.2 ◆ Improved Neubauer's chamber. Counting areas for WBCs, RBCs and platelets are depicted by different colours diagrammatically though the improved Neubauer's chamber does not have any such colours.

◆ Allow the cells to settle down for 2 minutes.
◆ Count the WBCs under low power (10x) in 4 large corner squares (Fig. 48.2). Count the cells lying on left and lower lines while ignoring those on its right and upper lines.

*Calculations**

Volume of area in which WBCs counted in 4 corner squares	$= [(1{\times}1{\times}0.1) \times 4]$ mm^3
	$= 0.4$ mm^3
Number of WBCs in 0.4 mm^3	$= n$
Number of WBCs in 1 mm^3	$= \dfrac{n}{0.4}$
Dilution factor	$= 20$
$\therefore$ Number of WBCs per mm^3 (μl)	$= \dfrac{n}{0.4} \times 20$
	$= n \times 50$

Where n is the total number of WBCs counted in 4 corner squares.

―――――――――――

*For calculation of count of WBCs, RBCs and platelets using Neubauer's chamber, please remember the dimensions of corner squares of the chamber as 1 mm each side and depth 0.1 mm.
Volume = Length × Breadth × Depth

Precautions
   i. The workbench must be free of vibrations and chamber should not be exposed to heat.
  ii. The cover glass should be of special thickness and should have perfectly flat surface.
 iii. The chamber area should be completely filled leaving no air bubbles or debris in the chamber area.
  iv. The fluid should not overflow to the moat surrounding the ruled area on the chamber.

Electronic Method

Electronic counter is based on the principle of aperture impedance method, or light scattering technology, or both. In this, particles passing through a chamber in single file scatter the light and convert by a detector into pulses proportionate to the size of the cells, which are then counted electronically. A lysate is used to lyse red cells so as to count WBCs.

Advantages
   i. Easy and rapid method.
  ii. Time saving method.
 iii. Very large number of cells are counted rapidly.
  iv. There is high level of precision.

Disadvantages
  i. Costly equipment.
 ii. Calibration error.
iii. Nucleated RBCs are counted as leucocytes.
 iv. Platelet clumps counted as leucocytes.

NORMAL RANGE FOR WBC COUNT

Adults   :   4,000–11,000/µl
Infants at birth   :   10,000–26,000/µl
Children under 1 year   :   6,000–18,000/µl

CAUSES OF ABNORMAL LEUCOCYTE COUNT

Increased leucocyte count: Leucocytosis
Decreased leucocyte count: Leucopenia
    The conditions causing *leucocytosis* and *leucopenia* are given in Exercise 51.

RBC Count

This is defined as determination of the number of RBCs per µl of blood.

METHODS FOR RBC COUNTS

1. Visual haemacytometer method
2. Electronic method

Visual Haemacytometer Method

Principle. This is counting of RBCs in a calibrated chamber by dilution of blood to 1 in 200 dilution with a diluent which is isotonic to blood. The diluent used prevents clotting, clumping and rouleaux formation and does not destroy WBCs.

Diluting fluids
Two types of diluting fluids are used for RBC counting: Hayem's fluid and Dacie's fluid.

Composition of Hayem's fluid
  Mercuric chloride   :   0.25 g
  Sodium chloride   :   0.5 g
  Sodium sulphate   :   2.5 g
  Distilled water   :   100 ml

Composition of Dacie's fluid
  40% Formaldehyde   :   5 ml
  3% Trisodium citrate   :   495 ml

Procedure
- Draw anticoagulated blood or blood from finger prick up to mark 0.5 in RBC pipette (Fig. 48.1,B).

- Wipe tip and outside of the pipette.
- Draw diluting fluid up to mark 101 in the RBC pipette.
- Mix well by rotating the pipette for 2-3 minutes.
- Charge the Neubauer's chamber after discarding 1-2 drops of mixture from the RBC pipette.
- Allow the cells to settle down for 2 minutes.
- Count RBCs under high power 40X in 80 tiny squares (5 × 16 tiny squares) in the centre of the chamber as shown in Figure 48.2.

Calculations

Volume of area in which RBCs counted in 5 squares

$$= \left[\left(\frac{1}{5} \times \frac{1}{5} \times 0.1 \right) \times 5 \right] mm^3$$

$$= \frac{1}{50} mm^3$$

∴ Number of RBCs in volume $\frac{1}{50} mm^3$ = n

Number of RBCs in 1 mm³   = n × 50
Dilution factor   = 200
∴ RBC count per mm³ (µl)   = n × 50 × 200
                                 = n × 10,000

Where n is the number of RBCs counted in 5 small squares.

Electronic Method

Principle. Principle of electronic method for counting RBCs is the same as for WBCs. But unlike WBC counting, no lysate is used; instead anticoagulated blood is diluted with particle-free diluting fluid such as physiological saline or phosphate buffer saline.

Advantages
  i. Easy and rapid method.
 ii. Many thousands of cells are counted compared to fewer cells counted in manual method.

Disadvantages
  i. Costly equipment.
 ii. Calibration error.
iii. Altered composition of diluent causes erroneous results.
 iv. Giant platelets are counted as RBCs.
  v. High WBC count alters results.

NORMAL RANGE FOR RBC COUNT

Males   :   5.0–6.0 million/µl (5.5 ± 0.5 million/µl)
Females :   4.5–5.5 million/µl (5 ± 0.5 million/µl)
Children :   4.0–5.0 million/µl (4.5 ± 0.5 million/µl)

CAUSE OF DECREASED RBC COUNT

i. Anaemia

CAUSE OF INCREASED RBC COUNT

i. Polycythemia

Platelet Count

Platelets are thin discs 2-4 μm in diameter. They function in haemostasis, in maintaining vascular integrity and in the process of blood coagulation. Their lifespan is 7-10 days.

METHODS FOR COUNTING PLATELETS

1. Visual method
2. Electronic method

Visual Method

Type of blood used. Use only venous blood as the blood obtained from finger prick causes clumping of platelets.

Diluting fluid. 1% ammonium oxalate is prepared as under:
Ammonium oxalate : 1 g
Distilled water : 100 ml

Filter it and keep in a refrigerator at 4°C.

Procedure

♦ Using an RBC pipette, prepare a 1:200 dilution as for RBC method (Fig. 48.1,B).
♦ Mix for 2 minutes, charge the Neubauer's counting chamber.
♦ Place the charged Neubauer's chamber into a petri dish having a moist filter paper at bottom for allowing the platelets to settle down.
♦ Count the platelets as for red cell count using 40x objective with reduced condenser aperture.
♦ If platelet count is low, then a WBC pipette can be used for charging the Neubauer's chamber.

Calculations

Volume of area in which platelets counted in 5 squares

$$= \left[\left(\frac{1}{5}\times\frac{1}{5}\times0.1\right)\times5\right]mm^3$$

$$= \frac{1}{50}mm^3$$

∴ Number of platelets in volume $\frac{1}{50}mm^3$ = n

Number of platelets in 1 mm^3 = n × 50

Dilution factor = 200
∴ Platelet count per mm^3 (μl) = n × 50 × 200
= n × 10,000

A phase-contrast microscope can be used for platelet counting which gives better results.

Rough Visual Method for Platelet Counting

Prepare a thin peripheral blood film, stain it with any of the Romanowsky stain. Dry it and examine under high power. If you find one clump of platelet per high power field, then number of platelets is adequate; roughly each platelet under high power represents count of 25,000 platelets per mm^3.

Electronic Method

Platelets can be counted by electronic particle counter method which implies electrical impedance principle as for counting RBCs.

Disadvantages

i. Equipment is costly.
ii. Calibration error.
iii. Debris counted as platelets.
iv. Heinz bodies and Howell-Jolly bodies can be counted as platelets.

NORMAL PLATELET COUNT

1,50,000-400,000/μl

Conditions causing abnormal platelet counts

i. Decreased count is termed thrombocytopenia.
ii. Increased count is termed thrombocytosis.

CONDITIONS CAUSING THROMBOCYTOPENIA

1. *Impaired platelet production:*
   i. Aplastic anaemia
   ii. Acute leukaemias
   iii. Myelofibrosis
   iv. Marrow infiltration by malignancy
   v. Drugs (e.g. chloramphenicol, thiazides, anti-cancer drugs)
   vi. Chronic alcoholism
2. *Accelerated platelet destruction:*
   i. ITP
   ii. SLE
   iii. AIDS
   iv. CLL
   v. DIC
   vi. Giant haemangioma
   vii. Drug-induced (e.g. sulfonamides, quinine, gold)

viii. Microangiopathic haemolytic anaemia
  ix. Splenomegaly
   x. Massive transfusion of blood.

CONDITIONS CAUSING THROMBOCYTOSIS

   i. Essential thrombocytosis
  ii. Chronic infection
 iii. Haemorrhage
  iv. Postoperative state
   v. Malignancy
  vi. Postsplenectomy.

Absolute Eosinophil Count (AEC)

AEC is required for knowing the number of circulating eosinophils in blood in allergic conditions and other causes of eosinophilia.

METHODS

There are two methods:
1. Improved Neubauer chamber method
2. Fuchs-Rosenthal counting chamber method

Diluting fluid
For both methods, Dunger's diluting fluid is used with the following composition:

Eosin	:	200 mg
Distilled water	:	90 ml
Acetone	:	10 ml

Eosin stains the eosinophil granules bright red, water is used to lyse red cells and acetone is meant for fixation of eosinophils.

Improved Neubauer Chamber Method

Principle. This is counting of eosinophils in a calibrated chamber by diluting of blood to 1:10 dilution with diluent which causes lysis of RBCs and stains WBCs.

Procedure
- Suck anticoagulated blood up to mark 1 in WBC pipette (Fig. 48.1,A).
- Wipe tip and outside of the pipette.
- Draw diluting fluid up to mark 11 in the WBC pipette to get dilution of 1:10.
- Mix well by rotating the pipette for 2-3 minutes.
- Charge the Neubauer's chamber after discarding 1-2 drops of the mixture from the WBC pipette.
- Allow the cells to settle down for 2 minutes.
- Count the eosinophils under low power (10x) in 4 large corner squares as for TLC (Fig. 48.2). Eosinophils are identified by having brightly red granules.

Calculations

$$\text{Number of eosinophils in 1 mm}^3 \quad = \quad \frac{n \times 10}{4}$$

Dilution factor $\quad = \quad 10$
$\therefore$ Number of eosinophils per mm^3 (μl)$= \quad$ n $\times$ 10
$\quad\quad\quad\quad = \quad$ n $\times$ 25

Where n is the total number of eosinophils counted in 4 corner squares.

Fuchs-Rosenthal Counting Chamber Method

This is a preferred method in which the ruled area for counting is 16 small squares (one mm each) and depth of chamber is 0.2 mm. Hence more cells are counted and gives more accurate result. Rest of the method including diluting fluid are similar.

NORMAL RANGE FOR AEC

Adults   :   40-400/μl

CAUSES OF ABNORMAL AEC

Increased AEC: Eosinophilia
Decreased AEC: Eosinopenia

The conditions causing eosinophila and eosinopenia are given in Exercise 51.

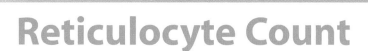

Reticulocyte Count

Objectives
➤ To learn various reticulocyte counting methods.
➤ To know their normal values and conditions causing abnormal counts.

Reticulocytes

Reticulocytes are juvenile or immature non-nucleated red cells which still contain the remains of RNA protein and continue to synthesise haemoglobin after loss of nucleus. Their number in the peripheral blood is an accurate reflection of erythropoietic activity in the bone marrow. An increased erythropoietic stimulus leads to premature release of juvenile RBCs (reticulocytes) into the circulation. Time taken by reticulocytes to mature into RBCs is approximately 1-2 days.

Methods for Counting of Reticulocytes

1. Visual method
2. Automated method

VISUAL METHOD

Principle. When blood is briefly incubated in a solution of supravital dye (new methylene blue or brilliant cresyl blue), the RNA is precipitated as dye-RNA protein complex. This reaction takes place only in vitally stained unfixed preparations, i.e. *supravital staining* is done on living cells rather than on air-dried blood smears.

Preparation of staining solution. 1% new methylene blue is prepared as under:

New methylene blue	:	1.0 g
Iso-osmotic phosphate buffer (pH 7.4)	:	100 ml

Dissolve in a dark bottle and filter before use.

Procedure
◆ Take 2-3 drops of new methylene blue in a small tube.
◆ Add 4-8 drops of patient's EDTA blood and mix.
◆ Incubate at 37°C for 15-20 minutes.
◆ Remix the tube contents.
◆ Place a drop of stained blood on a clean glass slide and make a thin blood film.
◆ Dry and examine under oil immersion.

Counting of Reticulocytes

Microscopically, reticulocytes have dark blue network or dark blue granules while RBCs appear pale blue or blue green (Fig. 49.1). Select a well spread portion of the smear in which the red cells are just overlapping. Count at least 100 reticulocytes. For counting of reticulocytes present per 100 RBCs, the visual field is restricted to manageable counts. This is achieved by either using Ehrlich's eyepiece having adjustable square window in it, or alternatively a round piece of thick paper of the diameter of eyepiece with a small square window of 4 mm diameter in it can be used (Fig. 49.2).

Calculations

Number of reticulocytes in n fields	=	x
Average number of cells/field	=	y
Total number of cells in n fields	=	$n \times y$

$$\text{Reticulocyte count (\%)} = \frac{x}{n \times y} \times 100$$

Absolute number of reticulocytes per µl =

$$\frac{\text{Reticulocyte count}}{100} \times \text{RBC count}$$

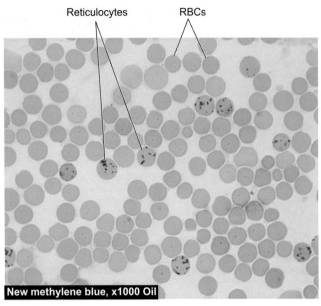

FIGURE 49.1 ◆ Reticulocytes contrasted with mature RBCs (New methylene blue, x 1000 oil).

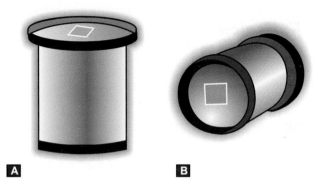

FIGURE 49.2 ◆ Ehrlich's eyepiece as viewed from top **(A)** and as viewed from below **(B)**.

AUTOMATED METHOD

Reticulocytes can be counted by automated reticulocyte analyser or by flow cytometry by using fluorescent dyes (e.g. auramine O, thiazole orange, acridine orange and thioflavine T) or non-fluorescent dyes (e.g. oxazine). Advantage of automatic equipment is that it is superior to that of manual counts since many more cells are counted and the subjectivity in recognition of reticulocytes is eliminated. However, automated equipment is costly and Howell-Jolly bodies, Heinz bodies, Pappenheimer bodies and giant platelets are counted as reticulocytes.

NORMAL VALUES

Infants	:	2-6%
Adults and children	:	0.5–2.5%
Absolute reticulocyte count	:	25,000-75,000/µl

ABNORMAL COUNTS

Increased count (Reticulocytosis)
  i. After haemorrhage.
 ii. Haemolysis.
iii. Haematopoietic response of anaemia to treatment.

Decreased counts (Reticulocytopenia)
  i. Ineffective erythropoiesis.
 ii. Aplastic anaemia.
iii. Thalassemia.
iv. Myelosclerosis.

Preparation and Staining of Peripheral Blood Film

Objectives

➢ To learn the technique of making thin and thick blood film and their significance.
➢ To know and perform various routine stains used for staining blood films.

The peripheral blood film (PBF) is of two types:
1. Thin blood film
2. Thick blood film

Thin Blood Film

Thin PBF can be prepared from anticoagulated (EDTA) blood obtained by venepuncture or from free flowing finger prick blood by any of the following three techniques:
1. Slide method
2. Cover glass method
3. Spin method

SLIDE METHOD

Procedure

◆ Place a drop of blood in the centre of a clean glass slide 1 to 2 cm from one end.
◆ Place another slide (spreader) with smooth edge at an angle of 30-45° near the drop of blood.
◆ Move the spreader backward so that it makes contact with drop of blood.
◆ Then move the spreader forward rapidly over the slide.
◆ A thin peripheral blood film is thus prepared (Fig. 50.1).
◆ Dry it and stain it.

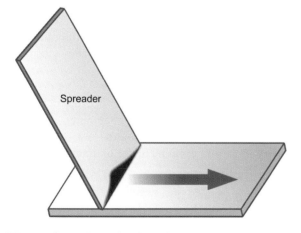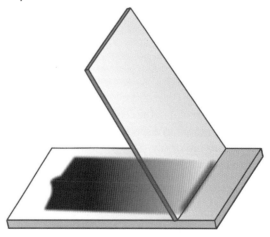

FIGURE 50.1 ◆ Method of making thin PBF by slide method.

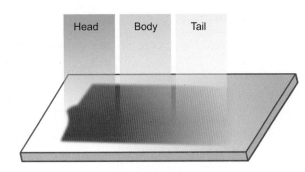

FIGURE 50.2 ◆ Parts of a thin blood film.

Qualities of a Good Blood Film

   i. It should not cover the entire surface of slide.
  ii. It should have smooth and even appearance.
 iii. It should be free from waves and holes.
 iv. It should not have irregular tail.

Parts of a Thin Blood Film

A PBF consists of 3 parts (Fig. 50.2):
1. *Head,* i.e. the portion of blood film near the drop of blood.
2. *Body,* i.e. the main part of the blood film.
3. *Tail,* i.e. the tapering end of the blood film.

COVER GLASS METHOD

Procedure

◆ Take a number 1 (22 mm square) clean cover glass.
◆ Touch it on to the drop of a blood.
◆ Place it on another similar cover glass in crosswise direction with side containing drop of blood facing down.
◆ Pull the cover glass quickly.
◆ Dry it and stain it.
◆ Mount it with a mountant, film side down on a clean glass slide.

SPIN METHOD

This is an automated method.

Procedure

◆ Place a drop of blood in the centre of a glass slide.
◆ Spin at a high speed in a special centrifuge, cytospin.
◆ Blood spreads uniformly.
◆ Dry it and stain it.

Thick Blood Film

This is prepared for detecting blood parasites such as malaria and microfilaria.

Procedure

◆ Place a large drop of blood in the centre of a clean glass slide.
◆ Spread it in a circular area of 1.5 cm with the help of a stick or end of another glass slide.
◆ Dry it and you should be able to just see the printed matter through the smear, when kept on printed paper.

Stains for Blood Film

Romanowsky stains are universally employed for staining of blood films. All Romanowsky combinations have two essential ingredients, i.e. methylene blue and eosin or azure. Methylene blue is the basic dye and has affinity for acidic component of the cell (i.e. nucleus) and eosin/azure is the acidic dye and has affinity for basic component of cell (i.e. cytoplasm).

Most Romanowsky stains are prepared in methyl alcohol so that they combine fixation and staining.

Various stains included under Romanowsky groups of dyes are as under:
   i. Leishman stain
  ii. Giemsa stain
 iii. Wright stain
 iv. Field stain
  v. Jenner stain
 vi. JSB stain

STAINING OF THIN BLOOD FILM

Leishman Stain

Preparation. Dissolve 0.2 g of powdered Leishman's dye in 100 ml of acetone-free methyl alcohol in a conical flask. Warm it to 50°C for half an hour with occasional shaking. Cool it and filter it.

Procedure for staining
◆ Pour Leishman's stain dropwise (counting the drops) on the slide and wait for 2 minutes. This allows fixation of the PBF in methyl alcohol.
◆ Add double the quantity of buffered water dropwise over the slide (i.e. double the number of drops of stain).
◆ Mix by rocking or blowing for 8 minutes.
◆ Wash in water for 1 to 2 minutes.
◆ Dry in air and examine under oil immersion lens of the microscope.

Giemsa Stain

Preparation. Stock solution of Giemsa stain is prepared by mixing 0.15 g of Giemsa powder in 12.5 ml of glycerine and

12.5 ml of methyl alcohol. Before use, dissolve one volume of stock solution in nine volumes of buffered water (dilution 1:9).

Procedure

- Pour diluted stain over slide or immense blood film in staining trough.
- Wait for 15-60 minutes.
- Wash in water.
- Dry it and examine under oil immersion lens of the microscope.

STAINING OF THICK SMEAR

It can be stained with any of the Romanowsky stains listed above except that before staining, the smear is dehaemoglobinised by putting it in distilled water for 10 minutes.

AUTOSTAINERS

Currently, automatic staining machines are available which enable a large batch of slides to be stained with a uniform quality.

PRECAUTIONS IN STAINING OF PBF

1. *Dark blue blood film.* It can be due to overstaining, inadequate washing or improper pH of the buffer. In this, RBCs are blue, nuclear chromatin is black, granules of the neutrophils are overstained and granules of the eosinophils are blue or grey.

2. *Light pink blood film.* In this, RBCs are bright red, the nuclear chromatin is pale blue and granules of the eosinophils are dark red. It can be due to understaining, prolonged washing, mounting the film before drying and improper pH of the buffer.

3. *Precipitate on the blood film.* This could be due to inadequate filtration of the stain, dust on the slide, drying during staining and inadequate washing.

Differential Leucocyte Count

Objectives

➢ To learn the method of examination of blood film for differential leucocyte count (DLC) and morphologic features of mature leucocytes.

➢ To know various techniques for DLC and to perform DLC by manual methods.

➢ To know normal range of mature leucocytes in blood and various conditions producing their variations in diseases.

Examination of PBF for DLC

Choose an area near the junction of body with the tail of the smear where there is slight overlapping of RBCs, i.e. neither rouleaux formation which occurs in head and body, nor totally scattered RBCs as occurs at the tail. By moving the slide in horizontal directions under oil immersion (Fig. 51.1), start counting the types of WBCs and go on entering P, L, M, E, B in a box having 100 cubes as shown in Figure 51.2. Alternatively, 100 leucocytes can be counted by pressing the keys of the automated DLC counter (Fig. 51.3). Zigzag counting of WBCs is discouraged. WBCs are then expressed as percent in the following sequence: polymorphonuclear leucocytes (P), lymphocytes (L), monocytes (M), eosinophils (E), basophils (B), i.e. P, L, M, E, B. Invariably, normal range is expressed alongside the results (Table 51.1).

L	P	P	L	P	L	P	P	L	P
P	L	P	P	L	P	P	L	P	P
P	P	P	L	P	P	L	P	P	L
P	P	P	L	P	P	P	L	P	P
L	P	L	P	M	L	L	P	M	P
P	B	E	P	P	L	P	E	P	P
P	M	P	L	L	P	L	P	L	L
L	P	E	P	P	P	L	L	P	P
P	P	P	L	P	L	P	P	L	P
P	L	L	P	P	M	P	L	P	L

Result of DLC				
P	L	M	E	B
60%	32%	4%	1%	3%

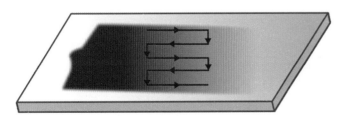

FIGURE 51.1 ◆ Counting of cells in PBF by moving in horizontal direction at the junction of the body with the tail of PBF.

FIGURE 51.2 ◆ Counting of WBCs for DLC in squares and expressing result of DLC.

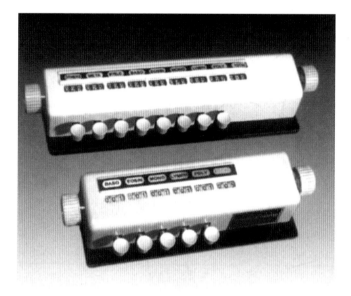

TABLE 51.1: Normal values for leucocytes in health in adults.		
	Normal range	Absolute value
Polymorphs (P)	40-75%	2,000-7,500/µl
Lymphocytes (L)	20-40%	1,500-4,000/µl
Monocytes (M)	2-10%	200-800/µl
Eosinophils (E)	1-6%	40-400/µl
Basophils (B)	0-1%	10-100/µl

FIGURE 51.3 ◆ Counting of WBCs for DLC in DLC counters with pressing keys (Photograph by courtesy of Yorco Sales Pvt. Ltd., Delhi).

Morphologic Identification of Mature Leucocytes

POLYMORPH (NEUTROPHIL)

A polymorphonuclear neutrophil (PMN), commonly called polymorph or neutrophil, is 12-15 µm in diameter. It consists of a characteristic dense nucleus, having 2-5 lobes and pale cytoplasm containing numerous fine violet-pink granules.

TABLE 51.2: Morphology of mature leucocytes.					
Feature	Neutrophil	Lymphocytes (small and large)	Monocyte	Eosinophil	Basophil
Morphology					
Cell diameter	12-15 µm	SL: 9-12 µm LL: 12-16 µm	12-20 µm	12-15 µm	12-15 µm
Nucleus	2-5 lobed, clumped chromatin	Large nucleus, round to indented, fills the cell, clumped chromatin	Large, lobulated, indented, with fine chromatin	Bilobed, clumped chromatin	Bilobed, clumped chromatin
Cytoplasm	Pink or violet granules	Peripheral rim of basophilic cytoplasm, no granules	Light basophilic, may contain fine granules or vacuoles	Coarse crimson red granules	Large coarse purplish granules obscuring the nucleus
Normal %	40-75	20-40	2-10	1-6	0-1
Absolute count per µl	2,000-7,500	1,500-4,000	200-800	40-400	10-100

LYMPHOCYTE

Majority of lymphocytes in the peripheral blood are small (9-12 μm in diameter) but large lymphocytes (12-16 μm in diameter) are also found. Both small and large lymphocytes have round or slightly indented nucleus with coarsely clumped chromatin and scanty basophilic and agranular cytoplasm.

MONOCYTE

The monocyte is the largest mature leucocyte in the peripheral blood measuring 12-20 μm in diameter. It possesses a large, central, oval, notched or indented or horseshoe-shaped nucleus which has characteristically fine reticulated chromatin network. The cytoplasm is abundant, pale blue and contains many fine granules and vacuoles.

EOSINOPHIL

Eosinophil is similar to segmented neutrophil in size (12-15 μm in diameter) but has coarse, deep red staining granules in the cytoplasm and has usually two nuclear lobes in the form of a spectacle.

BASOPHIL

Basophil resembles the other mature granulocytes but is distinguished by coarse, intensely basophilic granules which usually fill the cytoplasm and often overlap and obscure the nucleus.

Morphological features of different leucocytes are summarised in Table 51.2.

Methods of DLC

Differential leucocyte count (DLC) can be performed by two methods:
1. Visual counting
2. Automated counting

VISUAL COUNTING

This is counting of WBCs after identifying them by their morphologic features described above (Fig. 51.2).

AUTOMATED COUNTING

It is done by electronic counting method. There are three types of electronic methods—by cell size analysis, by flow cytometry, and by high resolution pattern recognition. In addition to counting, these methods also provide additional information on cell size, shape, nuclear size and density. Automated DLC counters have a differential counting capacity of counting either 3-part DLC (granulocytes, lymphocytes and monocytes) or 5-part DLC (P, L, M, E, B). However, automated method of DLC suffers from the disadvantage that normoblasts are counted as lymphocytes and these counters are quite expensive.

Pathologic Variations in DLC

NEUTROPHILS

Increase in neutrophil count above 7,500/μl is called *neutrophilia* (Fig. 51.4) while fall in neutrophil count below 2,000/μl is termed neutropenia. The causes for neutrophilia and neutropenia are given in Table 51.3.

LYMPHOCYTES

When the absolute lymphocyte count increases to more than 4,000/μl it is termed *lymphocytosis* (Fig. 51.5) while absolute lymphocyte count below 1,500/μl is called *lymphopenia;* causes for these are given in Table 51.4.

MONOCYTES

A rise in absolute monocyte count above 800/μl is called monocytosis (Fig. 51.6). Causes of monocytosis are given in Table 51.5.

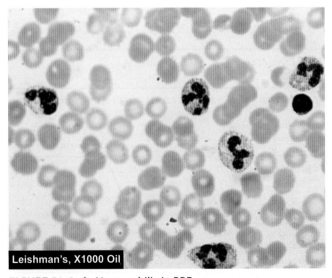

Leishman's, X1000 Oil

FIGURE 51.4 ◆ Neutrophilia in PBF.

TABLE 51.3: Causes of neutrophilia and neutropenia.

Neutrophilia	Neutropenia
1. *Acute infections* (By bacteria, fungi, parasites and some viruses)	1. *Infections*
i. Pneumonia	i. Typhoid
ii. Acute appendicitis	ii. Brucellosis
iii. Acute cholecystitis	iii. Measles
iv. Salpingitis	iv. Malaria
v. Peritonitis	v. Kala azar
vi. Abscess	vi. Miliary tuberculosis
vii. Acute tonsillitis	2. *Drugs and chemicals and physical agents*
viii. Actinomycosis	i. Antimetabolites
ix. Poliomyelitis	ii. Benzene
x. Furuncle	iii. Nitrogen mustard
xi. Carbuncle	iv. Irradiation
2. *Intoxication*	3. *Haematological and other diseases*
i. Uraemia	i. Aplastic anaemia
ii. Diabetic ketosis	ii. Pernicious anaemia
iii. Poisoning by chemicals	iii. SLE
iv. Eclampsia	iv. Gaucher's disease
3. *Inflammation from tissue damage*	v. Cachexia
i. Burns	vi. Anaphylactic shock
ii. Ischaemic necrosis	
iii. Gout	
iv. Hypersensitivity reaction	
4. *Acute haemorrhage*	
i. Acute haemolysis	
5. *Neoplastic conditions*	
i. Myeloid leukaemia (CML)	
ii. Polycythaemia vera	
iii. Myelofibrosis	
iv. Disseminated cancers	
6. *Miscellaneous conditions*	
i. Administration of corticosteroids	
ii. Idiopathic neutrophilia	

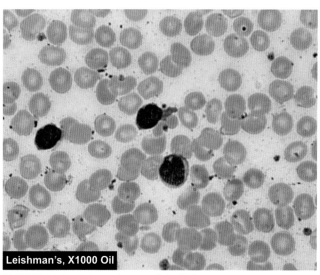

Leishman's, X1000 Oil

FIGURE 51.5 ◆ Lymphocytosis in PBF.

TABLE 51.4: Causes of lymphocytosis and lymphopenia.

Lymphocytosis	Lymphopenia
1. *Acute Infections*	i. Aplastic anaemia
i. Pertussis	ii. High dose of steroid administration
ii. Infectious mononucleosis	iii. AIDS
iii. Viral hepatitis	iv. Hodgkin's disease
2. *Chronic Infections*	v. Irradiation
i. Tuberculosis	
ii. Brucellosis	
iii. Secondary syphilis	
3. *Haematopoietic Disorders*	
i. CLL	
ii. NHL	

TABLE 51.5: Monocytosis.

1. *Bacterial infections*
   i. Tuberculosis
   ii. SABE
   iii. Syphilis
2. *Protozoal infections*
   i. Malaria
   ii. Kala azar
   iii. Trypanosomiasis
3. *Haematopoietic disorders*
   i. Monocytic leukaemia
   ii. Hodgkin's disease
   iii. Multiple myeloma
   iv. Myeloproliferative disorders
4. *Miscellaneous conditions*
   i. Sarcoidosis
   ii. Cancer of ovary, breast, stomach

EOSINOPHILS

Increase in the absolute eosinophil count above 400/µl is termed *eosinophilia* (Fig. 51.7) while the fall in number is called *eosinopenia*; the causes for abnormal eosinophil count are given in Table 51.6.

BASOPHIL

Basophilia refers to an increase in the absolute basophil count above 100/µl (Fig. 51.8). Causes of basophilia are given in Table 51.7.

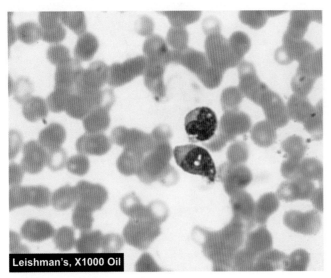

Leishman's, X1000 Oil

FIGURE 51.6 ◆ Monocytes in PBF.

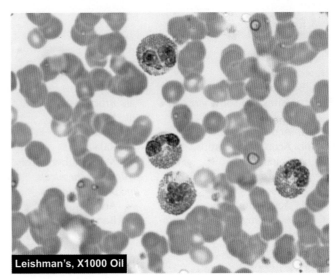

Leishman's, X1000 Oil

FIGURE 51.7 ◆ Eosinophilia in PBF.

TABLE 51.6: Causes of eosinophilia and eosinopenia.

Eosinophilia	Eosinopenia
1. Allergic disorders	Steroid administration
i. Bronchial asthma	
ii. Urticaria	
iii. Hay fever	
iv. Drug hypersensitivity	
2. Parasitic infestations	
i. Roundworm	
ii. Hookworm	
iii. Tapeworm	
iv. Echinococcosis	
3. Skin diseases	
i. Pemphigus	
ii. Dermatitis herpetiformis	
iii. Erythema multiforme	
4. Pulmonary diseases	
i. Löeffler's syndrome	
ii. Tropical eosinophilia	
5. Haematopoietic diseases	
i. Chronic myeloid leukaemia	
ii. Polycythaemia vera	
iii. Hodgkin's disease	
iv. Pernicious anaemia	
6. Miscellaneous conditions	
i. Rheumatoid arthritis	
ii. Polyarteritis nodosa	
iii. Sarcoidosis	
iv. Irradiation	

TABLE 51.7: Basophilia.

   i. Chronic myeloid leukemia
   ii. Polycythaemia vera
  iii. Myxoedema
  iv. Ulcerative colitis
   v. Hodgkin's disease
  vi Urticaria pigmentosa

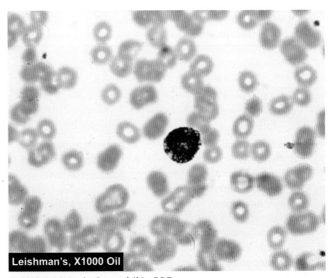

Leishman's, X1000 Oil

FIGURE 51.8 ◆ Basophil in PBF.

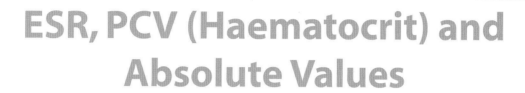

ESR, PCV (Haematocrit) and Absolute Values

Objectives

➢ To learn the principle, technique and interpretation of erythrocyte sedimentation rate (ESR) and packed cell volume (PCV or haematocrit).

➢ To understand the method of finding absolute haematological values and their significance.

Erythrocyte Sedimentation Rate

Erythrocyte sedimentation rate (ESR) is used as an index for presence of an active disease which could be due to many causes.

PRINCIPLE

When well mixed anticoagulated blood is placed in a vertical tube, the erythrocytes tend to fall towards the bottom of the tube/pipette till they form a packed column in the lower part of the tube in a given time.

MECHANISM OF ESR

Fall of RBCs depends upon following factors:

   i. Rouleaux formation
   ii. Concentration of fibrinogen in plasma
   iii. Concentration of α and β globulins
   iv. Ratio of red cells to plasma
   v. Length of the tube
   vi. Bore of the tube
   vii. Position of the tube

i) Rouleaux formation. The erythrocytes sediment in the tube/pipette because their density is greater than that of plasma. When a number of erythrocytes aggregate in the form of rouleaux and settle down, their area is much less than that of the sum of the area of constituent corpuscles. The rouleaux formation is very important factor which increases the ESR.

ii) Concentration of fibrinogen. It leads to colloidal changes in plasma which cause increased viscosity of plasma. Concentration of fibrinogen parallels ESR. If concentration of fibrinogen is raised, ESR is increased. In defibrinated blood, ESR is very low.

iii) Concentration of α and β globulins. These protein molecules have a greater effect than other proteins in decreasing the negative charge of the RBCs that tends to keep them apart thus promoting rouleaux formation. Albumin retards the ESR; thus conditions where albumin is low ESR is more.

iv) Ratio of red cells to plasma. The change in the ratio of RBCs to plasma affects ESR. When plasma is more, ESR will be increased, and vice versa.

v) Length of the tube. If length of the tube/pipette is more, RBCs will have to travel a longer distance and thus ESR is low than when length of the tube is short, and vice versa.

vi) Bore of the tube. If bore of the tube is more the negative charge which keeps the RBCs apart will be less and ESR will be more, and vice versa.

vii) Position of the tube. If the tube/pipette is not vertical, the RBCs will have to travel less distance and ESR will be more.

PHASES IN ESR

ESR takes place in the following three phases which are carried out in sequence within one hour:

♦ *Phase of rouleaux formation:* In the initial period of 10 minutes, the process of rouleaux formation occurs and there is little sedimentation.

♦ *Phase of settling:* In the next 40 minutes, settling of RBCs occurs at a constant rate.

♦ *Phase of packing:* In the last 10 minutes, sedimentation slows and packing of the RBCs to the bottom occurs.

That is why ESR by all methods is expressed as mm first hour rather than per hour.

METHODS OF ESR

1. Westergren's method
2. Wintrobe's method
3. Micro ESR method
4. Automated methods

1. WESTERGREN'S METHOD

Owing to its simplicity this method used to be the most commonly employed standard method prior to the AIDS-era. Westergren's pipette is a straight pipette 30 cm long open at both ends with internal bore diameter of 2.5 mm and is calibrated from 0-200 mm from top to bottom (Fig. 52.1,A).

Anticoagulant. Trisodium citrate as 3.8 g/dl liquid anticoagulant is used. It is used in the concentration of 1:4 between anticoagulant and blood.

Procedure

♦ The patient is advised to come in the morning fasting (as heavy protein diet affects concentration of plasma proteins).

♦ Take 1.6 ml of patient's blood and mix it with 0.4 ml of citrate as anticoagulant already put in a tube. The test should be done within two hours of taking blood.

♦ Fill the pipette up to mark 0 with citrated blood with the help of rubber teat by vacuum filling and fix it in a rack vertically away from sun light or vibrations.

♦ Let it stand for one hour after which reading is taken at the upper meniscus of the RBCs.

Normal values

Males	3-5 mm 1st hour
Females	4-7 mm 1st hour

Advantages

i. It is a more sensitive method.

ii. It is easy to fill and clean the Westergren's pipette.

Disadvantages

i. Requires more amount of blood.

ii. Dilution of blood in anticoagulant affects ESR.

iii. Filling of blood by mouth pipetting should be strictly discouraged.

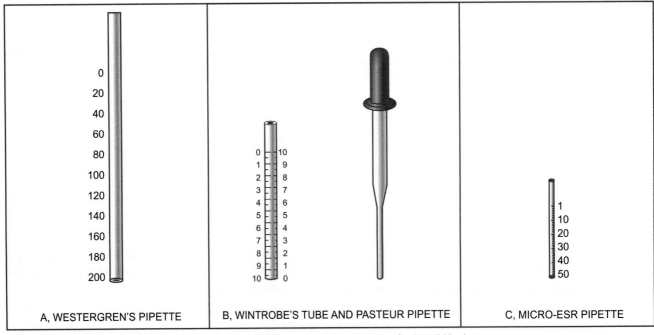

A, WESTERGREN'S PIPETTE   B, WINTROBE'S TUBE AND PASTEUR PIPETTE   C, MICRO-ESR PIPETTE

FIGURE 52.1 ♦ Westergren's pipette, Wintrobe's tube with Pasteur pipette and micro ESR pipette.

2. WINTROBE'S METHOD

The Wintrobe tube is a glass tube closed at one end. The tube is 110 mm long and has an internal bore diameter of 2.5 mm. The tube is graduated on both sides : from 0 to 10 cm on one side and 10 to 0 cm on the otherside (Fig. 52.1,B).

Anticoagulants. Either of the following two anticoagulants can be used:
   i. Ethylene diamine tetra-acetic acid (EDTA) solid crystals 1-2 mg/ml.
   ii. Double oxalate (solid) 2-3 mg/ml (ammonium oxalate and sodium or potassium oxalate in the ratio of 3:2; the former causes swelling and the latter causes shrinkage of RBCs and hence RBC shape is retained).

Procedure
   ◆ The patient is called in the morning fasting.
   ◆ Draw 2 ml of blood into the anticoagulant.
   ◆ Fill the Wintrobe tube up to mark 0 with anticoagulated blood with the help of a Pasteur pipette having a long stem so as to fill the tube free of air bubbles (Fig. 52.1,B).
   ◆ Place the tube vertically in a stand and note the ESR after one hour.

Normal values
Males	0-7 mm 1st hour
Females	0-15 mm 1st hour

Advantages
   i. It is simple method and requires small amount of blood.
   ii. There is no dilution with anticoagulant.
   iii. Packed cell volume (PCV) can also be done by the same tube.
   iv. Filling of tube with Pasteur pipette eliminates chance of any infection due to handling of blood.

Disadvantages
   i. Because of short column and choice of anticoagulant, it is not as sensitive index of diseases.
   ii. Addition of more anticoagulant can lower ESR.
   iii. ESR of more than 100 mm cannot be measured.

3. MICRO ESR METHOD

This method is used in pediatric patients or in patients where venepuncture is not possible. In this method a capillary 160 mm long with an internal bore diameter of 1 mm is used. The capillary is graduated with 1 mm markings for 50 mm, with two red lines on it. Alternatively, nongraduated heparinised capillary may be used and the reading is taken by measurement of length of column (Fig. 52.1,C).

Anticoagulant. Mixture of sodium citrate and EDTA is used.

Procedure
   ◆ Fill the microsedimentation pipette up to first red mark with anticoagulant.
   ◆ Fill the pipette with free flowing capillary blood up to second red mark.
   ◆ Invert it several times and allow it to stand for one hour in the sedimentation rack.
   ◆ Take the reading and results are given as that for Westergren's method.

4. AUTOMATED ESR METHOD

Automated closed systems use either blood collected in special evacuated tubes containing citrate or EDTA. It is taken up through a pierceable cap and then automatically diluted in the system.

CLINICAL SIGNIFICANCE OF ESR

ESR is a non-specific test of evaluating diseases. It is seldom used for diagnostic purpose but its use is limited to monitoring the prognosis of disease process.

Diagnostic Uses

   i. Rheumatoid arthritis
   ii. Chronic infections
   iii. Collagen diseases
   iv. Multiple myeloma
   v. Macroglobulinaemia

Monitoring Prognosis of Diseases

To see the response to treatment in:
   i. Tuberculosis
   ii. Temporal arteritis
   iii. Polymyalgia rheumatica
   iv. In patients of Hodgkin's disease, ESR of < 10 mm 1st hour indicates good prognosis while ESR of > 60 mm 1st hour indicates poor prognosis.

Table 52.1 sums up the list of conditions causing raised and lowered ESR.

Packed Cell Volume or Haematocrit

Packed cell volume (PCV) or haematocrit is defined as ratio of volume of RBCs to that of whole blood and is expressed as percentage.

TABLE 52.1: Causes of abnormal ESR.	
Diseases causing raised ESR	*Diseases causing low ESR*
i. Tuberculosis	i. Polycythaemia
ii. SABE	ii. Spherocytosis
iii. Acute myocardial infarction	iii. Sickle cell anaemia
iv. Rheumatoid arthritis	iv. Congestive heart failure
v. Shock	v. Newborn infant
vi. Anaemias	vi. Hypofibrinogenaemia
vii. Liver disease	
viii. Multiple myeloma	
ix. Pregnancy	
x. Ankylosing spondylitis	

METHODS FOR ESTIMATION OF PCV

1. Macro method (Wintrobe's method)
2. Microhaematocrit method
3. Electronic method

1. MACRO (WINTROBE'S) METHOD

In this method PCV is measured by Wintrobe tube which has a length of 110 mm and internal bore of 2.5 mm and graduated from 0–10 cm on both directions. PCV by Wintrobe's method can be done on the same blood after ESR by the same tube has been done.

Procedure
♦ Fill the Wintrobe tube upto mark 10 with well mixed anticoagulated blood (EDTA) by Pasteur's pipette free of air bubbles.
♦ Centrifuge the tube at 2000-2300 g for 30 minutes.
♦ After centrifugation layers are noted in the wintrobe tube as under (Fig. 52.2):
   i. Uppermost layer of *plasma.*
   ii. Thin white layer of *platelets.*
   iii. Greyish-pink layer of *leucocytes.*
   iv. Lowermost is the layer of *RBCs.*
   v. Grey-white layer of leucocytes and platelets interposed between plasma above and packed RBCs below is called *buffy coat.*
♦ Note the lowermost height of column of packed RBC layer and express it as percentage.

Advantages of macro method
   i. PCV and ESR can be measured simultaneously.
   ii. Buffy coat can be prepared for other tests.
   iii. By seeing the colour of plasma we can know about some of the pathological conditions, e.g. in jaundice it is yellow, in haemolysis it is pink, in hyperlipidaemia it is milky.

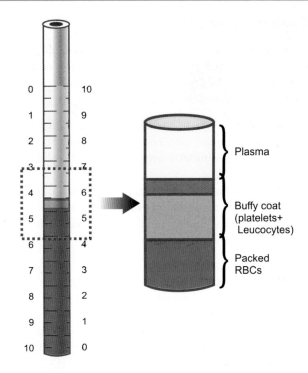

FIGURE 52.2 ♦ Haematocrit by Wintrobe's tube method.

2. MICROHAEMATOCRIT METHOD

In this method a capillary tube 70 mm long with an internal bore of 1 mm is used and blood from skin puncture is directly taken into heparinised capillary tube.

Procedure
♦ Take a heparinised capillary tube.
♦ Fill it with blood by capillary action leaving 10 mm unfilled.
♦ Seal the empty end by plastic seal or by heating on flame.
♦ Centrifuge it in microhaematocrit centrifuge at 10,000 g for 5 minutes (Fig. 52.3).
♦ Measure the blood column by using a reading device which is usually a part of centrifuge.

Advantages of micro method
   i. Less amount of blood is required.
   ii. Results are available within 5 minutes.
   iii. Method is more accurate, trapping of plasma is less.

Sources of errors in macro and micro methods
   i. Improper handling of sample.
   ii. Calibration error.
   iii. Unclean and contaminated tube.
   iv. Improper centrifugation time.

3. ELECTRONIC METHOD

Electronic methods employ automated counters where derivation of RBC count, PCV and MCV are closely interrelated.

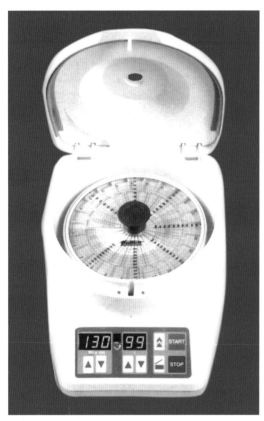

FIGURE 52.3 ◆ Microhaematocrit method for PCV. Haematocrit 20 model (Photograph courtesy of Hetlich, Germany through Global Medical System, Delhi).

CLINICAL SIGNIFICANCE OF PCV

PCV reflects the concentration of red cells and not the total red cell mass. PCV is generally three times the haemoglobin value. Table 52.2 lists the conditions causing raised and lowered PCV.

Absolute Values

Based on normal values of RBC count, haemoglobin and PCV, a series of absolute values or red cell indices can be derived which have diagnostic importance in various haematologic disorders. These are as under:

TABLE 52.2: Causes of abnormal PCV.

Diseases causing raised PCV	*Diseases causing low PCV*
i. Polycythaemia	i. Anaemia
ii. Dehydration due to severe vomitings, diarrhoea, profuse sweating	ii. Pregnancy
iii. Burns	
iv. Shock	

1. MEAN CORPUSCULAR VOLUME (MCV)

$$= \frac{\text{PCV in L/L}}{\text{RBC count/L}}$$

The normal value is 85 ± 8 fl (77-93 fl).

2. MEAN CORPUSCULAR HAEMOGLOBIN (MCH)

$$= \frac{\text{Hb/L}}{\text{RBC count/L}}$$

The normal range is 29.5 ± 2.5 pg (27-32 pg).

3. MEAN CORPUSCULAR HAEMOGLOBIN CONCENTRATION (MCHC)

$$= \frac{\text{Hb/dl}}{\text{PCV in L/L}}$$

The normal value is 32.5 ± 2.5 g/dl (30-35 g/dl).

Since MCHC is independent of red cell count and size, it is considered to be of greater clinical significance as compared with other absolute values. It is low in iron deficiency anaemia but is usually normal in macrocytic anaemia.

Significance

1. In iron deficiency and thalassaemia, MCV, MCH and MCHC are reduced.
2. In anaemia due to acute blood loss and haemolytic anaemias, MCV, MCH and MCHC are all within normal limits.
3. In megaloblastic anaemias, MCV is raised above the normal range.

Screening Tests for Haemostasis

Objectives
➢ To learn the principle, technique and interpretation of screening tests for haemostasis— bleeding time (BT) and clotting time (CT).
➢ To know the normal range of BT and CT and abnormal values in diseases.

Haemostasis is the process by which the bleeding from an injured site is arrested by formation of haemostatic plug, followed by removal of that plug spontaneously in due course of time. Following five components are involved in arrest of such a bleeding and subsequent removal of haemostatic plug:
1. Integrity of vascular wall
2. Platelets—abnormalities in count and function
3. Coagulation system—various plasma coagulation factors
4. Fibrinolytic mechanism
5. Inhibitors of coagulation

Normally, a delicate balance is maintained in these factors (Fig. 53.1). Anything that interferes with any of these components results in abnormal bleeding. For investigation of a case for haemostatic function, following scheme is followed:
A. *Clinical evaluation* that includes patient's history including intake of drugs, family history, details of sites of bleeding, frequency, and character of haemostatic defect.
B. *Screening tests* for assessment of abnormalities of various components of haemostasis.
C. *Specific tests* to pinpoint the cause of abnormality.

While clinical evaluation and specific tests can be learnt from textbook, following screening tests are carried out routinely to assess above-mentioned components of haemostasis:
1. *Disorders of vascular haemostasis:* Bleeding time (BT), Hess capillary test (tourniquet test).
2. *Disorders of platelets:* count, bleeding time

3. *Coagulation system:* Whole blood clotting (coagulation) time (CT), activated partial thromboplastin time with kaolin (APTTK), one-stage prothrombin time (PT), thrombin time (TT)
4. *Fibrinolytic system:* Fibrinogen, fibrin degradation products (FDP)
5. *Inhibitors of coagulation:* FDPs

Two of the commonly used screening tests, bleeding time (as a screening test of bleeding from platelet disorders and vascular integrity) and whole blood clotting time (as a

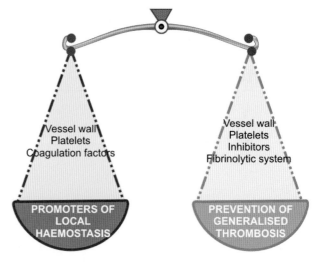

FIGURE 53.1 ◆ The haemostatic balance.

screening test for bleeding from coagulation disorders), are discussed below.

But before that, a few words about the method of collection of blood for coagulation studies are essential. Blood for coagulation studies is colleted by venepuncture in 3.8% trisodium citrate in the ratio of 1:9, i.e. 4.5 ml of blood is added to a clean collection tube containing 0.5 ml of citrate. Care must be taken that the sample is neither haemolysed nor clotted.

Bleeding Time

Bleeding time is duration of bleeding from a standard puncture wound on the skin which is a *measure of the function of the platelets as well as integrity of the vessel wall*. This is one of the most important preliminary indicators for detection of bleeding disorders. This is also the most commonly done preoperative investigation in patients scheduled for surgery.

Principle. A small puncture is made on the skin and the time for which it bleeds is noted. Bleeding stops when platelet plug forms and breach in the vessel wall has sealed.

METHODS FOR BLEEDING TIME

1. Finger tip method
2. Duke's method
3. Ivy's method

1. Finger Tip Method

Procedure
- Clean the tip of a finger with spirit.
- Prick with a disposable needle or lancet.
- Start the stop-watch immediately.
- Start gently touching the pricked finger with a filter paper till blood spots continue to be made on the filter paper.
- Stop the watch when no more blood spot comes on the filter paper and note the time.

Disadvantages
  i. It is a crude method.
  ii. Bleeding time is low by this method.

Normal bleeding time 1-3 minutes.

2. Duke's Method

Procedure
- Clean the lobe of a ear with a spirit swab.
- Using a disposable lancet/needle, puncture the lower edge of the earlobe to a depth of approximately 3 mm.

- Start the stop-watch immediately.
- Allow the drops of blood to fall on a filter paper without touching the earlobe and then slowly touching the blood drop gently on a new area on the filter paper.
- Stop the watch when no more blood comes over the filter paper and note the time.

Advantages of the method
  i. The ear lobule has abundant subcutaneous tissue and is vascular.
  ii. Flow of blood is quite good.

Normal bleeding time 3-5 minutes.

3. Ivy's Method

Procedure
- Tie the BP apparatus cuff around the patient's upper arm and inflate it upto 40 mmHg which is maintained throughout the test.
- Clean an area with spirit over the flexor surface of forearm and allow it dry.
- Using a disposable lancet or surgical blade, make 2 punctures 3 mm deep 5-10 cm from each other taking care not to puncture the superficial veins.
- Start the stop-watch immediately.
- Go on blotting each puncture with a filter paper as in Duke's method.
- Stop the watch, note the time in each puncture and calculate average bleeding time (Fig. 53.2).

Advantages of the method
  i. This is the method of choice.
  ii. It is a standardised method.
  iii. Bleeding time is more accurate.

Normal bleeding time 3-8 minutes.

Clinical Application of Bleeding Time

The bleeding time is *prolonged* in following conditions:
  i. Thrombocytopenia
  ii. Disorders of platelet functions
  iii. Acute leukaemias
  iv. Aplastic anaemias
  v. Liver disease
  vi. von Willebrand's disease
  vii. DIC
  viii. Abnormality in the wall of blood vessels
  ix. Administration of drugs prior to test, e.g. aspirin

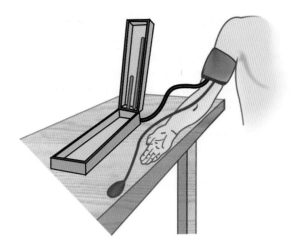
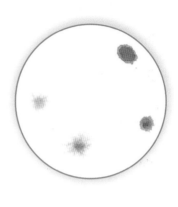

FIGURE 53.2 ◆ Ivy's method for bleeding time.

Clotting Time

This is also known as whole blood clotting time and is a *measure of the plasma clotting factors.* It is a screening test for coagulation disorders.

Various other tests for coagulation disorders include: prothrombin time (PT), partial thromboplastin time with kaolin (PTTK) or activated partial thromboplastin time with kaolin (APTTK), and measurement of fibrinogen.

METHODS FOR CLOTTING TIME

There are two methods of whole blood clotting time:
1. Capillary tube method
2. Lee and White method

1. Capillary Tube Method

Procedure
◆ Clean the tip of a finger with spirit.
◆ Puncture it upto 3 mm deep with a disposable needle.
◆ Start the stopwatch.
◆ Fill two capillary tubes with free flowing blood from the puncture after wiping the first drop of blood.
◆ Keep these tubes at body temperature.
◆ After 2 minutes, start breaking the capillary tube at 1 cm distance to see whether a thin fibrin strand is formed between the two broken ends.
◆ Stop the watch and calculate the time from average of the two capillary tubes.

Disadvantages
i. Method is insensitive.
ii. Method is unreliable.

Advantages
It can be performed when venous blood cannot be obtained.

Normal clotting time 1-5 mintues.

2. Lee and White Method

Procedure
◆ After cleaning the forearm, make a venepuncture and draw 3 ml of blood in a siliconised glass syringe or plastic syringe.
◆ Start the stopwatch.
◆ Transfer 1 ml of blood each into 3 glass tubes which are kept at 37°C in a water bath (Fig. 53.3).
◆ After 3 minutes tilt the tubes one by one every 30 seconds.
◆ The clotting time is taken when the tubes can be tilted without spilling of their contents.
◆ Calculate the clotting time by average of 3 tubes.

Advantages
i. More accurate and standard method.
ii. Test can be run with control.

Disadvantages
i. It is also a rough method.
ii. There can be contamination of syringe or tubes.

Normal clotting time 5-10 mintues.

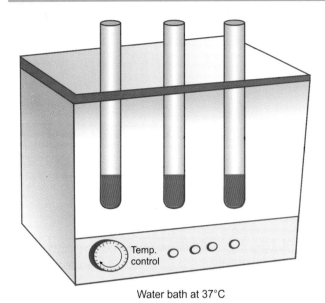

Water bath at 37°C

FIGURE 53.3 ◆ Lee and White method for clotting time.

Sources of error

i. The temperature should be maintained because higher temperature accelerates clotting.
ii. The diameter of the glass tubes should be uniform because clotting is accelerated in narrow tubes.
iii. Vigorous agitation of the tubes should be avoided as it shortens the clotting time.

Clinical Applications of Clotting Time

Clotting time is prolonged in following conditions:

i. Severe deficiency of coagulation factors.
ii. Afibrinogenaemia.
iii. Administration of heparin.
iv. Disseminated intravascular coagulation (DIC).
v. Administration of drugs such as anticoagulants.

Blood Grouping and Cross-matching

Objectives
➢ To learn the principle, technique and interpretation of ABO-Rh blood group system and routine cross-matching.

There are more than 300 blood group systems but ABO and rhesus (Rh) systems are of greatest importance from clinical point of view. These are inherited characters which give rise to antigen-antibody reactions.

ABO System

ABO system was discovered by Landsteiner in 1900 and was conferred Nobel Prize for his discovery belatedly in 1930.

H gene causes secretion of a blood group precursor substance H, which under influence of A and B gene, is majorly converted to either of the two major blood group antigens—A and B present on red cells, while a minor component remains unconverted. Thus ABO system results in 4 major blood groups: A, B, AB and O.

Principle. The red cells contain different types of antigens (agglutinogen), while plasma contains naturally-occurring antibodies (agglutinins). In order to determine the blood group of an individual, the red cells are allowed to react with a sera containing known antibody (agglutinin).

INCIDENCE OF ABO BLOOD GROUPS IN INDIA

Incidence of ABO blood groups varies in different parts of the world and in different ethnic groups. Generally reported data in India are as under:

A	=	22-27%
B	=	31-33%
O	=	34-40%
AB	=	5-8%

METHODS FOR ABO GROUPING

1. Slide method
2. Tube method

1. SLIDE METHOD

◆ Take a clean glass slide (Fig. 54.1).
◆ Divide the slide into two halves with a glass marking pencil and mark these areas as A and B.
◆ Place a drop of serum anti-A (blue) on the slide in area marked A and a drop of serum anti-B (yellow) in the area marked B.
◆ Make a finger prick with a disposable needle after cleaning the area.
◆ Place a drop of blood near anti-A and anti-B serum and mix them with a stick or with the end of a glass slide.
◆ Wait for 5 minutes and look for agglutination.

Observations. If any agglutination occurs it is visible with naked eyes as dark reddish clumps of different sizes. If agglutination is minimal, it can be confirmed by examining it under a microscope.

2. TUBE METHOD

In this method cells and serum of the unknown blood sample to be tested are separated. Cells as well as serum grouping is done (Fig. 54.2).

Cell Grouping (Fig. 54.2,A)

◆ Prepare a 2-5% cell suspension in saline from the unknown blood sample.

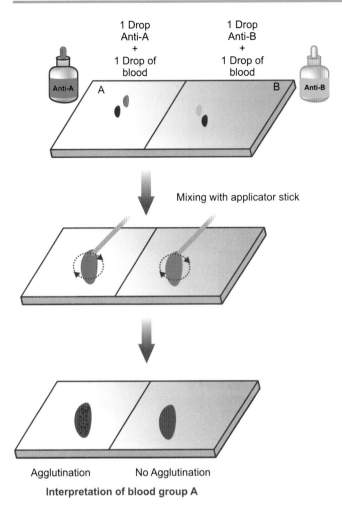

1 Drop
Anti-A
+
1 Drop of
blood

1 Drop
Anti-B
+
1 Drop of
blood

Anti-A   A

B   Anti-B

Mixing with applicator stick

Agglutination   No Agglutination

Interpretation of blood group A

FIGURE 54.1 ◆ Slide method for ABO blood grouping.

Table 54.1: Results of ABO grouping.		
Blood group of person	*Agglutination with anti-A serum*	*Agglutination with anti-B serum*
A	+	–
B	–	+
AB	+	+
O	–	–

Advantages of Tube Method Over Slide Method

Tube method is more accurate because both red cell and serum grouping is done.

The interpretation of ABO grouping by any of the above methods is given in Table 54.1.

NOTE

◆ Red blood cells from a person with *blood group O* contain no antigen; so no agglutination occurs; such a person is a *universal donor.*

◆ Red blood cells from persons with *blood group AB* contain both A and B antigens, so agglutination occurs in both as no antibodies are present in their serum; such individual is a *universal recipient.*

◆ *Bombay blood group* individuals lack H gene and hence no H substance is formed. In the absence of precursor substance H, no A or B antigens are formed (but may have AB genes). Thus, "Bombay blood group" individuals have blood group O but besides having anti-A and anti-B, also possess anti-H antibodies (compared from blood group O persons who have only anti-A and anti-B).

Rhesus (Rh) System

Rh blood group system was first reported by Landsteiner and Weiner in 1940. In contrast to ABO system, Rh antigens are present on red blood cells only while Rh antibodies develop in response to a known stimulus (e.g. blood transfusion, or after first pregnancy). Rh factor is present in 85-95% of human beings.

METHODS FOR Rh GROUPING

1. Slide method
2. Tube method

1. SLIDE METHOD

◆ Take a clean glass slide.
◆ Place a drop of anti-D serum on the slide.

◆ Take 3 test tubes 1,2,3 and put a drop of anti-A (blue), anti-B (yellow) and anti-AB serum (pink) to them.
◆ Add one drop of red cell suspension in each test tube.
◆ Centrifuge at 1500 rpm for one minute.
◆ Look for agglutination either with naked eye or under the microscope.

Serum Grouping (Fig. 54.2,B)

◆ Let the unknown blood sample stand for some time and separate the serum.
◆ Add 2 drops of unknown serum in test tubes 4,5,6.
◆ Add 1 drop of 2-5% cell suspension of known blood of A, B and O group into these test tubes.
◆ Centrifuge at 1500 rpm for one minute.
◆ Look for agglutination either with naked eye or under the microscope.

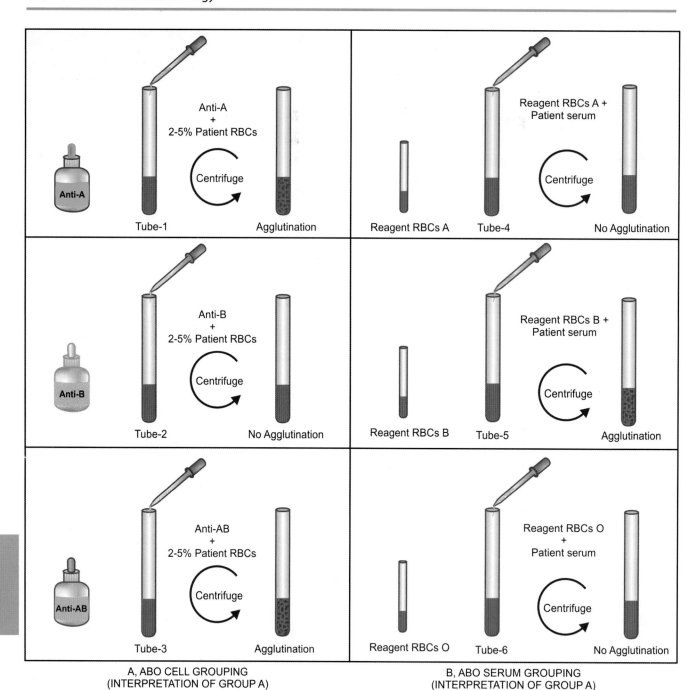

A, ABO CELL GROUPING
(INTERPRETATION OF GROUP A)

B, ABO SERUM GROUPING
(INTERPRETATION OF GROUP A)

FIGURE 54.2 ◆ ABO blood grouping by tube method.

- Place a drop of blood near anti-D serum and mix them as for ABO grouping.
- Wait for 5 minutes and see for agglutination (Fig. 54.3).

2. TUBE METHOD

- Prepare a 2-5% cell suspension in saline from the blood to be tested.

- Take a test tube and put a drop of anti-D serum.
- Add one drop of red cell suspension in the tube.
- Centrifuge at 1500 rpm for 1 minute.
- Look for agglutination either with naked eye or under the microscope (Fig. 54.4).

The interpretation of Rh grouping is given in Table 54.2.

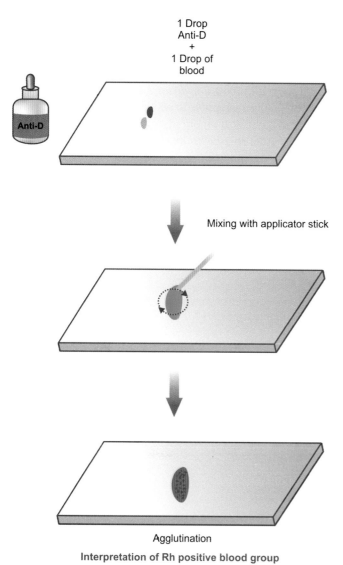

Agglutination

Interpretation of Rh positive blood group

FIGURE 54.3 ◆ Rh grouping by slide method.

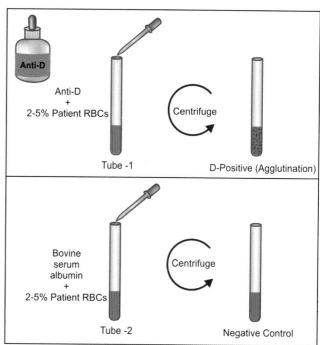

FIGURE 54.4 ◆ Rh grouping by tube method.

Table 54.2: Results of Rh grouping.	
Agglutination	*Rh group*
Present	+
Absent	–

NOTE

◆ Rh-positive subjects have Rh antigen on their red blood cells but no Rh antibody in their serum.

◆ Rh-negative subjects have neither Rh antigen on their red blood cells nor Rh antibody in their serum. The most common Rh antigen is D.

Cross-matching

Before blood transfusion, a cross match is a prerequisite so as to avoid untoward reactions of mismatched transfusion. The donor-recipient compatibility is tested by matching recipient's serum and donor red cells.

PROCEDURE

◆ In a small test tube, place a drop of recipient's serum.
◆ Add washed donor red cells suspended in 5% saline.
◆ Mix the two and incubate at 37° for 30 minutes.
◆ Centrifuge it at 3000 rpm for one minute.
◆ After dislodging the cell palette gently from the centrifuge tube, examine it for presence or absence of agglutination and haemolysis, first grossly and then under the low power of the microscope.

INTERPRETATION

◆ If there is no agglutination or haemolyis, the donor-recipient blood groups are *matched*.

◆ In a *mismatch*, there is either haemolysis or agglutination, or both.

Importance of Blood Grouping

1. *Blood transfusion.* Blood grouping and cross matching are always done prior to blood transfusion to any person.
2. *Haemolytic disease of newborn (HDN).* There is a role of Rh and ABO blood grouping in HDN.
3. *Paternity disputes.* ABO and Rh blood grouping are used as a routine test in such cases. It is possible to disprove parentage but impossible to prove parent-hood.
4. *Medicolegal use.* In criminal cases, whether a stain is blood or not and its blood group can be detected.
5. *Usefulness of blood groups,* in immunology, genetics and anthropology.
6. *Susceptibility to various diseases.* Persons with blood group O are more susceptible to peptic ulcer while persons with blood group A are more susceptible to gastric cancer.
7. As a part of routine *health check-up* and routine licensing for driving, job, etc.

Peripheral Smear Examination in Anaemias

Objectives

➢ To have knowledge for systematic planning of investigations in a case of anaemia.
➢ To learn the skill of systematic approach to examine a stained peripheral blood film.
➢ To learn the skill of examination of blood film for typing of anaemia into 3 major types: microcytic-hypochromic (iron deficiency), macrocytic (megaloblastic) and haemolytic (thalassaemia).

Anaemia is defined as a haemoglobin concentration in blood below the lower limit of the normal range for the age and sex of the individual:

◆ *In adults*, the lower extreme of the normal haemoglobin is taken as 13 g/dl for males and 11.5 g/dl for females.

◆ *In pregnancy* due to haemodilution the lower limit of Hb is taken as 10.5 g/dl.

◆ *For newborn infants*, 15 g/dl is taken as the lower limit at birth and 9.5 g/dl at 3 months.

However, according to WHO criteria, haemoglobin less than 12 gm/dl in males and less than 10.5 gm/dl in females is taken as anaemia.

After obtaining the full medical history pertaining to different general and specific signs and symptoms, the patient is examined for evidence of anaemia. Special emphasis is placed on colour of skin, conjunctivae, sclerae and nails. Changes in the retina, atrophy of the papillae of the tongue, rectal examination for evidence of bleeding, and presence of hepatomegaly, splenomegaly, lymphadenopathy and bony tenderness are looked for.

Plan of Investigation for Anaemia

In order to confirm or deny the presence of anaemia, its type and its cause, the following plan of investigations is generally followed:

I. *Screening tests:*
  A. Haemoglobin estimation
  B. Peripheral blood film examination
  C. Red cell indices
  D. Leucocyte and platelet count
  E. Reticulocyte count
II. *Confirmatory tests:*
  A. Bone marrow examination
  B. Biochemical tests

HAEMOGLOBIN ESTIMATION

The first and foremost investigation in any suspected case of anaemia is to carry out the haemoglobin estimation. Several methods are available but most reliable and accurate is the cyanmethaemoglobin (HiCN) method employing Drabkin's solution and a spectrophotometer (Exercise 47). If the haemoglobin value is below the lower limit of the normal range for particular age and sex, the patient is said to be anaemic.

PERIPHERAL BLOOD FILM EXAMINATION

The haemoglobin estimation is invariably followed by examination of a peripheral blood film for morphologic features after staining it with the Romanowsky dyes (e.g. Leishman's stain, May-Grunwald-Giemsa's stain, Jenner-Giemsa's stain, etc). The blood smear is evaluated in an area where there is neither rouleaux formation nor so thin as to cause red cell distortion. Such an area can usually be found towards the tail of the film, but not actually at the tail (Exercise 50). The following abnormalities in erythroid series of cells are particularly looked for in a blood smear:

Variation in Size (Anisocytosis)

Normally, there is slight variation in diameter of the biconcave disc shaped red cells from 6.7-7.7 mm (mean value 7.2 mm). Increased variation in size of the red cell is termed anisocytosis. Anisocytosis may be due to the presence of cells larger than normal (macrocytosis) or cells smaller than normal (microcytosis). Sometimes both microcytosis and macrocytosis are present (dimorphic).

- *Macrocytes* are classically found in megaloblastic anaemia; other causes are aplastic anaemia, other dyserythropoietic anaemias, chronic liver disease and in conditions with increased erythropoiesis.
- *Microcytes* are present in iron-deficiency anaemia, thalassaemia and spherocytosis. They may also result from fragmentation of erythrocytes such as in haemolytic anaemia.

Variation in Shape (Poikilocytosis)

Increased variation in shape of the red cells is termed poikilocytosis. The nature of the abnormal shape determines the cause of anaemia. Poikilocytes are produced in various types of abnormal erythropoiesis, e.g. in megaloblastic anaemia, iron-deficiency anaemia, thalassaemia, myelosclerosis and microangiopathic haemolytic anaemia.

Inadequate Haemoglobin Formation (Hypochromasia)

Normally, the intensity of pink staining of haemoglobin in a Romanowsky-stained blood smear gradually decreases from the periphery to the centre of the cell. Increased central pallor is referred to as *hypochromasia*. It may develop either from lowered haemoglobin content (e.g. in iron-deficiency anaemia, chronic infections), or due to thinness of the red cells (e.g. in thalassaemia, sideroblastic anaemia). Unusually deep pink staining of the red cells due to increased haemoglobin concentration is termed hyperchromasia and may be found in megaloblastic anaemia, spherocytosis and in neonatal blood.

Compensatory Erythropoiesis

A number of changes are associated with compensatory increase in erythropoietic activity. These are as under:

i. *Polychromasia* is defined as more than one type of colour in the red cells. Polychromatic red cells are slightly larger, generally stain bluish-grey and represent reticulocytes and, thus, correlate well with reticulocyte count.

ii. *Normoblastaemia* is presence of nucleated red cells in the peripheral blood film. A small number of normoblasts (or erythroblasts) may be normally found in cord blood at birth. They are found in large numbers in haemolytic disease of the newborn, other haemolytic disorders and in extramedullary erythropoiesis. They may also appear in the blood in various types of severe anaemias except in aplastic anaemia. Normoblastaemia may also occur after splenectomy.

iii. *Punctate basophilia* or *basophilic stippling* is diffuse and uniform basophilic granularity in the cell which does not stain positively with Perl's reaction (in contrast to Pappenheimer bodies which stain positively). Classical punctate basophilia is seen in aplastic anaemia, thalassaemia, myelodysplasia, infections and lead poisoning.

iv. *Howell-Jolly bodies* are purple nuclear remnants, usually found singly, and are larger than basophilic stippling. They are present in megaloblastic anaemia and after splenectomy.

Miscellaneous Changes

In addition to the morphologic abnormalities of red cells described above, several other abnormal red cells may be found in different haematological disorders. Some of these are as follows (Fig. 55.1):

i. *Spherocytosis* is characterised by presence of spheroidal rather than biconcave disc-shaped red cells. Spherocytes are seen in hereditary spherocytosis, autoimmune haemolytic anaemia and in ABO haemolytic disease of the newborn.

ii. *Schistocytosis* is identified by fragmentation of erythrocytes. Schistocytes are found in thalassaemia, hereditary eliptocytosis, megaloblastic anaemia, iron-deficiency anaemia, microangiopathic haemolytic anaemia and in severe burns.

iii. *Irregularly contracted red cells* are found in drug- and chemical-induced haemolytic anaemia and in unstable haemoglobinopathies.

iv. *Leptocytosis* is the presence of unusually thin red cells. Leptocytes are seen in severe iron deficiency and thalassaemia. *Target cell* is a form of leptocyte in which there is central round stained area and a peripheral rim of haemoglobin. Target cells are found in iron deficiency, thalassaemia, chronic liver disease, and after splenectomy.

v. *Sickle cells or drepanocytes* are sickle-shaped red cells found in sickle cell disease.

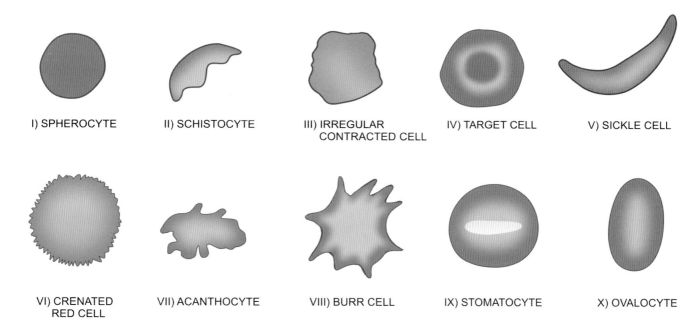

I) SPHEROCYTE II) SCHISTOCYTE III) IRREGULAR CONTRACTED CELL IV) TARGET CELL V) SICKLE CELL

VI) CRENATED RED CELL VII) ACANTHOCYTE VIII) BURR CELL IX) STOMATOCYTE X) OVALOCYTE

FIGURE 55.1 ◆ Some of the common morphologic abnormalities of red cells (The serial numbers in the illustrations correspond to the sequence in which they are described in the text).

vi. *Crenated red cells* are the erythrocytes which develop numerous projections from the surface. They are present in blood films due to alkaline pH, presence of traces of fatty substances on the slides and in cases where the film is made from blood that has been allowed to stand overnight.

vii. *Acanthocytosis* is the presence of coarsely crenated red cells. Acanthocytes are found in large number in blood film made from splenectomised subjects, in chronic liver disease and in abetalipoproteinaemia.

viii. *Burr cells* are cell fragments having one or more spines. They are particularly found in uraemia and in pyruvate kinase deficinecy.

ix. *Stomatocytosis* is the presence of stomatocytes which have central area having slit-like or mouth-like appearance. They are found in alcoholism or as an artefact.

x. *Ovalocytosis* or *elliptocytosis* is the oval or elliptical shape of red cells. Their highest proportion (79%) is seen in hereditary ovalocytosis and elliptocytosis; other conditions showing such abnormal shapes of red cells are megaloblastic anaemia and hypochromic anaemia.

RED CELL INDICES

An alternative method to diagnose and detect the severity of anaemia is by measuring the red cell indices (Exercise 52):

1. In iron deficiency and thalassaemia, MCV, MCH and MCHC are reduced.
2. In anaemia due to acute blood loss and haemolytic anaemias, MCV, MCH and MCHC are all within normal limits.
3. In megaloblastic anaemias, MCV is raised above the normal range.

LEUCOCYTE AND PLATELET COUNT

Measurement of leucocyte and platelet count helps to distinguish pure anaemia from pancytopenia in which red cells, granulocytes and platelets are all reduced. In anaemias due to haemolysis or haemorrhage, the neutrophil count and platelet counts are often elevated. In infections and leukaemias, the leucocyte counts are high and immature leucocytes appear in the blood (Exercise 51).

RETICULOCYTE COUNT

Reticulocyte count (normal 0.5-2.5%) is done in each case of anaemia to assess the marrow erythropoietic activity (Exercise 49). In acute haemorrhage and in haemolysis, the reticulocyte response is indicative of impaired marrow function.

BONE MARROW EXAMINATION

Bone marrow aspiration is done in cases where the cause for anaemia is not obvious. The procedures involved for marrow aspiration and trephine biopsy and their relative advantages and disadvantages have been discussed in Exercise 58.

BIOCHEMICAL TESTS

In addition to these general tests, certain specific tests are done in different types of anaemias which include biochemical tests, radio-assay and others.

PBF in Microcytic Hypochromic Anaemia (Iron Deficiency Anaemia)

The degree of anaemia in iron deficiency varies. It is usually mild to moderate but occasionally it may be marked (haemoglobin less than 6 g/dl) due to persistent and severe blood loss. The salient haematological findings in these cases are as under:

i. *Haemoglobin.* The essential feature is a fall in haemoglobin concentration up to a variable degree.

ii. *Red cells.* The red cells in the blood film are hypochromic and microcytic, and there is anisocytosis and poikilocytosis. Hypochromia generally precedes microcytosis. Hypochromia is due to poor filling of the red cells with haemoglobin so that there is increased central pallor (Fig. 55.2). In severe cases, red cells reveal only a thin rim of haemoglobin at the periphery (ring or pessary cell). Target cells, elliptical forms and polychromatic cells are often present. Normoblasts are uncommon. RBC count is below normal but is generally not proportionate to the

fall in haemoglobin value. When iron deficiency is associated with severe folate or vitamin B12 deficiency, a dimorphic blood picture occurs with dual population of red cells, macrocytic as well as microcytic-hypochromic.

iii. *Reticulocyte count.* The reticulocyte count is normal or reduced but may be slightly raised (2-5%) in cases after haemorrhage.

iv. *Absolute values.* The red cell indices reveal a diminished MCV (below 50 fl), diminished MCH (below 15 pg) and diminished MCHC (below 20 g/dl).

v. *Leucocytes.* The total and differential white cell counts are usually normal. However, in cases in which iron deficiency is due to parasitic infestations such as hookworm infestation, there may be associated eosinophilia.

vi. *Platelets.* Platelet count is usually normal but may be slightly to moderately raised in patients who have had recent bleeding.

PBF in Macrocytic Anaemia (Megaloblastic Anaemia)

The investigations of a suspected case of megaloblastic anaemia are aimed at 2 aspects:

A. ***General laboratory investigations of anaemia*** which include blood picture, red cell indices, bone marrow findings, and biochemical tests.

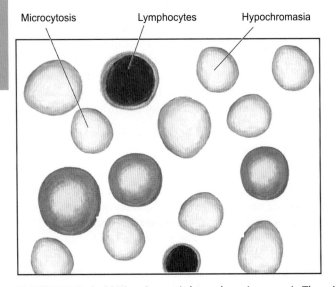

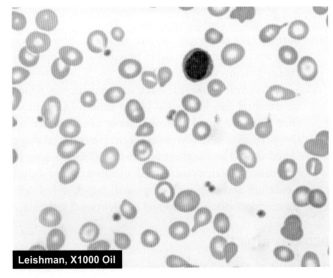

Leishman, X1000 Oil

FIGURE 55.2 ◆ PBF in microcytic hypochromic anaemia. There is moderate microcytosis and hypochromasia and a few target cells.

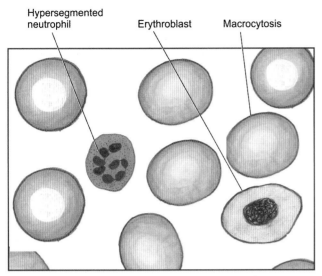

Hypersegmented neutrophil   Erythroblast   Macrocytosis

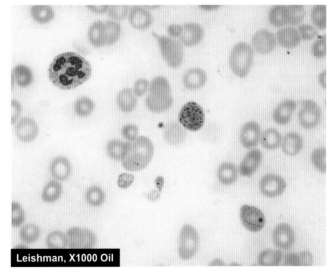

Leishman, X1000 Oil

FIGURE 55.3 ◆ PBF in megaloblastic anaemia. There is prominent macrocytosis, oval red cells and hypersegmented neutrophil.

B. *Special tests* to establish the cause of megaloblastic anaemia as to know whether it is due to deficiency of vitamin B12 or folate.

The estimation of haemoglobin, examination of a blood film and evaluation of absolute values are essential preliminary investigations.

   i. *Haemoglobin.* The haemoglobin estimation reveals values below the normal range. The fall in haemoglobin concentration may be of a variable degree.

   ii. *Red cells.* The red blood cell morphology in a blood film shows the characteristic macrocytosis. However, macrocytosis can also be seen in several other disorders such as: haemolysis, liver disease, alcoholism, hypothyroidism, aplastic anaemia, myeloproliferative disorders and reticulocytosis. In addition, the blood smear demonstrates marked anisocytosis, poikilocytosis and presence of macro-ovalocytes. Basophilic stippling, Howell-Jolly bodies, Cabot ring and occasional normoblast may also be seen (Fig. 55.3).

   iii. *Reticulocyte count.* The reticulocyte count is generally low to normal in untreated cases.

   iv. *Absolute values.* The red cell indices reveal an elevated MCV (above 120 fl) proportionate to the severity of macrocytosis, elevated MCH (above 50 pg) and normal or reduced MCHC.

   v. *Leucocytes.* The total white blood cell count may be reduced. Presence of characteristic hypersegmented neutrophils (5% neutrophils having more than 5 nuclear lobes) in the blood film should raise the suspicion of

megaloblastic anaemia. An occasional myelocyte may also be seen.

   vi. *Platelets.* Platelet count may be moderately reduced in severely anaemic patients. Bizarre forms of platelets may be seen.

PBF in Haemolytic Anaemia (Thalassaemia)

The thalassaemias are a diverse group of hereditary disorders in which there is reduced rate of synthesis of one or more of the globin polypeptide chains. Thus, thalassaemias, unlike haemoglobinopathies which are qualitative disorders of haemoglobin, are *quantitative abnormalities of polypeptide globin chain synthesis.**

A classification of various types of thalassaemias along with the clinical syndromes produced and salient laboratory findings is given in Table 55.1.

β-thalassaemia major, also termed Mediterranean or Cooley's anaemia, is the most common form of congenital haemolytic anaemia. More commonly, β-thalassaemia major is a homozygous state with either complete absence of β-chain synthesis (β° thalassaemia major) or only small amounts of β-chains are formed (β+ thalassaemia major).

---

*In a normal adult, distribution of haemoglobin is as under: HbA ($\alpha_2\beta_2$) = 95-98%, HbA$_2$ ($\alpha_2\delta_2$) (a minor variant of HbA) = 1.5-3.5%, HbF ($\alpha_2\gamma_2$) = less than 1%. But the level of HbF in children under 6 months is slightly higher.

	TABLE 55.1: Classification of thalassaemias.			
Type	Hb	Hb-electrophoresis	Genotype	Clinical syndrome
α-Thalassaemias				
1. Hydrops foetalis	3-10 g/dl	Hb Barts (γ_4) (100%)	Deletion of four α-genes	Fatal in utero or in early infancy
2. Hb-H disease	2-12 g/dl	HbF (10%)	Deletion of three α-genes	Haemolytic anaemia
3. α-Thalassaemia trait	10-14 g/dl	Normal	Deletion of two α-genes	Microcytic hypochromic blood picture but no anaemia
β-Thalassaemias				
1. β-Thalassaemia major	< 5 g/dl	HbA (0-50%), HbF(50-98%)	$\beta^{thal}/\beta^{thal}$	Severe congenital haemolytic anaemia, requires blood transfusions
2. β-Thalassaemia intermedia	5-10 g/dl	Variable	Multiple mechanisms	Severe anaemia, but regular blood transfusions not required
3. β-Thalassaemia minor	10-12 g/dl	HbA$_2$ (4-9%) HbF (1-5%)	β^{A}/β^{thal}	Usually asymptomatic

These result in excessive formation of alternate haemoglobins, HbF ($\alpha_2 \gamma_2$) and HbA$_2$ ($\alpha_2 \delta_2$).

Clinical manifestations appear insidiously and are as under:

1. *Anaemia* starts appearing within the first 4-6 months of life when the switch from γ-chain to β-chain production occurs.
2. *Marked hepatosplenomegaly* occurs due to excessive red cell destruction, extramedullary haematopoiesis and iron overload.
3. *Expansion of bones* occurs due to marked erythroid hyperplasia leading to thalassaemic facies and malocclusion of the jaw.
4. *Iron overload* due to repeated blood transfusions causes damage to the endocrine organs resulting in slow rate of growth and development, delayed puberty, diabetes mellitus and damage to the liver and heart.

The haematological investigations reveal the following findings (Fig. 55.4):

i. *Anaemia*, usually severe.
ii. *Blood film* shows severe microcytic hypochromic red cell morphology, marked anisopoikilocytosis, basophilic stippling, presence of many target cells, tear drop cells and normoblasts.
iii. *Serum bilirubin* (unconjugated) is generally raised.
iv. *Reticulocytosis* is generally present.
v. *MCV, MCH and MCHC* are significantly reduced.

vi. *WBC count* is often raised with some shift to left of the neutrophil series, with presence of some myelocytes and metamyelocytes.
vii. *Platelet count* is usually normal but may be reduced in patients with massive splenomegaly.
viii. *Osmotic fragility* done by NESTROF (Naked Eye Single Tube Rapid Osmotic Fragility) test characteristically reveals increased resistance to saline haemolysis, i.e. decreased osmotic fragility.
ix. *Alkali denaturation test* for HbF reveals increased HbF levels in thalassaemia major.
x. *HbA$_2$ denaturation* may be carried out by Hb electrophoresis, column chromatography or high performance liquid chromatography (HPLC).
xi. *Haemoglobin electrophoresis* shows presence of increased amounts of HbF, increased amount of HbA$_2$ and almost complete absence or presence of variable amounts of HbA. The increased level of HbA$_2$ has not been found in any other haemoglobin abnormality except β-thalassaemia. The increased synthesis of HbA$_2$ is probably due to increased activity at both δ-chain loci.
xii. *Bone marrow aspirate examination* shows normoblastic erythroid hyperplasia with predominance of intermediate and late normoblasts which are generally smaller in size than normal. Iron staining demonstrates siderotic granules in the cytoplasm of normoblasts, increased reticuloendothelial iron but ring sideroblasts are only occasionally seen.

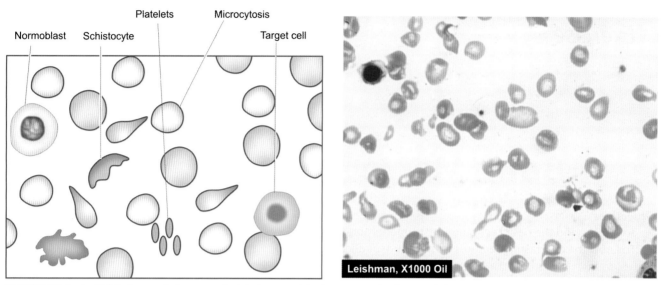

FIGURE 55.4 ◆ PBF in haemolytic anaemia (Thalassaemia). There is marked anisopoikilocytosis and presence of nucleated red cells.

Bone Marrow Examination

Objectives
➢ To understand the basic technique, instruments and applications of bone marrow aspiration and trephine biopsy.
➢ To know the contrasting features of marrow aspiration and trephine and to know normal myelogram.

Examination of the bone marrow provides an invaluable diagnostic help in some cases, while in others it is of value in confirming a diagnosis suspected on clinical examination or on the blood film. A peripheral blood examination, however, must always precede bone marrow examination.

Bone marrow examination may be performed by two methods: aspiration and trephine biopsy. A comparison of the two methods is summarised in Table 56.1 below.

Bone Marrow Aspiration

The method involves suction of marrow via a strong, wide bore, short-bevelled needle fitted with a stylet and an adjustable guard in order to prevent excessive penetration; for instance Salah bone marrow aspiration needle (Fig. 56.1,A) or Klima bone marrow needle. Smears are prepared immediately from the bone marrow aspirate and are fixed in 95% methanol after air-drying. The usual Romanowsky technique is employed for staining and a stain for iron is performed routinely so as to assess the reticuloendothelial stores of iron.

The marrow film provides assessment of the following features:

i. Cellularity
ii. Details of developing blood cells (i.e. normoblastic or megaloblastic, myeloid, lymphoid, macrophages and megakaryocytic)

TABLE 56.1: Comparison of bone marrow aspiration and trephine biopsy.		
Feature	Aspiration	Trephine
1. Site	Sternum, posterior iliac crest; tibial head in infants	Posterior iliac crest
2. Instrument	Salah BM aspiration needle	Jamshidi trephine needle
3. Stains	Romanowsky, Perls' reaction for iron on smears	Haematoxylin and eosin, reticulin on tissue sections
4. Time	Within 1-2 hours	Within 1-7 days
5. Morphology	Better cellular morphology of aspiration smears but marrow architecture is indistinct	Better marrow architectural pattern but cell morphology is not as distinct since tissue sections are examined and not smears
6. Indications	Anaemias, suspected leukaemias, neutropenia thrombocytopenia, polycythaemia, myeloma, lymphomas, carcinomatosis, lipid storage diseases, granulomatous conditions, parasites, fungi, and unexplained enlargements of liver, spleen or lymph nodes.	Additional indications are: myelosclerosis, aplastic anaemia and in cases with 'dry tap' on aspiration.

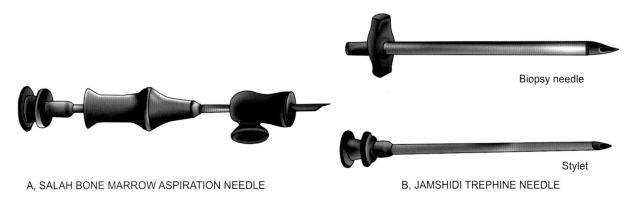

A, SALAH BONE MARROW ASPIRATION NEEDLE   B, JAMSHIDI TREPHINE NEEDLE

FIGURE 56.1 ◆ Needles used for bone marrow examination.

iii. Ratio between erythroid and myeloid cells in storage diseases

iv. For the presence of cells foreign to the marrow such as secondary carcinoma, granulomatous conditions, fungi (e.g. histoplasmosis) and parasites (e.g. malaria, leishmaniasis, trypanosomiasis).

Estimation of the proportion of cellular components in the marrow, however, can be provided by doing a differential count of at least 500 cells called myelogram. Parameters of normal myelogram are given in Table 56.2. In some conditions, the marrow cells can be used for more detailed special tests such as cytogenetics, microbiological culture, biochemical analysis, and immunological and cytological markers.

A few examples of application of bone marrow aspiration in iron deficiency anaemia (Fig. 56.2), megaloblastic anaemia (Fig. 56.3), sideroblastic anaemia (Fig. 56.4) and idiopathic thrombocytopenic purpura (ITP) (Fig. 56.5) are illustrated.

TABLE 56.2: Normal adult bone marrow counts (Myelogram).

Fat/cell ratio: 50 : 50

Myeloid/erythroid (M/E) ratio: 2-4:1 (mean 3:1)

Myeloid series: 30-45% (37.5%)
— Myeloblasts: 0.1-3.5%
— Promyelocytes: 0.5-5%

Erythroid series: 10-15% (mean 12.5%)

Megakaryocytes: 0.5%

Lymphocytes: 5-20%

Plasma cells: ≤ 3%

Reticulum cells: 0.1-2%

The format of bone marrow aspirate report in a case of iron deficiency anaemia is shown in Figure 56.6.

Trephine Biopsy

Trephine biopsy is performed by a simple Jamshidi trephine needle by which a core of tissue from periosteum to bone marrow cavity is obtained (Fig. 56.1,B). As the core of the bone marrow is obtained, it is rolled between two glass slides to obtain imprint smears. These smears can be used to study

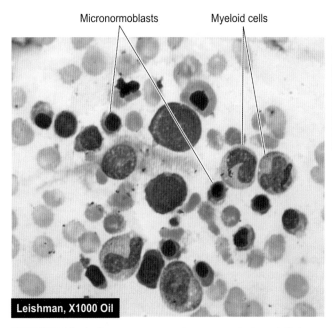

FIGURE 56.2 ◆ Bone marrow aspirate smear in iron deficiency anaemia showing micronormoblastic erythropoiesis.

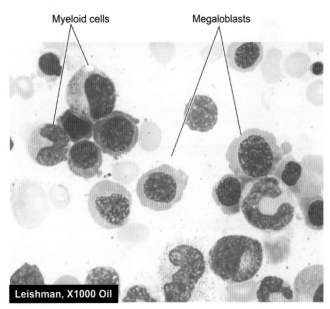

FIGURE 56.3 ◆ Bone marrow aspirate smear showing megaloblastic erythropoiesis.

the morphology and to perform special stains. The tissue is then fixed, decalcified and processed for histological sections and stained with haematoxylin and eosin and for reticulin (Fig. 56.7).

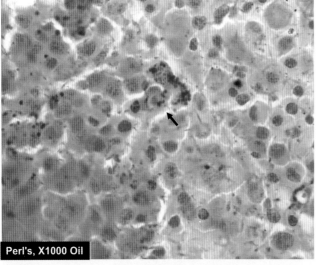

FIGURE 56.4 ◆ Bone marrow aspirate smear in sideroblastic anaemia (Perl's stain). It shows marked excess of reticular iron and a ringed sideroblast (arrow) having Prussian blue granules.

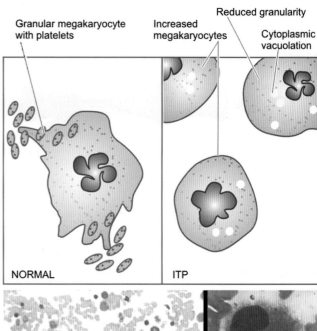

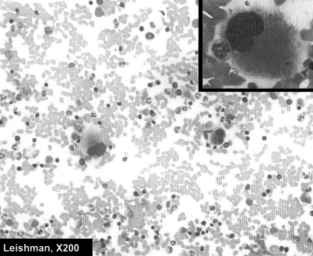

FIGURE 56.5 ◆ Bone marrow aspirated in immune thrombo-cytopenic purpura (ITP). It shows characteristic increase in number of megakaryocytes without budding of any platelets. These megakaryocytes have single non-lobulated nuclei and reduced cytoplasmic granularity (inbox).

Trephine biospy is useful over aspiration since it provides an excellent view of the overall marrow architecture, cellularity, and presence or absence of infiltrates, but is less valuable than aspiration as far as individual cell morphology is concerned, as summed up in Table 56.1.

BONE MARROW ASPIRATION REPORT

No.................

Date............................

Name ....Age......................Sex...

C.R.No/O.P.D. No..

Report.

Preparation/cellularity	:	Cellular preparation
M.E. ratio	:	Equal (Normal mean = 3:1)
Erythropoiesis	:	Micronormoblastic with inadequate haemoglobinisation
Myeloid cells	:	Normal in number, morphology and maturation
Megakaryocytes	:	Normal in number and morphology (Normal = 0.1-0.5%)
Plasma cells	:	Within normal limits (Normal = ≤ 3%)
Reticulum cells	:	Unremarkable (Normal = 0.3-0.9%)
Reticular iron	:	Grade zero (Normal = Grade III to IV)
Sideroblasts	:	None
Any other finding	:	Nil
Comments	:	IRON DEFICIENT ERYTHROPOIESIS

Signature

FIGURE 56.6 ◆ Format of bone marrow aspirate report.

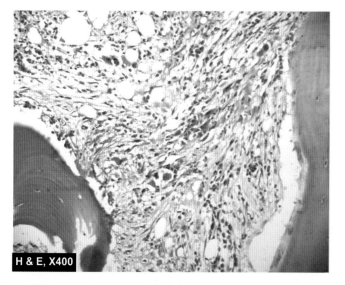
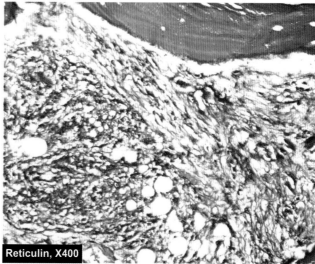

FIGURE 56.7 ◆ Trephine biopsy in myelofibrosis. The soft tissue enclosed in the marrow spaces is composed of rich fibrous tissue.

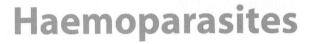

Haemoparasites

Objectives

➤ To learn to examine the peripheral smear for identification of various types of malarial parasites and microfilaria.

➤ To know the features of *Leishmania donovani* (LD) bodies in bone marrow aspirate smear.

Infection with blood parasites, particularly malaria and filaria, exacts an enormous toll of human suffering in the Indian subcontinent. While malaria and microfilaria can be easily diagnosed by careful examination of well-prepared and stained peripheral blood film (PBF) or smear, *Leishmania* is identified in bone marrow smears.

PBF in Malarial Parasite

Four species of malarial parasite (MP) are encountered in human disease: *Plasmodium vivax* and *P. ovale*, both of which cause benign tertian malaria (febrile episodes typically occurring at 48 hourly intervals); *P. falciparum*, which is

Table 57.1: Contrasting features of common forms of malarial parasite.		
Features	P. falciparum	P. vivax
1. **Schizogony period**	48 hours	48 hours or less
2. **Forms in peripheral blood**	Trophozoites, schizonts and gametocytes	Rings and crescents only; growing trophozoites and schizonts rarely seen
3. **Trophozoite and ring form**	Size 2.5 μ; cytoplasm opposite the nucleus is thicker	Size 1.25 to 1.5 μ; cytoplasm fine and regular in outline, often with 2 nuclei, may have accolé and multiple infection
4. **Growing forms**	Irregular with a vacuole; actively amoeboid	Assume a compact form; pigments collect into a single mass early
5. **Schizont**	Size 9 to 10 μ; regular, almost completely fills an enlarged red blood cell	Size 4.5 to 5 μ; fills two-thirds of a red cell mass which is not enlarged
6. **Merozoites**	12 to 24, arranged in an irregular grape-like cluster	18 to 24 or more, arranged in a grape-like cluster
7. **Haemozoin**	Yellowish-brown, fine granules	Dark brown or blackish, one solid block
8. **Changes in infected host RBCs**	Enlarged, pale, Schuffner's dots present	Usually unaltered, crenation, reddish violet colour and Maurer's dots
9. **Gametocyte**	Spherical or globular; much larger than a red blood cell; host cell enlarged with Schuffner's dots	Crescentic; larger than a red blood cell; host cell hardly recognisable

responsible for most fatalities; and *P. malariae*, which causes quartan malaria (febrile episodes typically occurring at 72 hourly intervals). The differences in appearances of various stages of *P. falciparum* and *P. vivax* are contrasted in Table 57.1.

M/E

1. Blood smears should be made within a few hours of peak of febrile paroxysms.
2. Thin and thick blood smears can be made to demonstrate the malarial parasite.
3. *Thick smear* is prepared by spreading a drop of blood on the slide in an area of about 2 cm diameter and allowing it to dry. The smear is then given a few dips in tap water until red coloured solution comes out (dehaemoglobinisation of the smear). The smear is then fixed in the methanol and stained with Leishman's or Giemsa or Field's stain. Thick smear is of use in quick detection of malarial parasite while thin smear is useful for studying morphology.
4. The detailed features in morphology of two main species of malarial parasite (*P. vivax* and *P. falciparum*) are given in Table 57.1 and shown in Figure 57.1.
5. Besides, PBF also shows monocytosis with moderate leucopenia. Two-thirds of patients infected with *P. falciparum* infection also show anaemia with increased reticulocyte count (due to haemolysis) and thrombocytopenia.

In addition to examination of PBF, malaria can also be detected by other methods as follows:

i. *Fluorescent microscopy.* Nucleic acids of the parasite are stained with fluorescent dyes and visualised by fluorescent microscopy.

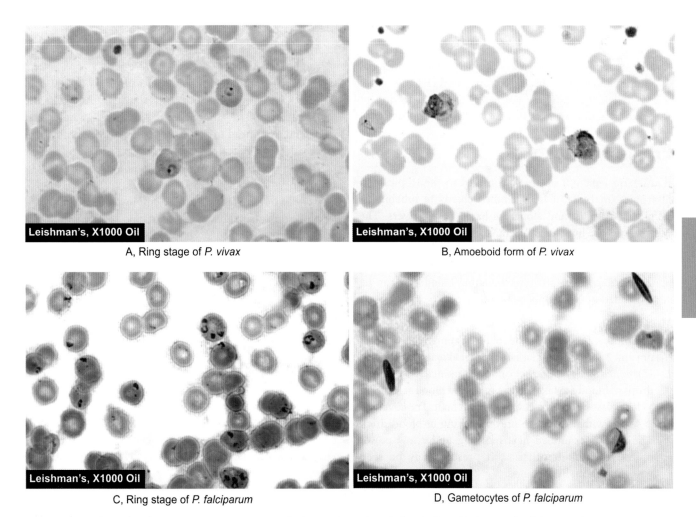

A, Ring stage of *P. vivax*

B, Amoeboid form of *P. vivax*

C, Ring stage of *P. falciparum*

D, Gametocytes of *P. falciparum*

FIGURE 57.1 ◆ Malarial parasite—various stages of two main species of *Plasmodium* (*P. vivax* and *P. falciparum*).

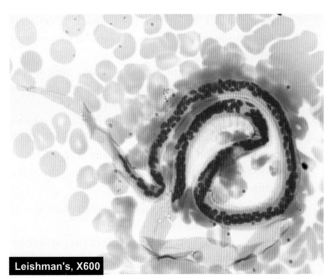

Leishman's, X600

FIGURE 57.2 ◆ Microfilariae in thick peripheral blood smear.

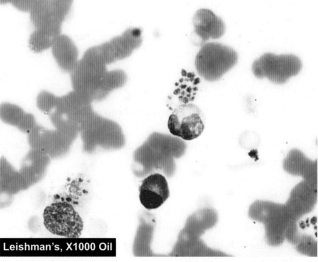

Leishman's, X1000 Oil

FIGURE 57.3 ◆ *Leishmania donovani* (LD) bodies in the reticulum cells of the bone marrow aspirate smear.

ii. *pLDH based immunochromatographic test.* Presence of *Plasmodium* LDH enzyme is detected using monoclonal antibodies against specific epitopes of pLDH.

iii. *PCR based test.* These are based on the detection of nucleic acid sequences specific to *Plasmodium* species.

PBF in Filariasis

Wuchereria bancrofti is largely confined to the tropics and subtropics. In India, it is distributed chiefly in inhabitants along the sea-coast and along the banks of big rivers. The adult worms are long hair like transparent nematodes which remain localised to lymphatic vessels and lymph nodes causing massive lymphoedema and elephantiasis. Embryonic forms (microfilariae) reach into the circulating blood and can be demonstrated in the peripheral blood.

M/E
1. The blood sample should be collected at night between 10 pm and 2 am as microfilariae exhibit *nocturnal periodicity*.
2. *Unstained wet preparation* can be examined. In this, 2-3 drops of blood are taken of the midnight blood sample on a clean glass slide and a coverslip is put on it. The coverslip is sealed with vaseline to prevent drying of blood drop. The slide is examined next morning under low power objective and microfilariae, if present, may be seen wriggling about in the blood.

3. *Thin and thick blood smears* as described for malaria above can be made.
4. *Morphologically*, microfilariae measures about 290 μ in length and 6 μ in breadth. A hyaline sheath engulfs the larval body. The somatic cells appear as granules and extend from head to tail except five percent terminal tail sheath (Fig. 57.2).
5. In addition, PBF shows *eosinophilia* as compared to monocytosis seen in case of malaria.
6. *Concentration methods* can be employed for higher yield of the organism. Five to ten ml of blood is taken in EDTA vial and centrifuged at 2000 rpm for 2 to 5 minutes. The supernatant fluid is decanted and the sediment is examined for microfilariae.

Bone Marrow in Leishmaniasis

The parasite *Leishmania donovani* (LD) causes visceral leishmaniasis or kala-azar. In India, it is endemic in the states of Bihar, Orissa, Chennai and eastern parts of Uttar Pradesh.

M/E
i. Amastigote forms or LD bodies are observed in reticuloendothelial cells of the bone marrow and spleen.
ii. LD body measures 2 to 4 μ in size having a nucleus and kinetoplast (Fig. 57.3).

Haematologic Malignancies: Leukaemias

Objectives

➢ To understand the current concept of common classification of haematologic malignancies (leukaemias-lymphomas) as myeloid and lymphoid neoplasms.

➢ To learn to diagnose leukaemias by routine haematologic tests into acute and chronic, and further subtyping of chronic leukaemias into chronic myeloid and chronic lymphoid (i.e. CML and CLL).

Common Classification of Leukaemias-Lymphomas

Neoplastic proliferations of white blood cells—leukaemias and lymphomas, are the most important group of leucocyte disorders.

Historically, leukaemias have been classified on the basis of cell types predominantly involved into *myeloid* and *lymphoid,* and on the basis of natural history of the disease, into *acute* and *chronic.* Thus, there are 4 main types of leukaemias:

◆ *Acute myeloblastic leukaemia (AML)*
◆ *Acute lymphoblastic leukaemia (ALL)*
◆ *Chronic myeloid leukaemia (CML)*
◆ *Chronic lymphocytic leukaemias (CLL).*

In general, acute leukaemias are characterised by predominance of undifferentiated leucocyte precursors or leukaemic blasts and have a rapidly downhill course. Chronic leukaemias, on the other hand, have easily recognisable late precursor series of leucocytes circulating in large number as the predominant leukaemic cell type and the patients tend to have more indolent behaviour.

Similarly, over the years, lymphomas which are malignant tumours of lymphoreticular tissues have been categorised into two distinct clinicopathologic groups: *Hodgkin's lymphoma* or *Hodgkin's disease (HD)* characterised by pathognomonic presence of Reed-Sternberg cells, and a heterogenous group of *non-Hodgkin's lymphomas (NHL).*

In the last 50 years, several classification systems have been proposed for leukaemias and lymphomas. Current classification scheme proposed by the World Health Organisation (WHO) in 2002 combines all tumours of haematopoietic and lymphoid tissues together. The basis of the WHO classification is the cell type of the neoplasm as identified by combined approach of clinical features and morphologic, cytogenetic and molecular characteristics, rather than location of the neoplasm (whether in blood or in tissues) because of the fact that haematopoietic cells are present in circulation as well as in tissues in general, and lymphoreticular tissues in particular.

Currently, therefore, neoplasms of haematopoietic and lymphoid tissues are considered as a unified group and are divided into 3 broad categories:

I. Myeloid neoplasms. This group includes neoplasms of myeloid cell lineage and, therefore, includes neoplastic proliferations of red blood cells, platelets, granulocytes and monocytes. There are 5 categories under myeloid series of neoplasms: myeloproliferative disorders, myeloproliferative/

myelodysplastic diseases, myelodysplastic syndromes (MDS), and acute myeloid leukaemia (AML), acute biphenotypic leukaemias.

II. Lymphoid neoplasms. Neoplasms of lymphoid lineage include leukaemias and lymphomas of B, T or NK cell origin. This group thus includes B cell neoplasms (including plasma cell disorders), T cell neoplasms, NK cell neoplasms and Hodgkin's disease.

III. Histiocytic neoplasms. This group is of interest mainly due to neoplastic proliferations of histiocytes in Langerhans cell histiocytosis.

Besides the WHO classification, the FAB (French-American-British) Cooperative Group classification of lymphomas and leukaemias based on morphology and cytochemistry is also widely used. These as well as other classification schemes have been tabulated and discussed in the textbook under separate headings of myeloid and lymphoid malignancies and are beyond the scope of Practical Pathology Book. In this exercise, a brief account of morphology of major forms of leukaemias is outlined, while morphology of major forms of lymphomas is discussed in Exercise 59.

The proliferation of leukaemic cells takes place primarily in the bone marrow, and in certain forms, in the lymphoid tissues. Ultimately, the abnormal cells appear in the peripheral blood raising the total white cell count to high level. In addition, features of bone marrow failure (e.g. anaemia, thrombocyto-penia, neutropenia) and involvement of other organs (e.g. liver, spleen, lymph nodes, meninges, brain, skin, etc.) may occur.

Leukaemias account for 4% of all cancer deaths. Generally, acute leukaemias have a rapidly downhill course, whereas chronic leukaemias tend to have more indolent behaviour. The incidence of both acute and chronic leukaemias is higher in men than in women. ALL is primarily a disease of children and young adults, whereas AML occurs at all ages. CLL tends to occur in the elderly, while CML is found in middle age.

Acute Leukaemia

Acute leukaemias are characterised by predominance of undifferentiated leucocyte precursors or leukaemic blasts. Acute leukaemias may be derived from the myeloid stem cells called acute myeloblastic leukaemia (AML), or from the lymphoid stem cells termed acute lymphoblastic leukaemia (ALL).

According to FAB classification of acute leukaemia, the label acute leukaemia is given to a case when the bone marrow contains more than 30% blasts. FAB classification divides AML into 8 subtypes (M0 to M7) and ALL into 3 subtypes (L1 to L3). However, as per WHO classification of acute leukaemias, which takes into account cytogenetic and molecular markers, the cut off of blasts in the bone marrow for diagnosis of acute leukaemia has been lowered to 20%. In the current WHO classification, AML is classified as one of the groups of myeloid neoplasms (i.e. myeloproliferative diseases, myelodysplasic diseases/syndromes, AML, and acute biphenotypic leukaemias) while ALL is grouped under lymphoid neoplasms (i.e. precursor B and T cell leukaemia or precursor B and T cell leukaemia-lymphoma). The contrasting features of AML and ALL are outlined in Table 58.1.

The diagnosis of acute leukaemia is made by a combination of routine blood picture and bone marrow examination, coupled with cytochemical stains and certain biochemical investigations.

Findings of routine haematologic investigations are as under:

Anaemia

Anaemia is almost always present in acute leukaemias. It is generally severe, progressive and normochromic in type. A moderate reticulocytosis up to 5% and a few nucleated red cells may be present.

Thrombocytopenia

The platelet count is usually moderately to severely decreased (below 50,000/μl) but occasionally it may be normal. Bleeding tendencies in acute leukaemia are usually correlated with the level of thrombocytopenia but most serious spontaneous haemorrhagic episodes develop in patients with fewer than 20,000/μl platelets. Acute promyelocytic leukaemia (M3) may be associated with a serious coagulation abnormality called disseminated intravascular coagulation (DIC).

White Blood Cells

The total WBC count ranges from subnormal-to-markedly elevated values. In 25% of patients, the total WBC count at presentation is reduced to 1,000-4,000/μl. More often, however, there is progressive rise in white cell count which may exceed 100,000/μl in more advanced disease. Majority of leucocytes in the peripheral blood are blasts and there is often neutropenia due to marrow infiltration by leukaemic cells. Some patients present with pancytopenia and have a few blasts (subleukaemic leukaemia) or no blasts (aleukaemic leukaemia) in the blood. Both these conditions are nowadays included under 'myelodysplastic syndrome'. The comparative morphologic features of myeloblasts and lymphoblasts are given in

TABLE 58.1: Contrasting features of AML and ALL.

Feature	AML	ALL
1. Common age	Adults between 15-40 years; comprise 20% of childhood leukaemias	Children under 15 years; comprise 80% of childhood leukaemias
2. Physical findings	Splenomegaly + Hepatomegaly + Lymphadenopathy + Bony tenderness + Gum hypertrophy +	Splenomegaly ++ Hepatomegaly ++ Lymphadenopathy ++ Bony tenderness + CNS involvement +
3. Laboratory findings	Low-to-high TLC; predominance of myeloblasts and promyelocytes in blood and bone marrow; thrombocytopenia moderate to severe	Low-to-high TLC, predominance of lymphoblasts in blood and bone marrow; thrombocytopenia moderate to severe.
4. Diagnostic criteria	FAB types M0-M7 WHO criteria = >20% blasts	FAB types L1-L3, WHO types Pre B (90%) Pre T (10%) WHO criteria = >20% blasts
5. Cytochemical stains	Myeloperoxidase +, Sudan black +, NSE + in M4 and M5, acid phosphatase (diffuse) + in M4 and M5	PAS +, acid phosphatase (focal) +
6. Specific therapy	Cytosine arabinoside, anthracyclines (daunorubicin, adriamycin) and 6-thioguanine	Vincristine, prednisolone, anthracyclines and L-asparaginase
7. Immunophenotyping	CD13, 33, 41, 42	Both B and T cell ALL TdT +ve Pre B: CD19, 20 Pre T: CD1, 2, 3, 5, 7
8. Cytogenetics	M3: t(15;17) M4: in(16)	Pre B: t(9;21)
9. Response to therapy	Remission rate low, duration of remission shorter	Remission rate high, duration of remission prolonged
10. Median survival	12-18 months	Children without CNS prophylaxis 33 months, with CNS prophylaxis 60 months; adults 12-18 months

TABLE 58.2: Morphologic characteristics of the blast cells in Romanowsky stains.

Feature	Myeloblast	Lymphoblast
1. Size	10-18 μm	10-18 μm
2. Nucleus	Round or oval	Round or oval
3. Nuclear chromatin	Fine meshwork	Slightly clumped
4. Nuclear membrane	Very fine	Fairly dense
5. Nucleoli	2-5	1-2
6. Cytoplasm	Scanty, blue, agranular, Auer rods may be seen	Scanty, clear blue, agranular

Table 58.2. In some instances, the identification of blast cells is greatly aided by the company they keep, i.e. by more mature and easily identifiable leucocytes in the company of blastic cells of myeloid or lymphoid series (Figs 58.1 and 58.2).

Chronic Myeloid Leukaemia

In the WHO classification of myeloid neoplasms, CML is currently classified as myeoild neoplasm under along with other myeloproliferative diseases due to common histogenesis from haematopoietic stem cells of the group of diseases.

Chronic myeloid (myelogenous, granulocytic) leukaemia comprises about 20% of all leukaemias and its peak incidence is seen in 3rd and 4th decades of life. A distinctive variant of

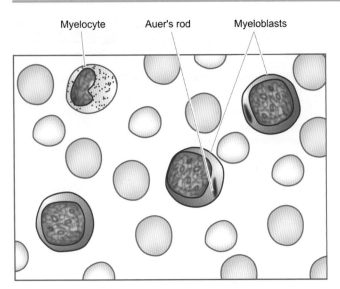
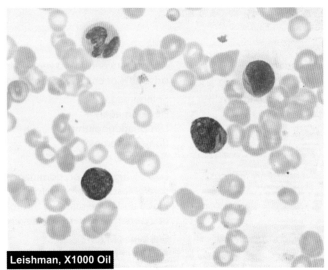

Leishman, X1000 Oil

FIGURE 58.1 ◆ PBF findings in AML showing numerous myeloblasts, accompanying myeloid precursor cells and reduced platelets.

CML seen in children under 3 years of age is called juvenile CML. Both the sexes are affected equally.

The diagnosis of CML is generally possible on blood picture alone. However, bone marrow, cytochemical stains and other investigations are of help. The characteristic Ph chromosome or BCR-ABL translocation between chromosome 9 and 22 can be detected using bone marrow or peripheral blood sample. Another important test is neutrophil alkaline phosphatase (NAP) score is low in cases of chronic phase of CML (compared from leukaemoid reaction in which

it is high) while it rises during accelerated phase and blast crisis.

The typical blood picture in a case of CML at the time of presentation shows the following features:

Anaemia

Anaemia is usually of moderate degree and is normocytic normochromic in type. Occasional normoblasts may be present.

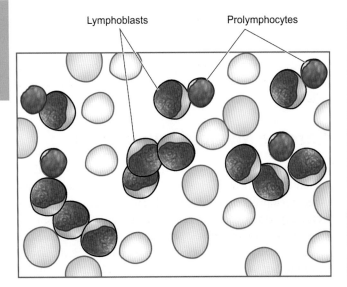
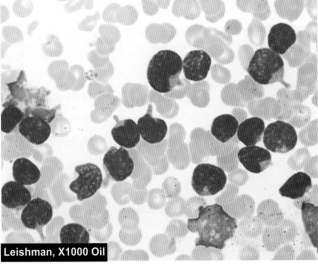

Leishman, X1000 Oil

FIGURE 58.2 ◆ PBF findings in ALL showing agranular cytoplasm of lymphoblasts and reduced platelets.

Metamyelocytes   Myelocytes   Eosinophil   Basophil

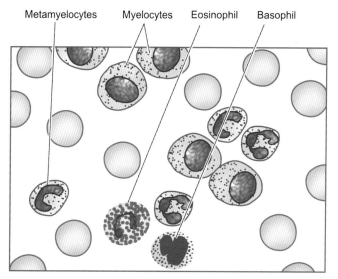

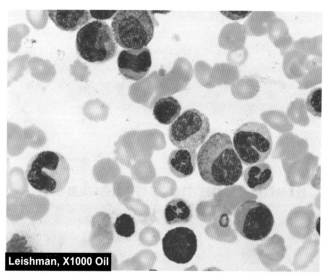

Leishman, X1000 Oil

FIGURE 58.3 ◆ PBF findings in chronic myeloid leukaemia. There is rise in leucocyte count consisting of immature myeloid precursor cells of various stages. It also shown prominent presence of eosinophils and basophils.

White Blood Cells

Characteristically, there is marked leucocytosis (approximately 200,000/µl or more at the time of presentation). The natural history of CML consists of 2 phases-chronic and blastic.

- The *chronic phase of CML* begins as a myeloproliferative disorder and consists of excessive proliferation of myeloid cells of intermediate grade (i.e. myelocytes and metamyelocytes) and mature segmented neutrophils (Fig. 58.3). Myeloblasts usually do not exceed 10% of cells in the

peripheral blood and bone marrow. An accelerated phase of CML is also described in which there is progressively rising leucocytosis associated with thrombocytosis or thrombocytopenia and splenomegaly.

- The *blastic phase or blast crisis in CML* may be myeloid or lymphoid in origin. An increase in the proportion of basophils up to 10% is a characteristic feature of CML. There may be associated eosinophilia. A rising basophilia (more than 20%) in peripheral blood is indicative of impending blastic transformation. Myeloid blast crisis in CML is more

Small lymphocytes   Platelets   Smudge cell

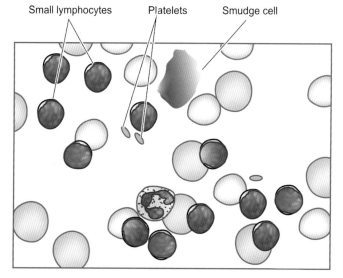

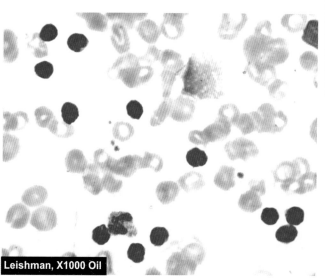

Leishman, X1000 Oil

FIGURE 58.4 ◆ PBF in chronic lymphocytic leukaemia. The white cell count is increased with predominance of small lymphocytes and a few degenerated forms which appear as bare smudged nuclei.

common (two-third cases) and resembles AML. However, unlike AML, Auer rods are rarely seen in myeloblasts of CML in blast crisis. Lymphoid blast crisis in CML having the characteristics of lymphoblasts such as presence of TdT is seen in one-third cases of blastic phase in CML.

Platelets

The platelet count may be normal but is raised in about half the cases.

Chronic Lymphocytic Leukaemia

Chronic lymphocytic leukaemia (CLL) constitutes about 25% of all leukamias and is predominantly a disease of the elderly (over 60 years of age in 80% of patients) with a male preponderance (male-female ratio 2:1). In the WHO classification of lymphoid neoplasm, CLL is a peripheral (mature) B cell malignancy used synonymously with B cell CLL-SLL. The diagnosis of CLL can usually be made on the basis of physical findings and blood smear examination. Bone marrow examination/ biopsy is generally not required for diagnosis of CLL but is useful to assess normal marrow reserve and the pattern of involvement by CLL which has prognostic significance.

The findings of routine blood picture are as under:

Anaemia

Anaemia is usually mild to moderate and normocytic normochromic in type. Anaemia in CLL is related to marrow replacement but in about 20% cases develop a Coomb's-positive autoimmune haemolytic anaemia. Mild reticulocytosis may be present. About 20% cases develop a Coomb's-positive autoimmune haemolytic anaemia.

White Blood Cells

Typically, there is marked leucocytosis but less than that seen in CML (50,000-200,000/μl). Usually, more than 90% of leucocytes are mature-appearing lymphocytes. Smear cells (smudge cells or basket cells) which are degenerated forms are frequently present (Fig. 58.4). The absolute neutrophil count is, however, generally within normal range. Granulocytopenia occurs in fairly advanced disease only.

Platelets

The platelet count is normal or moderately reduced. When thrombocytopenia is present in CLL, it is indicative of higher grade and worse prognosis.

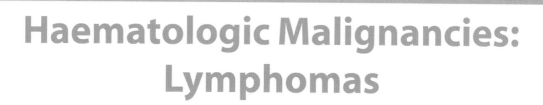

Haematologic Malignancies: Lymphomas

Objectives
➤ To understand the current concept of common classification of haematologic malignancies (leukaemias-lymphomas) as myeloid and lymphoid neoplasms.
➤ To learn to diagnose lymphomas as non-Hodgkin and Hodgkin's (i.e. NHL and HL), and learn the morphology of common forms of Hodgkin's lymphoma (i.e. nodular sclerosis type and mixed cellularity type).

As already discussed in previous exercise, the current concept of combined haematologic malignancies (leukaemias-lymphomas) in the WHO classification underscores the fact that the neoplastic proliferation of white blood cells results in myeloid and lymphoid malignancies.

WHO classification has categorised lymphoid malignancies or lymphomas into two distinct clinicopathologic groups: *Hodgkin's lymphoma* or *Hodgkin's disease (HD)* characterised by pathognomonic presence of Reed-Sternberg cells, and a heterogeneous group of *non-Hodgkin's lymphomas (NHL)*.

HD has further 2 subtypes:
♦ *nodular lymphocytic predominant;* and
♦ *classic HD,* which has further 4 variants: nodular sclerosis, lymphocytic rich classic, mixed cellularity and lymphocytic depletion type)

NHL has 2 major subgroups:
♦ *B cell malignancies;* and
♦ *T cell type malignancies.*

B and C cell cancers have several subtypes of both leukaemias and lymphomas.

Thus, there is a unifying classification of leukaemias-lymphomas. Various classification schemes of HD and NHL have been tabulated and discussed in the textbook and are beyond the scope of Practical Pathology Book. In this exercise,

a brief account of morphology of NHL and two major forms of HD is outlined, while morphology of major forms of leukaemias has already been discussed in Exercise 58.

Non-Hodgkin's Lymphoma (NHL)

NHL is more common than Hodgkin's disease. Majority (65%) arise in lymph nodes while the remaining 35% take origin in extranodal lymphoid tissues.

G/A The affected groups of lymph nodes are enlarged and matted due to infiltration into the surrounding connective tissue. Sectioned surface appears grey-white and fleshy (Fig. 59.1).

M/E The microscopic features of various prognostic groups are variable. Salient features of 2 prototypes of NHL, small lymphocytic lymphoma-chronic lymphocytic leukaemia (SLL-CLL) and follicular lymphoma are given below:

SLL-CLL
i. There is diffuse effacement of nodal architecture (Fig. 59.2,B).
ii. There is diffuse replacement of the node by mature, small and well-differentiated B lymphocytes, positive for CD 20 (Fig. 59.3).

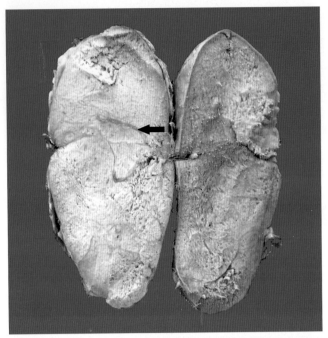

FIGURE 59.1 ◆ Non-Hodgkin's lymphoma. Lymph nodes are identified by bean-shaped contour, peripheral capsule and fat. Sectioned surface shows matted lymph nodes having homogeneous, grey-white and fleshy parenchyma (arrow).

iii. Infiltration by the tumour cells into perinodal soft tissue is common.

iv. Blood picture of these cases may show picture of CLL (Exercise 58).

FOLLICULAR LYMPHOMA

i. There is follicular pattern of entire nodal architecture (Fig. 59.2,C).

ii. Lymphoid cells comprising the follicles have small, cleaved to large cleaved cells positive for pan-B cell marker, CD 20.

iii. CLL-like picture in the blood, unlike SLL-CLL, is uncommon but bone marrow involvement may occur and shows paratrabecular involvement.

Hodgkin's Disease (HD)

HD arises primarily within the lymph nodes. As given above, classic HD has 4 subtypes: nodular sclerosis, lymphocytic rich classic, mixed cellularity and lymphocytic depletion type). Central to diagnosis of HD is the essential identification of Reed-Sternberg (RS) cell.

G/A The affected lymph nodes are matted together. The sectioned surface is homogeneous and fleshy and indistinguishable form that in NHL. *Nodular sclerosis type,*

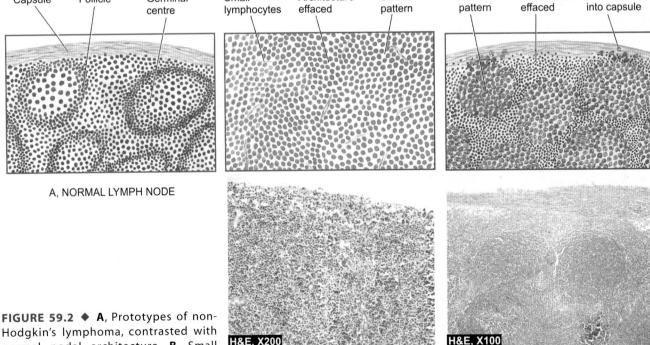

FIGURE 59.2 ◆ **A,** Prototypes of non-Hodgkin's lymphoma, contrasted with normal nodal architecture. **B,** Small lymphocytic lymphoma- (SLL-CLL). **C,** Follicular lymphoma intermediate grade.

A, NORMAL LYMPH NODE

B, SMALL LYMPHOCYTIC LYMPHOMA(SLL/CLL)

C, FOLLICULAR LYMPHOMA

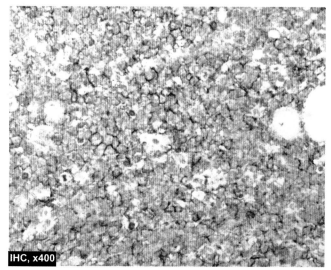

FIGURE 59.3 ◆ B cell NHL. Immunohistochemical (IHC) staining with CD20 (maker for B cells) shows membranous positivity.

however, shows nodular scarring while there is abundance of necrosis in *mixed cellularity type.*

M/E The characteristic microscopic feature of all types of HD is RS cell which has different morphologic variants. *Classic RS cell* is a large cell having bilobed nucleus appearing as mirror image of each other. Each lobe of the nucleus contains a prominent, eosinophilic, inclusion-like nucleolus with a clear halo around it giving it an owl-eye appearance. The cytoplasm of the cell is abundant and amphophilic. *Lacunar type RS cell* is characterised by pericellular halo due to shrinkage of cell.

The microscopic features of the two common types of HD are outlined below:

HD-NODULAR SCLEROSIS TYPE

It is characterised by two essential features:

   i. *Bands of collagen.* Variable amount of fibrous tissue is present in the involved lymph nodes.

   ii. *Lacunar type of RS cells.* Characteristic lacunar type of RS cells with distinctive pericellular halo are present (Fig. 59.4).

HD-MIXED CELLULARITY TYPE

The features are as under:

   i. Replacement of the entire affected lymph nodes by heterogeneous mixture of various types of apparently normal cells that include proliferating lymphocytes, histiocytes, eosinophils, neutrophils and plasma cells.

   ii. Some amount of fibrosis and focal areas of necrosis are generally present.

   iii. Typical or classic RS cells are frequent (Fig. 59.5).

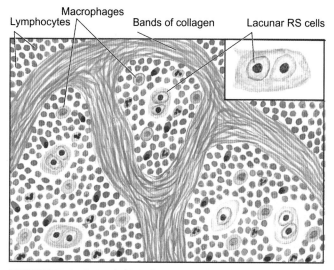

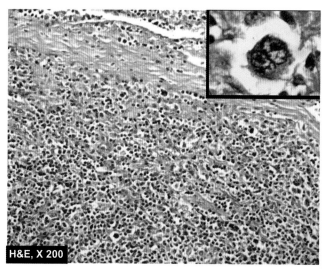

FIGURE 59.4 ◆ Hodgkin's disease, nodular sclerosis type. There are bands of collagen forming nodules and characteristic lacunar type RS cells (inbox).

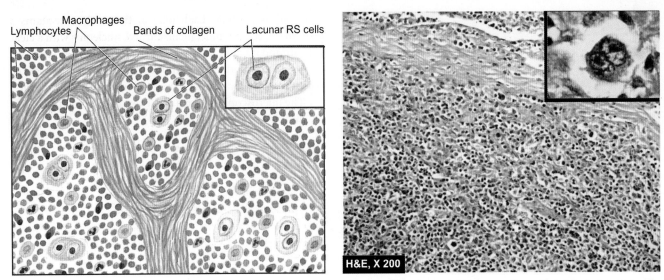

FIGURE 59.5 ◆ Hodgkin's disease, mixed cellularity. There is mixed infiltrate of lymphocytes, plasma cells, neutrophils and eosinophils and a classic RS cell (inbox).

Section Seven

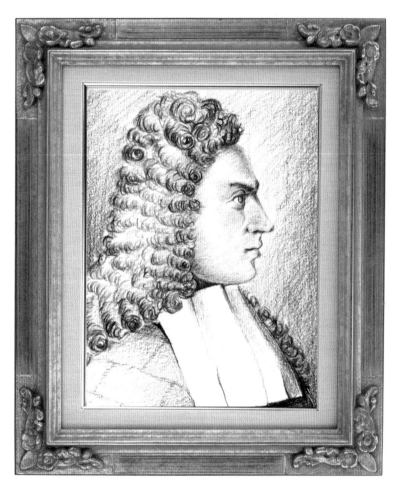

GIOVANNI B MORGAGNI (1682–1771)
'Founder of CPC'

**Italian anatomist and pathologist, who, for the first time made
correlation between pathology found at post-mortem
and clinical findings. Virchow believed that
Morgagni introduced modern pathology.**

Section Contents

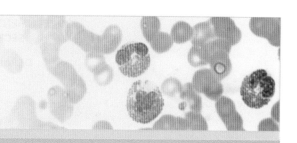

Autopsy Protocol— Request and Report

Objectives
➢ To learn the pathologic autopsy protocol.
➢ To prepare an *Autopsy Request* as clinician and *Autopsy Report* as pathologist.

Professor William Boyd in his inimitable style wrote 'Pathology had its beginning on the autopsy table'. The significance of study of autopsy in pathology is summed up in Latin inscription in an autopsy room reproduced in English as 'The place where death delights to serve the living'.

There is still no substitute for a careful postmortem examination that enlightens the clinician about the pathogenesis of disease, reveals hazardous effects of therapy administered, and settles the discrepancies finally between antemortem and postmortem diagnosis.

The study of autopsy throws new light on the knowledge and skills of both physician as well as pathologist. The main *purposes* of autopsy are as under:

1. *Quality assurance of patient-care* by:
   i. Confirming the cause of death;
   ii. establishing the final diagnosis; and
   iii. study of therapeutic response to treatment.
2. *Education of the entire team* involved in patient-care by the following:
   i. Making autopsy diagnosis of conditions which are often missed clinically, e.g. pneumonia, pulmonary embolism, acute pancreatitis, carcinoma prostate.
   ii. Discovery of newer diseases made at autopsy, e.g. Reye's syndrome, Legionnaire's disease.
   iii. Study of demography and epidemiology of diseases.
   iv. Affords education to students and staff of pathology.

Declining autopsy rate throughout the world in recent times are owing to the following reasons:
1. Higher diagnostic confidence made possible by advances in imaging techniques, e.g. CT, MRI, etc.
2. Physician's fear of legal liability on being wrong.

Continued support for advocating autopsy by caring physicians as well as by discernible pathologists in tertiary-care hospitals is essential for improved patient-care and progress in medical science.

Autopsy Protocol

Traditionally, there are two methods of carrying out autopsy, either of which may be followed:
1. Block extraction of abdominal and thoracic organs.
2. *In situ* organ-by-organ dissection.

In conditions where multiple organs are expected to be involved, complete autopsy should be performed. But if a particular organ-specific disease is suspected or limited consent is available, a mini-autopsy or limited autopsy may be sufficient.

For performing pathologic autopsy, also called clinical autopsy, there are two absolute essential requirements:
   i. To obtain permission for conducting autopsy including restrictions, if any.
   ii. To obtain as much history and laboratory data as possible about the deceased.

GOVERNMENT MEDICAL COLLEGE HOSPITAL
SECTOR-32, CHANDIGARH

DEPARTMENT OF PATHOLOGY

Referred by

Date of admission

Date of death

Name
Age/Sex
CR No.
Ward/OPD
Date   Income

HIV status

Autopsy No....................

Permission for autopsy: Yes/No

Restrictions on permission: Abdominal with brain or without brain
(tick mark √)   Thoracoabdominal with brain or without brain
                                                  Brain only
                                                  Spinal Cord/eyes/testes/others

Laboratory data and radiological findings:

Operative procedures:

Provisional diagnosis:

Previous cytology/histopathology number, if any:

Date and time   Requested by
                                                   Doctor's name & signature

AUTOPSY REQUEST

FIGURE 60.1 ◆ Specimen proforma for autopsy request

These two requirements can be incorporated in a standard *Autopsy Request Form* devised for the purpose so that the entire information has to be compulsorily filled by the clinical resident; a specimen proforma is shown in Figure 60.1.

A. PROSECTION

Prosection means carefully programmed dissection for demonstration of anatomic structures. The prosector on his part conducts the autopsy keeping the following sequenced checklist in mind:

1. Assessment of the body as regards age, sex, race, general physique and nutrition.
2. External examination including injuries (recent/old), if any.
3. Internal examination by thoracoabdominal midline incision from neck to pubis, but avoiding the umbilicus which has extensive fibrous tissue that may cause difficulty in sewing back (Fig. 60.2).
4. Examination of the peritoneal cavity for presence of fluid, blood or pus followed by examination of the bowel and organs in the pelvis.
5. Cutting through the structures in the neck up to the floor of mouth and base of the tongue.
6. Divide the sternoclavicular joints and cut with a saw from the costal margin upwards to the disarticulated sternoclavicular joints and lift the sternum.
7. Examine the pleural cavities for presence of fluid, blood or pus and visually assess the lungs.
8. Divide the diaphragm close to the costal margin all around.

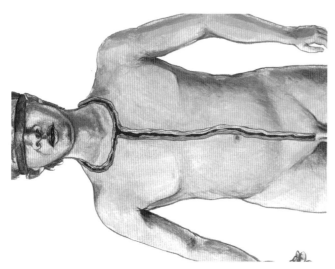

FIGURE 60.2 ◆ Thoracoabdominal midline incision from neck to the pubis but avoiding the umbilicus.

9. Move the kidneys medially and cut the tissue behind them to free the kidneys.
10. Now all the thoraco-abdominal organs are removed *en mass* and put on the dissecting table.
11. Incise the scalp behind the ears on to the posterior parts (bitemporal incision), peeling it forwards as well as backwards. Then with a handsaw or electric saw, the skull is cut circumferentially removing the skullcap by a V-shaped incision. Brain is then removed along with meninges, part of the brainstem and pituitary gland.

B. GROSS EXAMINATION OF ORGANS

Examination of the structures and organs so removed can be done by various methods but whatever plan is followed it should be adhered to so that no part remains unexamined. Briefly, systematic examination of the organs can be done as under:

1. Examination of the tongue, thyroid, oesophagus, larynx and other neck structures.
2. Examination of lungs by putting the hilum down on the cutting board and slicing them horizontally full length from apex to base.
3. The heart is examined next. It is weighed after removal of blood clots, from the chambers. Enzyme studies on gross specimen can be done at this stage before fixing.
4. The stomach is incised along the greater curvature down through the pylorus into the duodenum. At this stage gallbladder and ampulla of Vater are examined.
5. The adrenals are examined next.
6. The spleen is removed from the *en mass* and cuts given into the substance.
7. The kidneys are then removed by cutting from the hilum and the capsule and the capsule is stripped off. Transverse cut is made from outer border towards the hilum.
8. The urinary bladder and the other pelvic organs can be examined at this stage.
9. The liver is examined next. Parallel incisions are given to the liver after weighing the organ.
10. The brain is best examined after fixation in suspension in formation than to cut the soft and wet brain.

C. AUTOPSY REPORT

Lastly, the most important part in the autopsy is formulation of carefully worded Autopsy Report based on foregoing examination (external, internal and gross examination) (Fig. 60.3,A) followed by ancillary investigations that include histopathologic examination and other ancillary investigations (Fig. 60.3,B).

**GOVERNMENT MEDICAL COLLEGE HOSPITAL
SECTOR-32, CHANDIGARH**

DEPARTMENT OF PATHOLOGY

Referred by
Clinical diagnosis

HIV status

Date & time of death

Date & time of autopsy

Name
Age/Sex
CR No.
Ward/OPD
Date   Income

Autopsy No.....................

A. **EXTERNAL EXAMINATION**
(Body surface, nutritional status, height, weight, injuries if any, scars)

B. **INTERNAL EXAMINATION**

  1. INCISION

  2. EFFUSIONS
(Pericardial, pleural L/R, peritoneal)

  3. CENTRAL NERVOUS SYSTEM
(Meninges, cerebral vessels, brain, spinal cord)

  4. RESPIRATORY SYSTEM
(Larynx, trachea, bronchi, pleura, lungs)

  5. CARDIOVASCULAR SYSTEM
(Heart, valves, myocardium, pericardium, coronaries, great vessels)

  6. ALIMENTARY TRACT
(Mouth, tongue, oesophagus, stomach and its contents, duodenum, intestines, liver, gallbladder, pancreas, peritoneum)

  7. GENITOURINARY SYSTEM
(Kidneys, ureters, bladder, gonads)

  8. RETICULOENDOTHELIAL SYSTEM
(Spleen, lymph nodes, thymus)

  9. ENDOCRINE SYSTEM
(Adrenals, thyroid, pituitary)

  10. MUSCULOSKELETAL SYSTEM
(Skull, spine, rest of skeleton, muscles)

C. SAMPLE FOR ANCILLARY INVESTIGATIONS
(Toxicology/microbiology/virology/serology/EM)

Date & time

PROSECTOR
(Name & Signature)

AUTOPSY REPORT (A)

FIGURE 60.3 ◆ Specimen proforma for autopsy report (A).

**GOVERNMENT MEDICAL COLLEGE HOSPITAL
SECTOR-32, CHANDIGARH**

DEPARTMENT OF PATHOLOGY

Referred by
Clinical diagnosis

HIV status

| Name |
| Age/Sex |
| CR No. |
| Ward/OPD |
| Date   Income |

Autopsy No....................

MICROSCOPIC DESCRIPTION (ORGAN-WISE):

FINAL AUTOPSY DIAGNOSIS:

CAUSE OF DEATH:

Date of receiving......................
Date of reporting.......................   PATHOLOGIST

AUTOPSY REPORT (B)

FIGURE 60.3 (contd) ◆ Specimen proforma for autopsy report (B).

The autopsy report can be given in two formats:

i. A *printed proforma type* of report listing various body systems with space for writing the description against each. This pattern has the advantage that no organ is left out for describing and the standardised information can be used for coding purposes. However, this type of pattern has the disadvantage that the space provided for each organ and system is prefixed and cannot be accommodated according to the requirement of the specific case for which additional sheets may be attached.

ii. The *open type* of report is in the form of an essay, which can adjust any variation in the description of a particular organ or part of the body. But this pattern suffers from the disadvantage that description of some organs may be left out.

In general, the format of the Autopsy Report should consist of the following (Fig. 60.3):

1. *Permission* for autopsy.
2. *Data pertaining to the deceased*: Name, age, sex, address, serial number of autopsy, date of admission and date and time of death, clinical history and laboratory data including radiological findings, operative procedure and clinical diagnosis.

3. *Data pertaining to the pathologist*: Autopsy number, date and time of autopsy, name of prosector, initial gross autopsy findings including weights and measurements of organs, and gross autopsy diagnosis.

4. *Postmortem findings*: These should be listed in the following sequence:
   A. *External examination* as outlined above.
   B. *Internal examination* as explained above.
   C. *Pathologic examination* of formalin-fixed organs by description of gross and microscopic examination, with organs of interest in greater detail.

5. *Final autopsy diagnosis:* This is the conclusion of pathological findings of autopsy.

6. *Cause of death:* The final comment on the cause of death is of paramount importance. Summary and interpretation of causative sequence of various lesions observed by the pathologist about the case are given here.

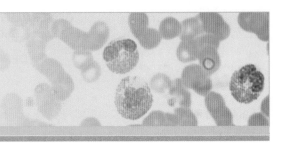

CD on Clinicopathological Conferences and Museum Review

Objectives
➢ To learn the role and significance of clinicopathological conference (CPC).
➢ To learn and write ten CPCs based on different clinical settings and pathologic diagnosis.
➢ To be acquainted with the CD containing the information on 10 CPCs and quick review of common museum specimens.

Clinicopathological Conference (CPC)

GB Morgagni in Italy (1682-1771) and THA Laennec (1781-1826) in France started collecting the case records of hospital cases and began correlation of clinical features with the lesions observed at autopsy and thus marked the beginning of clinicopathological correlation.

In the modern times, "Clinicopathological Conference" commonly known as "CPC", has about 100 years long history since its origin from Massachusetts General Hospital and Harvard Medical School, Boston. It started in 1890s as an informal discussion on case-based method of teaching medicine between two Harvard Internists, Dr Richard C Cabot and Walter B Cannon, who got the idea from another roommate in college who attended Harvard Law School where case method of teaching law was practiced. Cabot first published these case-based medical teaching exercises as the Cabot Case Records in the *Boston Medical and Surgical Journal* in 1924. In 1928, that journal became the *New England Journal of Medicine*, and has continued publication of the CPC since then regularly as *Case Records of the Massachusetts General Hospital*.

The purpose of the CPC is to teach anatomic-pathological correlation with the clinical sequence as it happened during

life in disease, and the principles of differential diagnosis and pathophysiology. The process of the CPC has been described as an exercise by reasoning, i.e. a logical and instructive analysis of the conditions involved.

Classically, CPC has a *Moderator* to direct the discussion and to maintain the time discipline between clinical and pathology discussants. The CPC involves presentation of clinical and laboratory data by a *Clinical Discussant* who is generally not a member of the treating unit of the selected case during life. The clinical discussant systematically analyses the data by suggesting various possible differential diagnosis and excluding one by one by giving diagnostic reasoning and pathophysiological sequence, and then he concludes by offering the most likely clinical diagnosis. This is followed by a discussion in the open house on the proposed diagnosis or other clinical possibilities. Then, the *Pathology Discussant* presents the autopsy findings on gross and microscopy of organs as well as results of some other ancillary studies which may have been carried out on autopsied organs. The pathologist also reconstructs the sequence as may have happened during life with autopsy findings to offer the pathophysiological aspect of the disease and assigns possible cause of death with reasoning. He concludes by providing autopsy diagnosis considered as "the final diagnosis". Moderator then invites the discussion for correlation of pathological findings at autopsy with the preceding clinical and laboratory data.

In general, CPC should not be allowed to become a forum for "Clinicopathological Competition" or a "Clinicopathological Contest" between the clinician and the pathologist but it should be taken essentially as an exercise in humility for learning lessons for all.

CD and its Contents

A user-friendly CD enclosed with this book contains following 2 sections:
1. Ten CPCs
2. Quick review of pathology museum.

SECTION I: TEN CPCs

CPC continues to be the most important form of clinical teaching activity in medical institutions worldwide. The curriculum of undergraduate students in medicine lays down this learning activity as part of pathology teaching towards the end of their MBBS-II, i.e. in the 5th semester. Not many institutions have access to CPC as teaching material due to dwindling rates of pathologic autopsies. Thus, it was considered prudent to present 10 structured CPCs based on common diseases (infective, inflammatory, neoplastic and non-neoplastic, etc.) pertaining to different organ systems for the students as learning exercises and put them on website. The pattern of presentation in the CD is in the conventional sequence as follows:
♦ ID of the deceased,
♦ Brief clinical signs and symptoms,
♦ Results of relevant laboratory data,
♦ Possible clinical diagnosis and
♦ Autopsy findings (i.e. external examination, internal examination that includes findings on gross and microscopic examination with greater emphasis on the organ or system of interest, final autopsy diagnosis and cause of death).

While the details of these 10 CPCs in the above sequence along with the representative photomicrographs are available in the CD, the final autopsy diagnosis of the 10 CPCs is given below which may serve as an index for ready reference:

CPC 1: Case of secondary systemic amyloidosis

♦ Bronchiectasis both lungs
♦ Secondary (Reactive) systemic amyloidosis involving the spleen, kidneys and the liver.

CPC 2: Case of septic shock with DIC

♦ Septic shock due to infected retained products of intrauterine gestation, myometrial and cervical abscesses, left pyosalpinx
♦ Disseminated intravascular coagulation (DIC) with acute tubular necrosis (ATN).

CPC 3: Case of HIV infection with miliary tuberculosis with tuberculous meningitis (TBM)

♦ Disseminated miliary tuberculosis involving both lungs, hilar lymph nodes, heart, liver, spleen, both kidneys, small intestines and tuberculous meningitis
♦ Senile emphysema both lungs.

CPC 4: Case of rheumatic heart disease (RHD) with infective endocarditis

♦ RHD
♦ Bacterial endocarditis
♦ Infarcts and abscesses in spleen, kidneys and brain.

CPC 5: Case of alcoholic cirrhosis with portal hypertension

♦ Alcoholic (micronodular) cirrhosis
♦ Portal hypertension (ascites, gastroesophageal varices with ulcerations, congestive splenomegaly).

CPC 6: Case of bronchogenic carcinoma

♦ Bronchogenic carcinoma, left main bronchus with left lung collapse
♦ Metastatic deposits in the hilar lymph nodes and both kidneys
♦ Complicated coronary atherosclerosis.

CPC 7: Case of long-standing inflammatory bowel disease

♦ Ulcerative colitis with features of toxic megacolon
♦ CMV colitis
♦ Fatty change liver.

CPC 8: Case of rapidly progressive glomerulonephritis (RPGN)

♦ Crescentric glomerulonephritis
♦ Thromboemboli multiple organs
♦ Pulmonary haemorrhages.

CPC 9: Case of type II diabetes mellitus with complications

♦ Diabetic nephropathy

- Coronary atherosclerosis with healed transmural myocardial infarcts
- Multiple lung abscesses.

CPC 10: Case of gestational choriocarcinoma

- Disseminated gestational choriocarcinoma of the uterus
- Metastatic deposits both lungs, liver, kidneys, heart and the brain.

SECTION II: QUICK REVIEW OF PATHOLOGY MUSEUM

This section of the CD contains images of specimens from pathology museum chosen from out of common diseases which a student of pathology "must know" (108 in all). Each of these images has a fairly detailed and complete legend describing the specimen in a systematic manner. The legend is also connected to the structures on the image with labeled number for easy understanding by a beginner. This method of museum review for students would emphasise self-learning of specimens and would also serve as a medium for quick recall of the specimens seen and learnt earlier in the museum.

Section Eight

APPENDICES

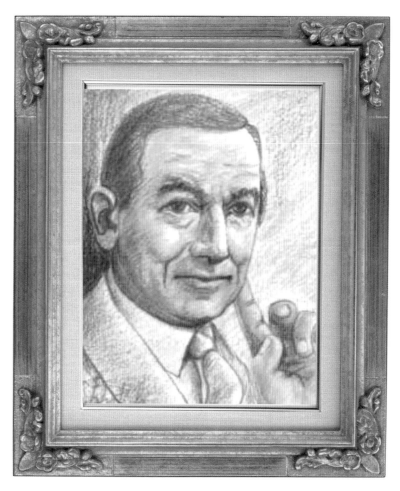

William Boyd (1885–1979)

Canadian pathologist and eminent teacher of pathology who was a
pioneering author of textbooks of pathology which have
been read all over the world by students of pathology
and surgery for over 50 years.

Section Contents

Common Instruments in Pathology

Objectives

➤ To hone skills at identification and applications of the major instruments used in pathology laboratories.
➤ To facilitate the student for viva voce on instruments in a short time.

In this section, a compilation of common instruments used in diagnostic laboratories in haematology, clinical pathology, histopathology and cytopathology (in that sequence) has been done. Each instrument has an image accompanied with its major application. An alphabetic order has been followed.

A. Haematology (1-20)

1. ANTISERA FOR BLOOD GROUPING

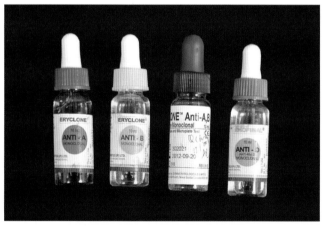

Colour-coded antisera bottles for ABO-Rh blood grouping. Blue=A, Yellow=B, Pink=AB, Colourless=anti-D (Rh) grouping.

2. BONE MARROW ASPIRATION (SALAH'S) NEEDLE

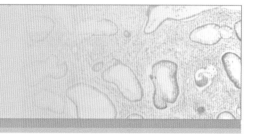

Used for bone marrow aspiration for study of haematopoiesis.

3. DLC COUNTER (MANUAL)

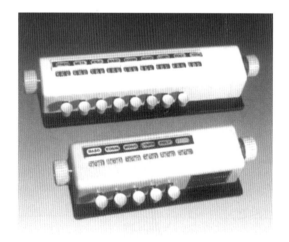

A manual counter with pressing keys for counting different cells in DLC.

4. EHRICH'S EYEPIECE

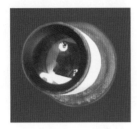

An eyepiece having a square window is fitted on the microscope; used for counting reticulocytes.

5. GRADUATED PIPETTE (1 ML)

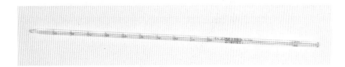

Glass pipette with etched markings of 0.1 each; used for dispensing liquids of required small volume.

6. LANCET

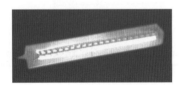

Metallic piece having a sharp-pointed end with fixed depth for blood collection by finger prick method.

7. NEUBAUER'S (IMPROVED) COUNTING CHAMBER (HAEMACYTOMETER)

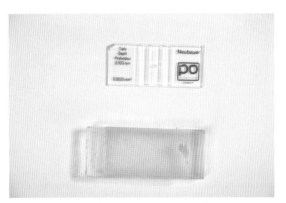

A counting chamber with markings used for counting RBCs, WBCs, absolute eosinophil count, platelets, cells in CSF and sperms.

8. PASTEUR PIPETTE

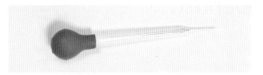

Glass pipette with capillary drawn at one end and a rubber teat at the other end; used for filling Wintrobe's tube with blood.

9. RBC PIPETTE

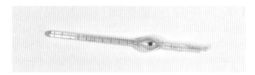

Used for RBC and platelet counting by manual method.

10. SAHLI'S COLOUR COMPARATOR

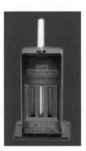

Glass colour comparator for reading haemoglobin value directly from the Hb tube after gradual dilution.

11. SAHLI'S HAEMOGLOBIN PIPETTE

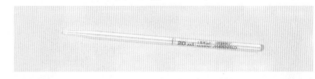

Used for taking 20 μl blood for haemoglobin estimation by Sahli's method.

12. SAHLI'S HAEMOGLOBIN TUBE

Calibrated tube used for making acid haematin by mixing N/10 HCl and blood in Sahli's method.

13. STOP WATCH

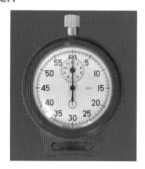

Used for determining the timing of the end point in tests for haemostasis.

14. THERMOMETER FOR WATERBATH

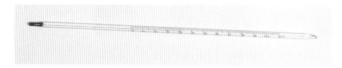

Mercury thermometer for placing in waterbath for taking temperature.

15. TREPHINE BIOPSY (JAMSHIDI'S) NEEDLE

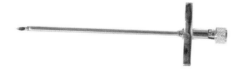

Used for bone marrow core biopsy for study of marrow components by paraffin-embedding technique.

16. VACUTAINERS WITH VACUPUNCTURE NEEDLE

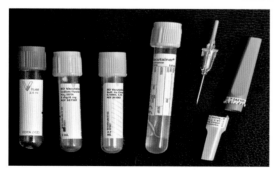

Colour-coded sealed tubes and vacupuncture needle, used for blood collection directly into tubes free of spillage. Purple=EDTA for haemogram, Blue= Sodium citrate for ESR, Grey=Fluoride tube for glucose, Yellow tube=Plain with gel for clotted blood.

17. WBC PIPETTE

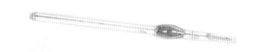

Used for TLC and sperm counting by manual method.

18. WESTERGREN'S PIPETTE

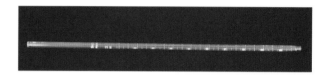

Glass pipette open at both ends, used for filling with citrated blood for reading ESR after one hour.

19. WINTROBE'S STAND

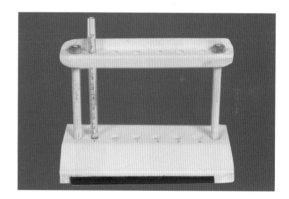

Used for keeping the Wintrobe's tube in upright position for ESR.

20. WINTROBE'S (HAEMATOCRIT) TUBE

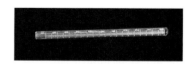

Glass tube closed at one end, used for filling with anticoagulated blood for testing for ESR and PCV (or haematocrit).

B. Clinical Pathology (21-25)

21. DIPSTIX FOR URINE

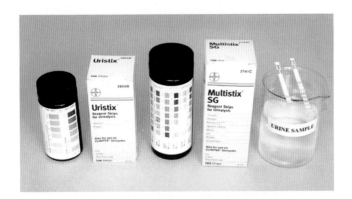

Reagent-coated strips for rapid testing of ingredients in urine.

22. ESBACH'S ALBUMINOMETER

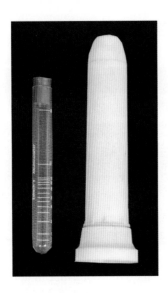

Used for quantitative estimation of albumin in the urine.

23. LUMBAR PUNCTURE NEEDLE

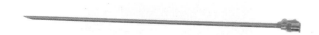

Used for aspiration of CSF by lumbar tap.

24. URINOMETER

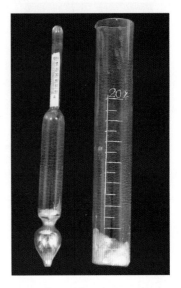

Used for estimation of specific gravity of urine.

25. VIM SILVERMAN'S NEEDLE

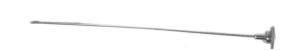

Used for tissue core biopsy from liver.

C. Histopathology (26-31)

26. BLOCK MOULDS (METAL), LEUCKHART'S (L)

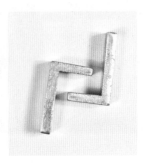

Used for making tissue blocks in wax.

27. BLOCK MOULDS (PLASTIC)

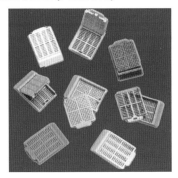

Used for placing and carrying the tissue through the tissue processor after grossing of the tissue.

28. MICROTOMY BLADES, HIGH AND LOW PROFILE

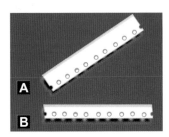

Disposable microtomy blades. A, High profile has wider edge. B, Low profile has narrower edge.

29. MICROTOMY KNIFE, PLAIN WEDGE TYPE

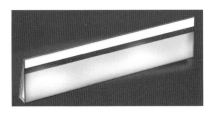

Fixed knife having wedge-shaped appearance when viewed from the side; used for cutting the wax block of tissue.

30. SLIDE CARRIER

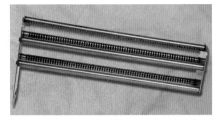

A metal carrier for carrying fixed number of slides for staining as a batch in staining troughs.

31. TISSUE CAPSULES (STAINLESS STEEL)

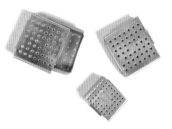

Used for placing and carrying the tissue through the tissue processor after gross examination.

D. Cytopathology (32-34)

32. AYRE'S SPATULA

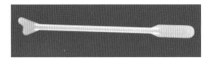

Used for cervical scrape (Pap) smear.

33. COPLIN JAR

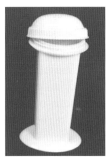

Glass/plastic jar for use in laboratory for Pap smear fixation and as staining jar.

34. FRANZEN HANDLE

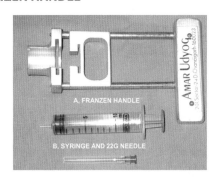

Used for fitting the syringe during FNA procedure for better grip.

Common Similes in Pathology

Objectives
- To be familiar with common terms used as a simile for a disease, organ, cell or a process.
- To know what these similes mean, how they look like, and where and why they are used in pathology.

Simile means "comparison of one thing to another". In this section of the Appendix, various commonly used similes for describing many diseases, processes, organ changes, appearance of cells, etc. have been compiled. An alphabetic order has been followed in the compilation. These include comparison with part of an animal and plant, food and eatable items, etc. Each of these similes is illustrated and is supplemented with its dictionary meaning, which is followed by its use in pathology. As they say 'an image is equal to a thousand words' and thus is the best form of learning.

The aim is to stimulate an inquisitive learner to explore '*why, what and how*' of these terms in learning and teaching of diseases.

1. ANCHOVY SAUCE

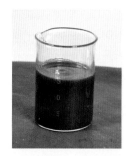

Sauce prepared from small Mediterranean fish of the herring family.

Term used in pathology for:
Appearance of chocolate-coloured pasty material found in cavities of amoebic liver abscess.

2. ANT-HILL

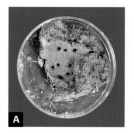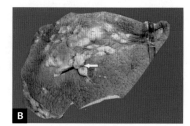

Pile of earth over an underground nest of white ants or termites (A).

Term used in pathology for:
Gross appearance of Madura foot (B).

3. BREAD AND BUTTER

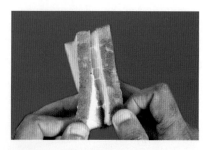

Thready appearance of butter between two slices when they are gently pulled apart.

Term used in pathology for:
Gross description of fibrinous pericarditis.

4. BUNCH OF GRAPES

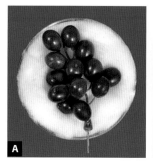
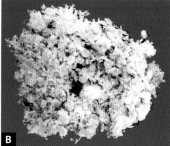

A cluster of grapes growing together (A).

Term used in pathology for:
1. Gross appearance of hydatidiform mole (B).
2. Sarcoma botyroides—a type of rhabdomyosarcoma.

5. BUTTON HOLE

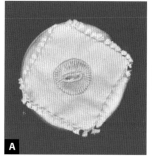
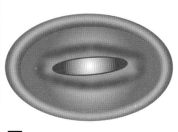

The oval hole in the shirt for closing button in it (A).

Term used in pathology for:
Mitral stenosis in chronic lesions of rheumatic heart disease (RHD) (B).

6. CATERPILLAR

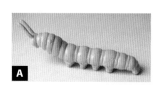
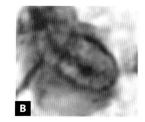

Larva of butterfly or moth (A).

Term used in pathology for:
Microscopic appearance of nuclei of modified histiocytes which form Aschoff bodies in rheumatic heart disease (RHD) (B).

7. CAULIFLOWER

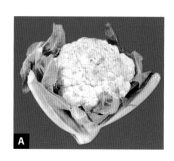
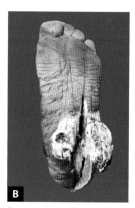

A kind of cultivated vegetable with a large white flower-head (A).

Term used in pathology for:
Gross description of exophytic growth pattern of epithelial tumours (B).

8. CIGAR-SHAPED

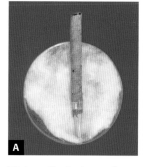
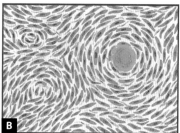

Tight roll of tobacco leaves with pointed ends for smoking (A).

Term used in pathology for:
Microscopic appearance of nuclei of smooth muscle cells (B).

9. CIGARETTES-IN-PACK

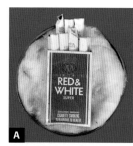
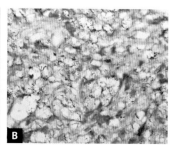

Cigarettes arranged in parallel rows in its packing (A).

Term used in pathology for:
Microscopic appearance of lepra bacilli in foamy macrophages revealed by lepra stain (B).

10. COFFEE-BEANS

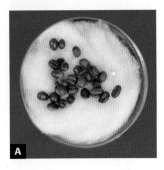 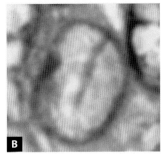

The seeds of coffee tree (A).

Term used in pathology for:
1. Microscopic appearance of tumour cells in granulosa cell tumour of the ovary (B).
2. Microscopic appearance of tumour cells in Brenner tumour of the ovary.

11. CORAL

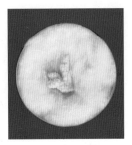

Hard, red, pink or white calcareous substance built on the seabed secreted by marine creatures, polyps, for support and habitation.

Term used in pathology for:
Description of a thrombus

12. CRAB

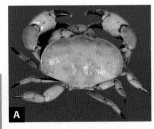 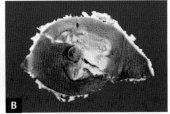

Ten-legged crustacean or shellfish used as food (A).

Term used in pathology for:
Sign for cancer which sticks to the organ like a crab (B).

13. FISH MOUTH

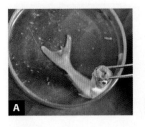 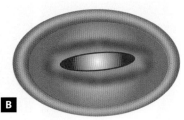

Fish having a small oval oral opening (A).

Term used in pathology for:
Mitral stenosis in chronic lesions of rheumatic heart disease (RHD) (B).

14. GALLSTONES*: COMBINED TYPE

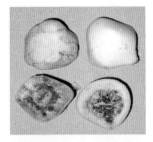

15. GALLSTONES*: PURE CALCIUM CARBONATE TYPE

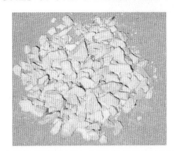

16. GALLSTONES*: PURE CHOLESTEROL TYPE

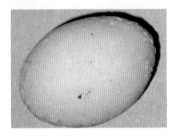

*Although various types of gallstones are not similes, their illustrations are included here since they are displayed in the museum alongside the similes.

17. GALL STONES*: MIXED TYPE

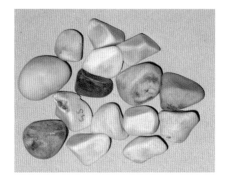

18. GALLSTONES*: PURE PIGMENT TYPE

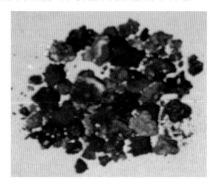

19. HERRINGBONE

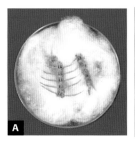 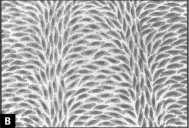

Herring is a sea fish used as food; herringbone is the spine of herring fish (A).

Term used in pathology for:
Microscopic arrangement of tumour cells in fibrosarcoma (B).

20. HONEYCOMB

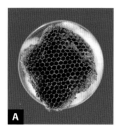 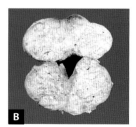

A wax structure of hexagonal (six-sided) cells made by bees for honey and eggs (A).

Term used in pathology for:
1. Cut-sectioned appearance of benign hyperplasia prostate (B).
2. Gross description of lung parenchyma on cut section in interstitial lung diseases.

21. HOURGLASS

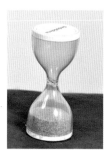

Two vertically connected glass bulbs containing sand taking an hour to pass from upper to lower bulb.

Term used in pathology for:
Description of cicatrical contracture around a saddle-shaped lesser curvature in peptic ulcer and in linitis plastica (scirrhous carcinoma of the stomach).

22. HOBNAIL

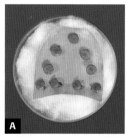 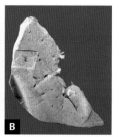

Short nail with a heavy head used for the soles of heavy shoes and boots (A).

Term used in pathology for:
Sectioned surface of the liver in alcoholic cirrhosis (B).

*Although various types of gallstones are not similes, their illustrations are included here since they are displayed in the museum alongside the similes.

23. HORSESHOE

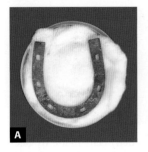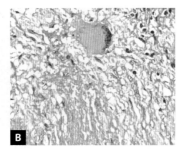

U-shaped iron shoe for a horse (A).

Term used in pathology for:
1. Microscopic appearance of peripheral arrangement of nuclei in Langhans' giant cells (B).
2. A form of congenital malformation of kidney called 'horseshoe kidney'.

24. LEATHER BOTTLE

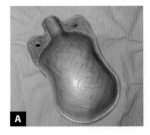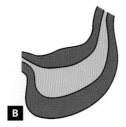

The appearance of bottle made of leather having narrow centre like the waist (A).

Term used in pathology for:
Gross appearance of cancer of the stomach in linitis plastica (B).

25. MILLET SEED

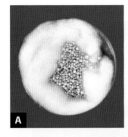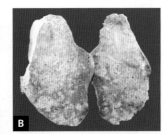

Spherical shaped seeds or grains of a cereal plant (A).

Term used in pathology for:
Gross appearance of small yellow-white firm lesions in military tuberculosis, measuring one to a few millimetres in diameter (B).

26. NUTMEG

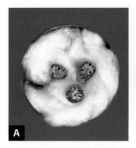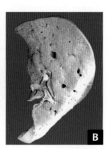

Hard, small, round aromatic seed of a nut used as an Indian spice (A).

Term used in pathology for:
Cut-sectioned appearance of chronic venous congestion (CVC) of the liver (B).

27. NAPKIN RING

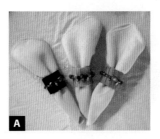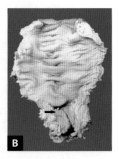

Arrangement of the napkin made of cloth in the form of a narrow waist and a ring put in the centre to keep it in place (A).

Term used in pathology for:
Gross appearance of left-sided colorectal carcinoma (B).

28. ONION-PEEL

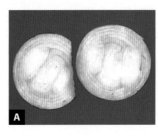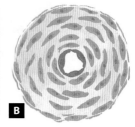

Cut onion showing concentric/multilayered appearance (A).

Term used in pathology for:
1. X-ray appearance of Ewing's sarcoma.
2. Concentric periarterial fibrosis in the spleen seen in systemic lupus erythematosis (SLE).
3. Histological appearance of intimal proliferation of arterioles in concentric manner in hypertension (B).

29. OWL-EYE

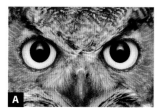 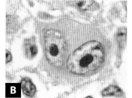

Night flying bird having large round eyes for night vision (A).

Term used in pathology for:
1. Microscopic appearance of nucleoli in Reed-Sternberg cell in Hodgkin disease and in Aschoff cells.
2. Intranuclear inclusions of cytomegalovirus (CMV) infection.

30. POTATO

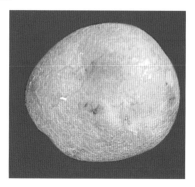

The plant with tubers used as vegetable.

Term used in pathology for:
Gross description of carotid body tumour.

31. PEAU-D'ORANGE

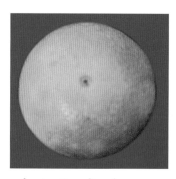

Peal of an orange having tiny dimples.

Term used in pathology for:
Description of oedematous skin of the breast over the tumour caused by lymphatic blockage.

32. SAGO GRAINS

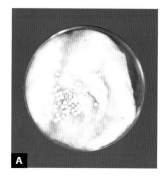 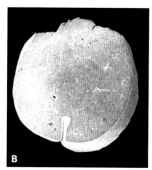

Starchy grains which appear as hard, white grains procured from a certain palm tree and is used in puddings, etc. (A).

Term used in pathology for:
Gross appearance of amyloidosis of the spleen limited to splenic follicles (B).

33. SICKLE-SHAPED

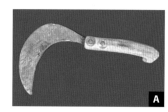 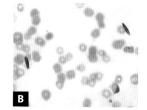

Short-handled tool with a semicircular or curved blade for cutting grass, grain, etc. (A)

Term used in pathology for:
1. Sickle-shaped blood cells found in sickle cell anaemia, a type of haemolytic anaemia.
2. Sickled-shaped appearance of gametocytes in *P. falciparum* (B).

34. SIGNET-RING

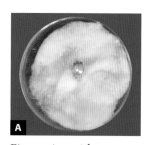 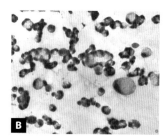

Finger ring with a stone set in it (A).

Term used in pathology for:
Appearance of tumour cells in signet ring cell adenocarcinoma of stomach, breast, etc. (B).

35. STAG-HORN

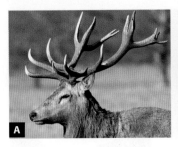 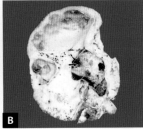

The antlers of a stag (male deer) having its paired terminal spikes (A).

Term used in pathology for:
Appearance of large renal stone of triple phosphate seen in the pelvicalyceal system of the kidney and taking its contour (B).

36. SWISS-CHEESE

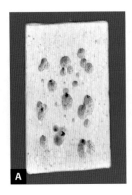 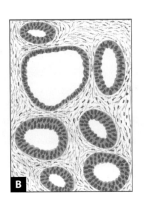

Cheese from Switzerland, frequently characterised by large holes (A).

Term used in pathology for:
1. Cut-sectioned appearance of juvenile papillomatosis breast.
2. Microscopic appearance of simple hyperplasia of the endometrium (B).
3. Cut-sectioned appearance of soft tissue in gas gangrene.

37. TREE-BARK

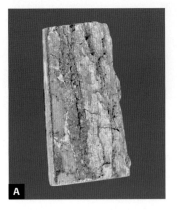 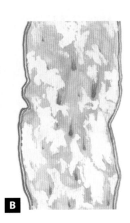

Thick outer skin of an old seasoned tree (A).

Term used in pathology for:
Gross appearance of intimal lesions in tertiary syphilitic aortitis (B).

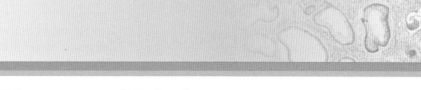

Appendix III

Normal Values

Objectives
➤ To know the normal weights and measurements of common organs.
➤ To know the normal values of common biochemical haematological and clinical pathological parameters.

Weights and Measurements of Normal Organs

In order to understand the significance of alterations in weight and measurement of an organ in disease, it is important to be familiar with the normal values. A comprehensive list of generally accepted normal weights and measurements of most of the normal organs in fully-developed, medium-sized individual are compiled in Table A-1.

Single value and value within brackets are indicative of the average figure for that organ. Measurements have been given as width × breadth (thickness) × length. An alphabetic order has been followed.

Table A-1: Weights and Measurements of Normal Organs.	
Organs	In Adults
Adrenal gland:	
Weight	4–5 gm
Brain:	
Weight (in males)	1400 gm
Weight (in females)	1250 gm
Volume of cerebrospinal fluid	120–150 ml
Heart:	
Weight (in males)	300–350 gm
Weight (in females)	250–300 gm
Thickness of right ventricular wall	0.3–0.5 cm
Thickness of left ventricular wall	1.3–1.5 cm
Circumference of mitral valve	10 cm
Circumference of aortic valve	7.5 cm
Circumference of pulmonary valve	8.5 cm
Circumference of tricuspid valve	12 cm
Volume of pericardial fluid	10–30 ml

Organs	In Adults
Intestines:	
Length of duodenum	30 cm
Total length of small intestine	550–650 cm
Length of large intestine	150–170 cm
Kidneys:	
Weight each (in males)	150 gm
Weight each (in females)	135 gm
Liver:	
Weight (in males)	1400–1600 (1500) gm
Weight (in females)	1200–1400 (1300) gm
Lungs:	
Weight (right lung)	375–500 (450) gm
Weight (left lung)	325–450 (400) gm
Volume of pleural fluid	< 15 ml
Oesophagus:	
Length (cricoid cartilage to cardia)	25 cm

Contd...

TABLE A-1: Weights and Measurements of Normal Organs. (contd...)	
Organs	*In Adults*
Distance from incisors to gastro-oesophageal junction	40 cm
Ovaries:	
Weight (each)	4–8 (6) gm
Pancreas:	
Total weight	60–100 (80) gm
Weight of endocrine pancreas	1–1.5 gm
Parotid glands:	
Weight (each)	30 gm
Pituitary gland (Hypophysis):	
Weight	500 mg
Placenta:	
Weight at term	400–600 gm
Prostate:	
Weight	20 gm
Spleen:	
Weight	125–175 (150) gm
Measurements	3.5 × 8.5 × 13 cm
Testis and epididymis:	
Weight each (in adults)	20–27 gm
Thymus:	
Weight	5–10 gm
Thyroid:	
Weight	15–40 gm
Uterus:	
Weight (in nonpregnant woman)	35–40 gm
Weight (in parous woman)	75–125 gm

Laboratory Values of Clinical Significance

Currently, the concept of 'normal values' and 'normal ranges' is replaced by 'reference values' and 'reference limits'. Reference ranges are valuable guidelines for the clinician. However, the following cautions need to be exercised in their interpretation:

♦ *Firstly,* they should not be regarded as absolute indicators of health and ill-health since values for healthy individuals often overlap with values for persons afflicted with disease.

♦ *Secondly,* laboratory values may vary with the method and mode of standardisation used; reference ranges given below are based on the generally accepted values by the standard methods in laboratory medicine.

The WHO as well as International Committee for Standardisation in Haematology (ICSH) have recommended adoption of SI system by the scientific community throughout world. In this section, laboratory values are given in both conventional and international units. Conversion from one system to the other can be done as follows:

$$mg/dl = \frac{mmol/L \times atomic\ weight}{10}$$

$$mmol/L = \frac{mg/dl \times 10}{atomic\ weight}$$

According to the SI system, the prefixes and conversion factors for metric units of length, weight and volume are given in Table A-2.

The laboratory values given here are divided into three sections: clinical chemistry of blood (Table A-3), other body fluids (Table A-4), and haematologic values (Table A-5). In general, an alphabetic order has been followed.

TABLE A-2: Prefixes and Conversion Factors in SI System.					
Prefix	*Prefix Symbol*	*Factor*	*Units of Length*	*Units of Weight*	*Units of Volume*
kilo-	k	10^3	kilometre (km)	kilogram (kg)	kilolitre (kl)
		1	metre (m)	gram (g)	litre (l)
deci-	d	10^{-1}	decimetre (dm)	decigram (dg)	decilitre (dl)
centi-	c	10^{-2}	centimetre (cm)	centigram (cg)	centilitre (cl)
milli-	m	10^{-3}	millimetre (mm)	milligram (mg)	millilitre (ml)
micro-	μ	10^{-6}	micrometre (μm)	microgram (μg)	microlitre (μl)
nano-	n	10^{-9}	nanometre (nm)	nanogram (ng)	nanolitre (nl)
pico-	p	10^{-12}	picometre (pm)	picogram (pg)	picolitre (pl)
femto-	f	10^{-15}	femtometre (fm)	femtogram (fg)	femtolitre (fl)
alto-	a	10^{-18}	altometre (am)	altogram (ag)	altolitre (al)

		Reference Value	
Component	Fluid	Conventional	SI Units
Aminotransferases (transaminases)			
aspartate (AST, SGOT)	Serum	12-38 U/L	0.20-0.65 μkat*/L
alanine (ALT, SGPT)	Serum	7-41 U/L	0.12-0.70 μkat/L
Ammonia	Plasma	19-60 μg/dl	11-35 μmol/L
Amylase	Serum	20-96 U/L	0.34-1.6 μkat/L
Bilirubin			
total	Serum	0.3-1.3 mg/dl	5.1-22 μmol/L
direct (conjugated)	Serum	0.1-0.4 mg/dl	1.7-6.8 μmol/L
indirect (unconjugated)	Serum	0.2-0.9 mg/dl	3.4-15.2 μmol/L
Calcium, total	Serum	8.7-10.2 mg/dl	2.2-2.6 mmol/L
Chloride (Cl⁻)	Serum	102-109 mEq/L	102-109 mmol/L
Cholesterol	Serum		
total desirable for adults		<200 mg/dl	<5.17 mmol/L
borderline high		200-239 mg/dl	5.17-6.18 mmol/L
high undesirable		≥240 mg/dl	>6.21 mmol/L
LDL-cholesterol, desirable range		<130 mg/dl	<3.34 mmol/L
borderline high		130-159 mg/dl	3.36-4.11 mmol/L
high undesirable		≥160 mg/dl	>4.11 mmol/L
HDL-cholesterol, protective range		>60 mg/dl	>1.55 mmol/L
low		<40 mg/dl	<1.03 mmol/L
triglycerides		<160 mg/dl	<2.26 mmol/L
Copper	Serum	70-140 μg/dl	11-22 μmol/L
C-reactive proteins	Serum	0.2-3.0 mg/L	0.2-3.0 mg/L
Creatine kinase (CK), total	Serum		
males		51-294 U/L	0.87-5.0 μkat/L
females		39-238 IU/L	0.66-4.0 μkat/L
Creatine kinase-MB (CK-MB)	Serum	0-5.5 ng/ml	0-5.5 μg/L
Creatinine	Serum	0.6-1.2 mg/dl	53-106 μmol/L
Gamma-glutamyl trans-peptidase (transferase) (γ-GT)	Serum	9-58 IU/L	0.15-1.00 μmol/L
Glucose (fasting)	Plasma		
normal		70-100 mg/dl	< 5.6 mmol/L
impaired fasting glucose (IFG)		101-125 mg/dl	5.6-6.9 mmol/L
diabetes mellitus		≥126 mg/dl	≥7.0 mmol/L
Glucose (2-hr post-prandial)	Plasma		
normal		<140 mg/dl	<7.8 mmol/L
impaired glucose tolerance (IGT)		140-200 mg/dl	7.8-11.1 mmol/L
diabetes mellitus		>200 mg/dl	>11.1 mmol/L
Haemoglobin A$_{1C}$	Whole blood	4-6%	0.04-0.06 Hb fraction
Lactate	Plasma (arterial)	4.5-14.4 mg/dl	0.5-1.6 mmol/L
Lactate dehydrogenase (LDH)	Serum	115-221 U/L	2.0-3.8 μkat/L
pH	Blood	7.35-7.45	7.35-7.45

*μkat (kat stands for katal, meaning catalytic activity) is a modern unit of enzymatic activity.

Contd...

TABLE A-3: Clinical Chemistry of Blood (Contd...)

Components	Fluid	Reference Value Conventional	SI Units
Phosphatases			
acid phosphatase	Serum	0-5.5 U/L	0.90 µkat/L
alkaline phosphatase	Serum	33-96 U/L	0.56-1.63 µkat/L
Phosphorus, inorganic	Serum	2.5-4.3 mg/dl	0.81-1.4 mmol/L
Potassium	Serum	3.5-5.0 mEq/L	3.5-5.0 mmol/L
Prostate specific antigen (PSA)	Serum	0-4.0 ng/ml	0-4.0 µg/L
Proteins	Serum		
total		6.7-8.6 g/dl	67-86 g/L
albumin		3.5-5.5 g/dl (50-60%)	35-55 g/L
globulins		2.0-3.5 g/dl (40-50%)	20-35 g/L
A/G ratio		1.5-3 : 1	
Pyruvate	Plasma (arterial)	0.35-1.14 mg/dl	40-130 µmol/L
Rheumatoid factor	Serum	< 30 IU/ml	< 30 kIU/L
Sodium	Serum	136-146 mEq/L	136-146 mmol/L
Thyroid function tests			
radioactive iodine uptake			
(RAIU) 24-hr		5-30%	
thyroxine (T_4) total	Serum	5.4-11.7 µg/dl	70-151 nmol/L
triiodothyronine (T_3) total	Serum	77-135 ng/dl	1.2-2.1 nmol/L
thyroid stimulating hormone (TSH)	Serum	0.4-5.0 µU/ml	0.4-5.0 mU/L
Troponins, cardiac (cTn)			
troponin I (cTnI)	Serum	0-0.08 ng/ml	0-0.8 µg/L
troponin T (cTnT)	Serum	0-0.01 ng/ml	0-0.1 µg/L
Urea	Blood	20-40 mg/dl	3.3-6.6 mmol/L
Urea nitrogen (BUN)	Blood	7-20 mg/dl	2.5-7.1 mmol/L
Uric acid	Serum		
males		3.1-7.0 mg/dl	0.18-0.41 µmol/L
females		2.5-5.6 mg/dl	0.15-0.33 µmol/L

TABLE A-4: Other Body Fluids.

Component	Fluid	Reference Value Conventional	SI Units
Cerebrospinal fluid (CSF)	CSF		
CSF volume		120-150 ml	
CSF pressure		60-150 mm water	
leucocytes		0-5 lymphocytes/µl	
pH		7.31-7.34	
glucose		40-70 mg/dl	
proteins		20-50 mg/dl	
Glomerular filtration rate (GFR)	Urine	180 L/day (about 125 ml/min)	
Seminal fluid	Semen		
liquefaction		Within 20 min	
sperm morphology		>70% normal, mature spermatozoa	
sperm motility		>60%	
pH		>7.0 (average 7.7)	

Contd...

TABLE A-4: Other Body Fluids (Contd...).

Components	Fluid	Reference Value Conventional	SI Units
sperm count		60-150 million/ml	60-150 × 10^6/ml
volume		1.5-5.0 ml	
Urine examination	24-hr volume	600-1800 ml (variable)	
pH	Urine	5.0-9.0	
specific gravity, quantitative	Urine (random)		1.002-1.028 (average 1.018)
protein excretion	24-hr urine	<150 mg/day	
glucose excretion, quantitative	24-hr urine	50-300 mg/day	
urobilinogen	24-hr urine	1.0-3.5 mg/day	
microalbuminuria (24 hour)		0-30 mg/24 hr	0-0.03 g/day
		(0-30 µg/mg creatinine)	(0-0.03 g/g creatinine)
Urobilinogen	Urine (random)	Present in 1: 20 dilution	

TABLE A-5: Normal Haematologic Values.

Component	Fluid	Reference Value Conventional	SI Units
Erythrocytes and Haemoglobin			
Erythrocyte count	Blood		
males		4.5-6.5 × 10^{12}/L (mean 5.5 × 10^{12}/L)	
females		3.8-5.8 × 10^{12}/L (mean 4.8 × 10^{12}/L)	
Erythrocyte diameter		6.7-7.7 µm (mean 7.2 µm)	
Erythrocyte thickness			
peripheral		2.4 µm	
central		1.0 µm	
Erythrocyte indices (Absolute values)	Blood		
mean corpuscular haemoglobin (MCH)		27-32 pg	
mean corpuscular volume (MCV)		77-93 fl	
mean corpuscular haemoglobin concentration (MCHC)		30-35 g/dl	
Erythrocyte life-span	Blood	120±30 days	
Erythrocyte sedimentation rate (ESR)	Blood		
Westergren 1st hr, males		0-15 mm	
females		0-20 mm	
Wintrobe, 1st hr, males		0-9 mm	
females		0-20 mm	
Ferritin	Serum		
males		30-250 ng/ml	30-250 µg/L
females		10-150 ng/ml	10-150 µg/L
Haematocrit (PCV)	Blood		
males		40-54%	0.47 ± 0.07 L/L
females		37-47%	0.42 ± 0.05 L/L
Haemoglobin (Hb)			
adult haemoglobin (HbA)	Whole blood		
males		13.0-18.0 g/dl	130-180 g/L
females		11.5-16.5 g/dl	115-165 g/L
plasma Hb (quantitative)		0.5-5 mg/dl	5-50 mg/L

Contd...

		Reference Value	
Components	*Fluid*	*Conventional*	*SI Units*
haemoglobin A$_2$ (HbA$_2$)		1.5-3.5%	
haemoglobin, foetal (HbF) in adults		<1%	
HbF, children under 6 months		<5%	
Iron, total	Serum	40-140 µg/dl	7-25 µmol/L
total iron binding capacity (TIBC)	Serum	250-406 µg/dl	45-73 µmol/L
iron saturation	Serum	20-45% (mean 33%)	0.20-0.45
Iron intake		10-15 mg/day	
Iron loss			
males		0.5-1.0 mg/day	
females		1-2 mg/day	
Osmotic fragility	Blood		
slight haemolysis		at 0.45 to 0.39 g/dl NaCl	
complete haemolysis		at 0.33 to 0.36 g/dl NaCl	
mean corpuscular fragility		0.4-0.45 g/dl NaCl	
Reticulocytes	Blood		
adults		0.5-2.5%	
infants		2-6%	
Transferrin	Serum	200-400 mg/dl	2-4 g/L
Leucocytes			
Differential leucocyte count (DLC)	Blood film/CBC counter		
P (polymorphs or neutrophils)		40-75% (2,000-7,500/µl)	
L (lymphocytes)		20-50% (1,500-4,000/µl)	
M (monocytes)		2-10% (200-800/µl)	
E (eosinophils)		1-6% (40-400/µl)	
B (basophils)		< 1% (10-100/µl)	
Total leucocyte count (TLC)	Blood		
adults		4,000-11,000/µl	
infants (full term, at birth)		10,000-25,000/µl	
infants (1 year)		6,000-16,000/µl	
Platelets and Coagulation			
Bleeding time (BT)			
Ivy's method	Prick blood	2-7 min	
template method		2.5-9.5 min	
Clotting time (CT)	Whole blood		
Lee and White method		4-9 min at 37°C	
Fibrinogen	Plasma	200-400 mg/dl	2-4 g/L
Fibrin split (or degradation) products (FSP or FDP)	Plasma	<10 µg/ml	<10 mg/L
Partial thromboplastin time with kaolin (PTTK or APTT)	Plasma	30-40 sec	
Platelet count	Blood	150,000-400,000/µl	
Prothrombin time (PT) (Quick's one-stage method)	Plasma	10-14 sec	
Thrombin time (TT)	Plasma	<20 sec (control ± 2 sec)	

Index

The letter "t" after page number in the index below denotes Table and the letter "f" stands for Figure on that page.